BIOLOGY OF IGF-1: ITS INTERACTION WITH INSULIN IN HEALTH AND MALIGNANT STATES

The Novartis Foundation is an international scientific and educational charity (UK Registered Charity No. 313574). Known until September 1997 as the Ciba Foundation, it was established in 1947 by the CIBA company of Basle, which merged with Sandoz in 1996, to form Novartis. The Foundation operates independently in London under English trust law. It was formally opened on 22 June 1949.

The Foundation promotes the study and general knowledge of science and in particular encourages international co-operation in scientific research. To this end, it organizes internationally acclaimed meetings (typically eight symposia and allied open meetings and 15–20 discussion meetings each year) and publishes eight books per year featuring the presented papers and discussions from the symposia. Although primarily an operational rather than a grant-making foundation, it awards bursaries to young scientists to attend the symposia and afterwards work with one of the other participants.

The Foundation's headquarters at 41 Portland Place, London W1B 1BN, provide library facilities, open to graduates in science and allied disciplines. Media relations are fostered by regular press conferences and by articles prepared by the Foundation's Science Writer in Residence. The Foundation offers accommodation and meeting facilities to visiting scientists and their societies.

Information on all Foundation activities can be found at http://www.novartisfound.org.uk

Novartis Foundation Symposium 262

BIOLOGY OF IGF-1: ITS INTERACTION WITH INSULIN IN HEALTH AND MALIGNANT STATES

2004

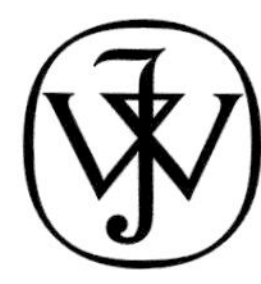

John Wiley & Sons, Ltd

Published in 2004 by John Wiley & Sons Ltd,
The Atrium, Southern Gate,
Chichester PO19 8SQ, UK

National 01243 779777
International (+44) 1243 779777
e-mail (for orders and customer service enquiries): cs-books@wiley.co.uk
Visit our Home Page on http://www.wileyeurope.com
or http://www.wiley.com

Other Wiley Editorial Offices

John Wiley & Sons Inc., 111 River Street, Hoboken, NJ 07030, USA

Jossey-Bass, 989 Market Street, San Francisco, CA 94103-1741, USA

Wiley-VCH Verlag GmbH, Boschstr. 12, D-69469 Weinheim, Germany

John Wiley & Sons Australia Ltd, 33 Park Road, Milton, Queensland 4064, Australia

John Wiley & Sons (Asia) Pte Ltd, 2 Clementi Loop #02-01, Jin Xing Distripark, Singapore 129809

John Wiley & Sons Canada Ltd, 22 Worcester Road, Etobicoke, Ontario, Canada M9W 1L1

Wiley also publishes its books in a variety of electronic formats. Some content that appears in print may not be available in electronic books.

Novartis Foundation Symposium 262
viii+280 pages, 33 figures, 8 tables

Library of Congress Cataloging-in-Publication

Biology of IGF-1 : its interaction with insulin in health and malignant states / [edited by]
Gregory Bock, Jamie Goode
p. cm. – (Novartis Foundation symposium ; 262)
Includes bibliographical references and index.
ISBN 0-470-86998-4 (alk. paper)
1. Somatomedin–Physiological effect–Congresses. 2.
Somatomedin–Pathophysiology–Congresses. 3. Carcinogenesis–Congresses. I. Bock, Gregory. II. Goode, Jamie. III. Series.

QP552.S65B566 2004
612′015756–dc22 2004048819

British Library Cataloguing in Publication Data

A catalogue record for this book is available from the British Library

ISBN 0 470 86998 4

Typeset in 10½ on 12½ pt Garamond by Dobbie Typesetting Limited, Tavistock, Devon.
Printed and bound in Great Britain by T. J. International Ltd, Padstow, Cornwall.
This book is printed on acid-free paper responsibly manufactured from sustainable forestry, in which at least two trees are planted for each one used for paper production.

Contents

Symposium on Biology of IGF-1: its interaction with insulin in health and malignant states, held at the Novartis Foundation, London, 14–16 October 2003

Editors: Gregory Bock (Organizer) and Jamie Goode

This symposium is based on a proposal made by Zvi Laron

Participants

David Carbone Vanderbilt University, Vanderbilt-Ingram Cancer Center, 2220 Pierce Ave, 685 PRB, Nashville, TN 37232-6838, USA

Jean-Louis Carpentier Department of Cell Physiology and Metabolism, Faculty of Medicine, University of Geneva, CH-1211 Geneva, Switzerland

Ross Clark Tercica Medica Inc., 651 Gateway Boulevard, Ste 950, South San Francisco, CA 94080-7111, USA

Pierre De Meyts Receptor Biology Laboratory, Novo Nordisk, Hagedorn Research Institute, Niels Steensens Vej 6, DK-2820 Gentofte, Denmark

Adam Denley (*Novartis Foundation Bursar*) Department of Molecular and Biomedical Sciences, The University of Adelaide, South Australia 5005, Australia

Diana Graus-Porta Oncology Research, Novartis Pharma AG, WKL-125.3.08, CH-4002 Basel, Switzerland

Adda Grimberg University of Pennsylvania School of Medicine, Division of Pediatric Endocrinology, The Children's Hospital of Philadelphia, Abramson Research Center, Room 802, 3615 Civic Center Blvd, Philadelphia, PA 19104-4318, USA

Jeff Holly Division of Surgery, Bristol Royal Infirmary, Marlborough Street, Bristol BS2 8HW, UK

Martin Holzenberger INSERM U-515, Hôpital Saint Antoine, F-75571, Paris Cedex 12, France

Paul Jenkins Department of Endocrinology, St Bartholomew's Hospital, West Smithfield, London EC1A 7BE, UK

Rudolf Kaaks International Agency for Research on Cancer, 150 cours Albert Thomas, F-69372 Lyon, France

Zvi Laron Schneider Children's Hospital, 14 Kaplan Street, Petah Tikva, 49202, Israel

Derek LeRoith (*Chair*) Diabetes Branch, Room 8D12, Building 10, NIH MSC 1758, Bethesda, MD 20892-1758, USA

Per Eystein Lønning Section of Oncology, Institute of Medicine, Haukeland Hospital, University of Bergen, N-5021 Bergen, Norway

Valentine Macaulay Cancer Research UK, Molecular Oncology Laboratories, Weatherall Institute of Molecular Medicine, Oxford OX3 9DS, UK

Rolf Ohlsson Department of Development & Genetics, Uppsala University, Norbyvägen 18A, 752 36 Uppsala, Sweden

Michael Pollak Cancer Prevention Centre, Pavilion C, Room C-107, Sir Mortimer B Davis-Jewish General Hospital, 3755 Côte Ste. Catherine Road, Montreal, Quebec, Canada H3T 1E2

Charles Roberts Department of Pediatrics (NRC5), Oregon Health & Science University, 3181 S.W. Sam Jackson Park Road, Portland, OR 97239-3098, USA

Ron Rosenfeld Lucile Packard Foundation for Children's Health, 770 Welch Road, Suite 350, Palo Alto, CA 94304, USA

George Thomas Friedrich Miescher Institute, PO Box 2543, Maulbeerstrasse 66, CH-4002 Basle, Switzerland

Haim Werner Department of Clinical Biochemistry, Sackler School of Medicine, Tel Aviv University, Tel Aviv, 69978, Israel

Doug Yee Department of Medicine and Pharmacology, University of Minnesota Cancer Center, MMC 80 b, 420 Delaware St SE, Minneapolis, MN 55455, USA

Yehiel Zick Department of Molecular Cell Biology, Weizmann Institute of Science, PO Box 26, Rehovot 76100, Israel

Chair's introduction

Derek LeRoith

Diabetes Branch, Room 8D12, Building 10, NIH MSC 1758, Bethesda, MD 20892-1758, USA

There are two main topics that will be covered by this meeting. The first is the biology of insulin and insulin-like growth factor (IGF)-1, which will be covered by several presentations. The other major theme is the role of IGF-1 in cancer, and since there are several new epidemiological studies on the potential relationship of insulin and cancer, this will also be covered.

There are four key questions that I'd like us to answer during this symposium. Perhaps we could revisit these at the end, and see how successful we have been in addressing them.

1. Are there truly differences between insulin and IGF-1 receptor signalling? This has been an ongoing discussion for many years now.
2. Is insulin a growth factor? This leads to question number 4 below.
3. Is IGF-1 causative in cancer progression or an 'innocent bystander'?
4. Is obesity/hyperinsulinaemia/type 2 diabetes associated with an increased risk of cancer, or do they affect cancer once it has developed?

One of the reasons for bringing up the question of insulin in addition to IGF-1 as being involved in cancer arises from recent epidemiological work. This has shown some relationship between cancer and factors that may involve hyperinsulinaemia, for example. One of many recent studies on this (Calle et al 2003), suggests that there is an effect on mortality from cancer in overweight and obese subjects. While this group didn't discuss hyperinsulinaemia, it was inherent in the paper that one should consider the possibility of insulin or IGF being involved in this situation. This is a question that we can bring up in the discussions.

When it comes to receptors, one of the recurrent questions is how do the differing biological functions of insulin and IGF-1 come about? Obviously, there are differences in the binding sites of the various receptors and there are differences in the C-terminal domains. But there is also the question of hybrid receptors. There are many combinations that are potentially possible. Again, there is a fair amount of recent work showing that some of the hybrid receptors between the insulin and the IGF receptors, between the A and B subtypes, have different interactions with hormones such as IGF-2. This could potentially explain some of the effects on the growth of tissues which then propagate cancer growth. So hybrid receptors and the various subtypes of insulin receptor should also be part of our discussions.

Reference

Calle EE, Rodriguez C, Walker-Thurmond K, Thun MJ 2003 Overweight, obesity, and mortality from cancer in a prospectively studied cohort of U.S. adults. N Engl J Med 348:1625–1638

Circulating IGF-1 and its role in cancer: lessons from the IGF-1 gene deletion (LID) mouse

Shoshana Yakar, Patricia Pennisi, Hong Zhao, Yang Zhang and Derek LeRoith[1]

Diabetes Branch, Room 8D12, Building 10, National Institutes of Health, MSC 1758, Bethesda MD 20892-1758, USA

Abstract. Recent epidemiological studies have suggested a statistical connection between serum IGF-1 levels in the upper quartile of the normal range and the relative risk of developing certain cancers. Our studies have focused on mouse models where circulating IGF-1 levels are reduced, while tissue expression of IGF-1 is normal. These mice show a lower risk for the development of colon and breast cancers and metastases when compared with control mice, and lend support to the hypothesis that circulating IGF-1 may be linked to cancer cell growth.

2004 Biology of IGF-1: its interaction with insulin in health and malignant states. Wiley, Chichester (Novartis Foundation Symposium 262) p 3–18

Tumour cells exhibit abnormally high levels of proliferation, which is promoted and controlled by a variety of growth factors. Among these, the insulin-like growth factors (IGFs) play a major role in regulating cell proliferation and inhibiting apoptosis. The IGFs are expressed ubiquitously and act in an autocrine/paracrine manner through binding to the IGF-1 receptor (IGF-1R). The bioactivity of IGF in tissues is determined by both local and systemic factors. The local factors include the levels of receptors that are expressed, various IGF binding proteins (IGFBPs) and IGFBP proteases. The systemic factors involved are mainly those that regulate the circulating levels of IGFs, such as growth hormone (GH) and various nutritional factors. Studies in cultured cells have demonstrated that the IGF-1R is frequently overexpressed in cancer cell lines. This has been attributed to mutations in certain tumour suppressor gene products, such as p53, the Wilms' tumour suppressor (WT-1),

[1]This paper was presented at the symposium by Derek LeRoith, to whom correspondence should be addressed.

BRAC1 and PTEN (Werner et al 1993, 1996, Abramovitch et al 2003). Under normal conditions, the wild-type tumour suppressor gene products typically suppress the expression of the IGF-1R promoter. IGF-2 is also commonly expressed by many tumours in culture and can act as an autocrine growth factor.

Recent epidemiological studies have suggested that there is an increased risk of developing breast, prostate, colon, lung and bladder cancer in individuals with circulating IGF-1 levels in the upper quartile of the normal range (Chan et al 1998, Hankinson et al 1998, Ma et al 1999, Yu et al 1999). Higher levels of IGF-1 were shown to be independently correlated with an increased risk of colorectal cancer. Subjects with adenomas designated as having a high risk for developing into cancer had significantly higher average levels of serum IGF-1 than normal subjects, although the levels were within the normal range. A prospective study among 397 women with breast cancer and 620 age-matched control women showed that among postmenopausal women, those in the top tertile of IGF-1 levels had a higher relative risk of developing breast cancer as compared to those in the bottom tertile. Based on these findings and the fact that the IGF system has long been implicated in cancer cell growth and metastases, we designed studies in mice to determine whether circulating IGF-1 levels represent a risk factor in tumour development and metastasis.

We have recently developed a mouse model that demonstrates a marked reduction in circulating IGF-1 levels, while exhibiting no significant retardation in growth and development, presumably because tissue IGF-1 production remains intact (Yakar et al 1999, 2001). In this review, we will first describe the creation and phenotype of this mouse model; we will then summarize the results of specific cancer-related studies.

Liver-specific IGF-1 gene-deleted (LID) mouse model

The purpose for creating this mouse model was to reduce or eliminate circulating IGF-1 levels and thereby study the role of tissue IGF-1 as compared to the role of 'endocrine' or circulating IGF-1. To achieve this, we utilized cre/*lox*P technology, which can be used to delete genes in a tissue-specific manner. A mouse line was created using homologous recombination to insert two *lox*P sequences flanking exon 3 of the *Igf-1* gene, while leaving the rest of the gene intact. This mouse was crossed with a second, transgenic mouse expressing the cre recombinase enzyme in the liver, utilizing the albumin promoter enhancer elements to drive cre expression. The resultant crossing led to recombination of the third exon of the *Igf-1* gene in liver only, and the resulting mice were designated as liver IGF-1 deficient (LID). LID mice exhibited >95% recombination and ~100% abrogation of IGF-1 mRNA in the liver, while expressing normal levels of IGF-1 in all other tissues. The total circulating levels of IGF-1 were reduced by 75%, as compared to control mice. Despite this marked reduction in circulating IGF-1 levels, post-natal growth and development was within normal limits. The reason for this normal growth in the face of markedly reduced serum IGF-1 levels is not clear, but might be a 'threshold effect', since further reductions in IGF-1 levels have resulted in growth retardation. An alternative explanation may be the normal levels of 'free' IGF-1 found in these mice. The elevated GH levels do not appear to be the cause of any compensatory growth effects, since IGF-1 expression, as measured by mRNA levels, is not elevated in non-hepatic tissues.

The LID mice do exhibit a metabolic phenotype, in that they display insulin insensitivity as early as 8 weeks of age (Yakar et al 2001). At this stage, insulin resistance occurs primarily at the level of skeletal muscle, with the liver largely escaping this effect until the age of 12–16 weeks. Studies have shown that the major cause for this insulin resistance is the elevated GH levels in LID mice, although there is some effect of the reduced circulating IGF-1 levels. Indeed, when mice expressing a GH antagonist are crossed with the LID mice, the insulin resistance virtually disappears. On the other hand, introduction of the acid labile subunit (ALS) null gene into LID mice, which results in a further reduction in serum IGF-1 levels, modestly improves the insulin resistance.

Using the LID mouse model, we designed experiments to determine the role of circulating IGF-1 levels in tumour growth and metastasis.

Previous studies related to the GH/IGF-1 system and cancer animal models

A number of studies have examined the potential role of the GH/IGF-1 axis in tumorigenesis. However, a direct causal relationship between circulating IGF-1 and/or IGFBPs and the initiation and development of tumours has not yet been established.

In rodent models, it was shown that energy-restricted diets, which significantly reduce the circulating levels of IGF-1, are correlated with a decrease in cancer incidence (Dunn et al 1997). *lit/lit* mice have a mutation in the GH releasing hormone receptor and, as a result, have only 10% of the normal circulating GH and IGF-1 levels. Experiments in *lit/lit* mice demonstrated a significant attenuation of neoplastic proliferation of human MCF7 cell xenografts (Yang et al 1996). Other studies showed that mice harbouring fibrosarcomas exhibited enhanced growth of the tumours in response to rhIGF-1 injection over a period of weeks. Transgenic mice that overexpress GH, and consequently have high levels of circulating IGF-1, display morphological evidence of mammary gland epithelial cell hyperplasia and a high frequency of breast cancer. On the other hand, transgenic mice overexpressing a GH antagonist exhibit ductal hypoplasia. When mammary tumours were induced in these mice with the

TABLE 1 Incidence of caecum tumour growth and caecum tumour weight

	Percentage of mice displaying tumours	*Tumour weight (g) (±SE)*
Control (plus saline)	57%[a]	1.6±0.4[a]
Control (plus rhIGF-1)	77%[b]	2.7±0.7[b]
LID (plus saline)	31%[c]	1.2±0.4[c]
LID (plus rhIGF-1)	65%	1.7±0.4

[a]Control (plus saline) versus LID (plus saline), $P<0.01$.
[b]Control (plus saline) versus control (plus rhIGF-1), $P<0.01$.
[c]LID (plus saline) versus LID (plus rhIGF-1), $P<0.01$.

carcinogen 7,12-dimethylbenz(a)anthracene (DMBA), the incidence of mammary tumour development was markedly reduced (Pollak et al 2001). Furthermore, overexpression of an IGF-1R agonist within the mammary gland was associated with increased rates of mammary gland cancer.

All of the studies described above were associated with whole body changes in either GH, IGF-1, or both, as well as significant alterations in growth and development. As such, these studies were unable to directly address the role played by circulating IGF-1 in tumour growth.

Serum IGF-1 and cancer

We utilized the LID mice to study the effect of reduced circulating IGF-1 levels (in the presence of normal tissue IGF-1 expression) to determine the effect of circulating IGF-1 on cancer growth. We used three models of cancer development and growth in these studies.

Murine colon 38 adenocarcinoma tissue fragments were implanted on the caecum of LID and control mice (Wu et al 2002). The growth of caecum tumours and the extent of liver metastasis were measured. Interestingly, the incidence of caecum tumour growth was significantly higher in control mice, as compared to the LID mice, which have circulating IGF-1 levels that are 75% lower than those in control mice (see Table 1 above). Administration of rhIGF-1 to both control and LID mice that harboured these caecal tumours similarly increased tumour growth in both groups.

Fewer liver metastases were present in LID mice, as measured by the number of nodules appearing in the liver. Furthermore, the metastatic process was enhanced by injection of rhIGF-1 in both control and LID mice (see Table 2 below). The results of this initial study suggest that reduced levels of circulating IGF-1 (despite the presence of normal expression of IGF-1 in tissues) are associated with reduced tumour development, tumour growth and metastases.

TABLE 2 Hepatic metastases: incidence and number of nodules

	Percentage of mice with metastases	*Number of nodules (±SE)*
Control (plus saline)	44%[a]	2.2±0.6[a]
Control (plus rhIGF-1)	57%[b]	4.9±2.9[b]
LID (plus saline)	31%[c]	1.2±0.4[c]
LID (plus rhIGF-1)	45%	1.6±0.5

[a]Control (plus saline) versus LID (plus saline), $P<0.05$.
[b]Control (plus saline) versus control (plus rhIGF-1), $P<0.05$.
[c]LID (plus saline) versus LID (plus rhIGF-1), $P<0.05$.

To expand on this initial study, we utilized the LID mouse model to study the role of endocrine IGF-1 in the development of mammary gland cancer (Wu et al 2003). Induction of mammary tumours was achieved in two ways: (a) by exposing mice to the DMBA carcinogen and (b) by crossing the LID mice with C3(1)/SV40 large T-antigen (LTA) transgenic mice. The latency period of mammary tumour development in the LID mice was markedly delayed in both models. In the DMBA-induced mammary tumour model, the incidence of palpable mammary tumours was significantly lower in LID mice (26% versus 56% in controls) and the onset of the tumours was delayed (74±1.2 days in LID mice versus 59.5±1.1 days in controls). Histologically, extensive squamous metaplasia was detected in late stage mammary tumours in control mice, whereas late stage tumours from LID mice demonstrated extensive hyperplasia, but little metaplasia. In the C3(1)/SV40-LTA-induced mammary tumours, the average age at the onset of tumour development in control mice was 21.6±1.8 weeks of age, whereas in the LID mice it was 30.2±1.7 weeks of age. In addition, 60% of the mice in the control group developed two or more mammary tumours per mouse, while only 30% of the LID mice developed more than one mammary tumour per mouse. These data demonstrate that in two established mammary tumour models, DMBA-induced mammary tumours and the C3(1)/SV40-LTA transgene, circulating IGF-1 levels represent a risk factor in the onset and development of mammary tumours.

Other related issues

These and other studies have focused on the possible role of the GH/IGF-1 axis and the risk of cancer as well as the progression of tumour growth. While there is adequate experimental evidence to demonstrate a direct effect of the IGF ligands, IGFBPs and IGF-1Rs on cancer growth, no causal relationship has yet been defined in humans. Trials of IGF-1R blockers, such as blocking peptides, blocking antibodies, or IGF-1R tyrosine kinase inhibitors will help to establish the level of involvement of the IGF-1R and cancer growth.

Meanwhile, there are related issues that need to be more fully studied. There are now reports that confirm the relationship of obesity, insulin resistance, type 2 diabetes and cancer. While earlier studies did not find this relationship, more recent long-term studies with larger cohorts positively identified diabetes and insulin resistance with hyperinsulinaemia as risk factors for cancer development and mortality from cancer (Calle et al 2003, Gapstur et al 2001, Levine et al 1990, Schoen et al 1999, Ragozzino et al 1982, Stengard et al 1992, Thompson et al 1989, Will et al 1998). The relationship of nutrition and obesity with circulating IGF-1 levels and the relationship of hyperinsulinaemia is compelling. These issues need to be addressed more fully using animal models and cell culture systems.

Conclusions

The number and rate of studies published on the topic of the IGFs and cancer is growing exponentially, and the interest in inhibiting the IGF-1R by biotech companies and the pharmaceutical industry attests to the importance of these issues. Thus, academic investigators would benefit from pursuing the link between the IGFs and cancer at a molecular level to further establish this connection and to delineate the mechanisms involved in these processes. Novel areas of research in this field should be approached using the most modern technology available to identify potential new targets for the treatment of this devastating disease.

References

Abramovitch S, Glaser T, Ouchi T, Werner H 2003 BRCA1-Sp1 interactions in transcriptional regulation of the IGF-1R gene. FEBS Lett 541:149–154

Calle EE, Rodriguez C, Walker-Thurmond K, Thun MJ 2003 Overweight, obesity, and mortality from cancer in a prospectively studied cohort of U.S. adults. N Engl J Med 348:1625–1638

Chan JM, Stampfer MJ, Giovannucci E et al 1998 Plasma insulin-like growth factor-I and prostate cancer risk: a prospective study. Science 279:563–566

Dunn SE, Kari FW, French J et al 1997 Dietary restriction reduces insulin-like growth factor I levels, which modulates apoptosis, cell proliferation, and tumor progression in p53-deficient mice. Cancer Res 57:4667–4672

Gapstur SM, Gann PH, Colangelo LA et al 2001 Postload plasma glucose concentration and 27-year prostate cancer mortality (United States). Cancer Causes Control 12:763–772

Hankinson SE, Willett WC, Colditz GA et al 1998 Circulating concentrations of insulin-like growth factor-I and risk of breast cancer. Lancet 351:1393–1396

Levine W, Dyer AR, Shekelle RB, Schoenberger JA, Stamler J 1990 Post-load plasma glucose and cancer mortality in middle-aged men and women. 12-year follow-up findings of the Chicago Heart Association Detection Project in Industry. Am J Epidemiol 131:254–262

Ma J, Pollak MN, Giovannucci E et al 1999 Prospective study of colorectal cancer risk in men and plasma levels of insulin-like growth factor (IGF)-I and IGF-binding protein-3. J Natl Cancer Inst 91:620–625

Pollak M, Blouin MJ, Zhang JC, Kopchick JJ 2001 Reduced mammary gland carcinogenesis in transgenic mice expressing a growth hormone antagonist. Br J Cancer 85:428–430

Ragozzino M, Melton LJ 3rd, Chu CP, Palumbo PJ 1982 Subsequent cancer risk in the incidence cohort of Rochester, Minnesota, residents with diabetes mellitus. J Chronic Dis 35:13–19

Schoen RE, Tangen CM, Kuller LH et al 1999 Increased blood glucose and insulin, body size, and incident colorectal cancer. J Natl Cancer Inst 91:1147–1154

Stengard JH, Tuomilehto J, Pekkanen J et al 1992 Diabetes mellitus, impaired glucose tolerance and mortality among elderly men: the Finnish cohorts of the Seven Countries Study. Diabetologia 35:760–765

Thompson MM, Garland C, Barrett-Connor E, Khaw KT, Friedlander NJ, Wingard DL 1989 Heart disease risk factors, diabetes, and prostatic cancer in an adult community. Am J Epidemiol 129:511–517

Werner H, Re GG, Drummond IA et al 1993 Increased expression of the insulin-like growth factor I receptor gene, IGF1R, in Wilms tumor is correlated with modulation of IGF1R promoter activity by the WT1 Wilms tumor gene product. Proc Natl Acad Sci USA 90:5828–5832

Werner H, Karnieli E, Rauscher FJ, LeRoith D 1996 Wild-type and mutant p53 differentially regulate transcription of the insulin-like growth factor I receptor gene. Proc Natl Acad Sci USA 93:8318–8323

Will JC, Galuska DA, Vinicor F, Calle EE 1998 Colorectal cancer: another complication of diabetes mellitus? Am J Epidemiol 147:816–825

Wu Y, Yakar S, Ling Z, Henninhausen L, LeRoith D 2002 Circulating insulin-like growth factor-I levels regulate colon cancer growth and metastasis. Cancer Res 62:1030–1035

Wu Y, Cui K, Miyoshi K, Hennighausen L et al 2003 Reduced circulating insulin-like growth factor I levels delay the onset of chemically and genetically induced mammary tumors. Cancer Res 63:4384–4388

Yakar S, Liu JL, Stannard B et al 1999 Normal growth and development in the absence of hepatic insulin-like growth factor I. Proc Natl Acad Sci USA 96:7324–7329

Yakar S, Liu JL, Fernandez AM et al 2001 Liver-specific IGF-1 gene deletion leads to muscle insulin insensitivity. Diabetes 50:1110–1118

Yang XF, Beamer WG, Huynh H, Pollak M 1996 Reduced growth of human breast cancer xenografts in hosts homozygous for the lit mutation. Cancer Res 56:1509–1511

Yu H, Spitz MR, Mistry J, Gu J, Hong WK, Wu X 1999 Plasma levels of insulin-like growth factor-I and lung cancer risk: a case-control analysis. J Natl Cancer Inst 91:151–156

DISCUSSION

De Meyts: I have a comment regarding signalling pathways that may be specific for insulin versus IGF-1. You didn't mention the new pathway described by Alan Saltiel and Jeff Pessin, the caveolin/lipid rafts pathway (TC10/APS/Cbl/CAP) that to my knowledge has only been described for insulin action in adipocytes (for review, see Saltiel & Pessin 2002). I don't think anyone has looked at its possible involvement in IGF-1 signalling.

LeRoith: That is my understanding: no one has looked at the TC10 pathway.

De Meyts: The crystal structure of one of the components of this pathway (APS) in complex with the phosphorylated activation loop of the tyrosine kinase domain of the insulin receptor has recently been reported (Hu et al 2003), which brings credence to a role for the postulated activation partners. What about the IRS5 and IRS6 that have been recently described (Grimm et al 2001, Hu et al 2003, Favre et al 2003, Cai et al 2003)?

LeRoith: I don't think anyone has looked at either of those in the context of IGF-1. Ideally, one would really have to make cell lines that are responsive to both insulin and IGF-1, and then see whether you could show the difference.

Roberts: In the array studies we described at the IGF Gordon Conference in March, 2003, we found that in human prostate epithelial cells that caveolin 1 was one of the most highly IGF-1-regulated genes. This suggests that it is also a component of IGF signalling. We didn't compare it with insulin.

Laron: In your microarray experiments you picked out two genes, Twist and TDAG. Are they also induced by insulin?

LeRoith: When we set up the microarray, we looked at IGF-1-specific genes. In those cells, even though they had a lot of insulin receptors and were stimulated with insulin, it did not stimulate those two genes. They were specifically induced by IGF-1 in that system.

Roberts: Were Twist and TDAG51 regulated by IGF-1 in cells that express a physiological level of IGF-1 receptors? The NWTb3 cells you used have 500 000 IGF-1 receptors per cell.

LeRoith: These cells express ∼150 000 receptors per cell, which is lower but still a higher level than the NIH 3T3 cells normally express. We haven't looked in cells that express 25–30 000 receptors.

Graus-Porta: I have a question concerning your last model, the caecal tumours. Is this a cell line that overexpresses the IGF-1 receptor?

LeRoith: It is not a cell line. It is actually a caecal tumour developed in mouse and propagated from mouse to mouse. We have to disperse the cells so we were able to measure the receptors—it is in the range of 20 000 per cell. Then we take a bunch of these cells and implant them in the next mouse.

Graus-Porta: So it is a model that depends not only on the IGF-1 receptor, but also on the presence of IGF-1.

LeRoith: That is what we would like to suggest.

Graus-Porta: Can you envision a situation in human tumours where the receptor is expressed at high levels and tumour growth proceeds independent of the ligand?

LeRoith: If you have very high expression of either the IGF-1 receptor or even the insulin receptor, you can get tumour growth in the absence of IGF-1. This has been done by Renato Baserga and colleagues (personal communication) either in culture or actually in mice. If you have tremendous overexpression of receptors you don't need to inject the ligand. We are talking about over 100 000 receptors per cell. Baserga showed that you need over a million in the case of the insulin receptor. If you bring enough receptors together you can activate the tyrosine kinase in the absence of the ligand.

Graus-Porta: Would there be a similar situation in human tumours?

LeRoith: Very few tumours express more than 50 000 receptors per cell.

Pollak: I think this is an interesting point. This came up in a more general way in your talk. IGF-1 receptor up-regulation might be important in cancers, but I would agree with the last point. This contrasts with overexpression of HER2/neu, for example, where a quarter of breast cancers have more than a million HER2/neu receptors which are pathophysiologically important in driving tumour growth. The IGF-1 receptor may be quite important in the malignant phenotype, but not because it is overexpressed. In other words, it is possible that even a modest receptor number might be pathophysiologically important. With other peptide receptors, there are examples where it is the ligand that is pathologically elevated and the receptor number is more conventional. I am not aware of an example where we have the kind of overexpression of the IGF-1 receptor that we see in human tumours analogous to the HER2/neu overexpression. I know that experimentally the million receptor per cell situation is interesting, but I would like to hear what other people's experience of this is.

Jenkins: You showed quite clearly that circulating IGF-1 is important. What about local IGF-1? We have been intrigued by this in colonic cancers, and using quantitative RT-PCR we find quite clearly that there is a subgroup of cancers that do not express IGF-1 at all. The IGF-1 receptor expression is pretty constant between them; it is the local expression that then seems to affect both tumour-associated gene expression and importantly, tumour angiogenesis.

LeRoith: 'Intrigued' is a very good word. The local expression of a ligand is important. In the case of the mice, IGF-2 is not a major ligand. There are only a few tissues that express it postnatally. We have also been intrigued as to what is affecting the metastases. In tumours that metastasize and have the same complement of IGF-1 receptors, what is the local attraction? Is it the local IGF that is attracting the tumour? We have shown that circulating levels are down and that is why there are fewer mestastases. We are intrigued but we don't know the local production and we don't have an answer to the question. The problem with local production is that one can either look at mRNA or protein. Protein is very hard to study in tissues. Again, there is a balance between how much of the protein is coming from the circulation and how much from the tissues. In these animals it seems like the mRNA is constant. Does this relate to normal protein levels? We assume so, but we don't know.

Grimberg: There is a potential mechanism to tie in the ligand with the receptor levels. You showed nice data about the IGF-1 receptor being repressed by p53 (Werner et al 1996). There is another paper showing that p53 also represses the expression of IGF-2 from the P3 promoter (Zhang et al 1996). So, if you lose p53, you derepress both IGF-2 and the IGF-1 receptor. This can constitute a nice system for autocrine growth stimulation.

Lønning: Turning to the issue of receptors, let's take the three hottest receptors in breast cancer today: ErbB2, IGF-1R and the oestrogen receptor (ER). In many ways the IGF-1R is more like the ER than ErbB2. In breast cancer ErbB2 is elevated by amplification. This is clearly a pathological process. If we look at the IGF-1R, similarly to ER, in the malignant tissue the expression is higher compared with the benign tissue, but we don't have an explanation for this. The IGF-1 receptor, similar to the ER receptor in general is correlated to a better differentiated tumour. This contrasts with the p53 mutation theory. p53 mutations in breast cancer are clearly associated with grade 3 highly malignant tumours.

LeRoith: There is a question of breast cancers having a more malignant phenotype if they have more insulin receptor, and a more differentiated phenotype if they have the IGF-1 receptor. This comes from studies by the Italian group (Belfiore et al 1996).

Roberts: That's right, although the German group argue that in advanced breast cancer there is a decrease in both type 1 receptor and IRS-1 (Schnarr et al 2000). It is still controversial.

LeRoith: It has become controversial in breast cancer and perhaps prostate cancer. There may be some differences from the standard theory of overexpression of the IGF-1R being relevant to more advanced tumour growth and worse prognosis.

Werner: I have a comment regarding the high levels of expression of IGF-1R. We have to distinguish between the different types of tumours. In solid tumours, and in particular in paediatric tumours, there is almost always an increase in the expression of the receptor. This is not true in tumours with a strong endocrine background, such as breast and prostate cancer. In this type of tumour, most reports showed an increased expression of IGF-1R at early stages and a significant decrease at advanced, metastatic stages.

LeRoith: It is only in those two tumours where there is some controversy. There was a recent publication in *Human Pathology* in which they looked at a dozen tumours. They found that in about 70% there was increased IGF-1R expression. One of the groups was breast cancer. Therefore I think there may be cancer-specific responses to IGF-1R overexpression.

Kaaks: I have a question about your cre-*lox* model and lethal knockouts of IGF-1. What happens to growth hormone (GH) secretion in these mice, and what happens to local synthesis of IGF-1 in tissues such as liver?

LeRoith: GH is increased fourfold. If you assume that the IGF-1 mRNA correlates with IGF-1 protein, then there is no increased production. Indeed, the production in those tissues is almost at a maximum anyway, because these are rapidly growing animals. They seem to have as much IGF-1 as the controls who are growing well. It seems to me that GH is not stimulating IGF-1 gene expression in those tissues even though it is raised fourfold, and in a second model 15-fold. I cannot exclude that there is no increased translation and that the protein is increased. Protein is hard to measure. We are assuming that the IGF-1 is at a maximum already in those tissues.

Kaaks: I have a related question from an epidemiological perspective. You started making the observation that elevated IGF in the circulation is associated with increased risk of a number of cancers. A number of studies have shown this. How do you interpret what you just said in the light of those other observations? The epidemiologists still seem to think that elevated IGF in the circulation might at the same time reflect higher GH levels and higher local synthesis as well—that it is not necessarily the circulating levels that determine this. Would you contradict this?

LeRoith: Yes. I would say that the increased levels of IGF-1 in the normal range suggests that these are not due to higher GH levels. If there were higher GH levels than normal, I would consider that an acromegalic patient. I think that high IGF-1 might be due to some nutritional effect. We know that IGF-1 is very closely regulated by nutrition. If you have a short fast or a low-calorie diet, your IGF-1 will go down. If you drink a good amount of milk your IGF-1 may go up, within the normal range. There are many people, including myself, who believe that high IGF-1 may be a marker for over-nutrition. I know this was potentially excluded in many of the studies, but it wasn't totally excluded. The NCI has an ongoing programme attempting to correlate nutrition and the IGF-1 level. This connection may explain the link between over-nutrition, higher IGF-1 within the normal range, and this increased relative risk for cancer. I don't think it is related to GH directly.

Holly: Related to the GH central or local effects, there is a paradigm that has come from a lot of people's work. In breast and prostate cancer, GH works on stromal cells to increase production of IGF-1, which then acts on the epithelial cells. Do you think your model discounts or disproves these?

LeRoith: I think GH on local tissues is only one of the stimuli to IGF-1 production. In our model, the animals are growing so well that IGF-1 is already up-regulated adequately: this is perhaps why GH can't increase its expression. I hate to discount other people's work, but our data speak against this in the tissues that we looked at. Also, in their studies they administered growth hormone, so this was more pharmacological. Here we are talking about a fourfold increase which is pathological but not pharmacological. Maybe this is the difference.

Holly: But there is no change in IGF-1 expression even in the tumours that you induced?

LeRoith: These are not making IGF-1, so there is no change.

Yee: How do you know that the tumour is a target for the reduction? How do you know it is not a host angiogenesis effect? For example, I have seen data like these presented for angiogenesis, in which breast cancer latency and multiplicity are decreased in the SV-40 Tag animals.

LeRoith: Are you suggesting that IGF-1 is affecting VEGF expression?

Yee: Or just directly affecting endothelial cell growth.

LeRoith: That's fine. What we have been able to show is that this is related to the IGF-1 level in the circulation. We have shown a change in VEGF but did not study angiogenesis *per se*. We have studied some of the immunology and there is no change.

Yee: Do you know that the epithelial cells themselves are IGF responsive? If you take these tumour cells out of the SV40-Tag animals, do they have an IGF response *in vitro*?

LeRoith: We have taken the colon cancer cells out, and they respond normally. We haven't studied the SV-40 cells.

Zick: I wanted to raise an issue we haven't touched on so far, which is the IGF-1 binding proteins. How do these fit in? Do you see changes in their levels? Might this affect the amount of IGF-1 bound versus active?

LeRoith: I don't think so. IGFBP3, the main binding protein, is markedly reduced in these animals. Free levels of IGF-1 seem to be normal. Is low IGFBP3 affecting tumour growth? You would have to say that in the absence of IGFBP3 there is less tumour, and this means that IGFBP3 is tumour promoting. There are some studies that suggest this, but there are a number of other groups who have suggested that IGFBP3 is pro-apoptotic. In this case we haven't entered the discussion of the binding proteins, but it is an important issue.

Thomas: An important experiment for you is a control, where you have rescue by putting back IGF-1. What happens to the controls in this condition, do they go up further? Is tumorigenesis increased?

LeRoith: They go up when they get IGF-1.

Thomas: Wouldn't it be better to do this experiment by conditional knockout of the receptor itself? Certainly, those animals exist already for the insulin receptor.

LeRoith: That's a good idea. The animals have been created but I'm not sure whether those experiments have been done.

Thomas: You might want to do this in a setting where you are not going to be dependent on development in the animal. For example, in your system you could do it with the MX-cre inducible system.

LeRoith: We have the IGF-1 conditional knockouts which we are starting to work on now, but we don't have the receptor conditional knockout. We are planning to do the more adult experiments with IGF-1 to see what happens if we knock it out in the adult stage.

Thomas: The other problem I see with knocking out IGF-1R is that you might induce apoptosis in those tissues. You might need IGF-1R to maintain those tissues. Is anyone trying to exploit some sort of hypomorphic approach to knock down IGF-1R levels?

Holzenberger: We have hypomorphic IGF-1R animals. So far we haven't studied them on a background that would allow us to evaluate the incidence of cancer and progression. Several projects are underway to consider this in a tissue-specific way.

Thomas: Apparently, Scott Lowe, Cold Spring Harbor, recently gave a talk. They have been using TVA technology involving a chicken retrovirus. They make a transgenic animal that only expresses the receptor in a specific tissue, and then you deliver your gene systemically. They did this with B cells. They delivered p53 sRNA systemically and it only induced lymphomas in the animal. Eric Holland has done the same thing at Sloan Kettering by taking an animal which has a flox PTEN and delivering cre systemically with the virus. This gives glioblastomas in the brain. This might be a good approach because then you could titrate this system.

Laron: Considering angiogenesis, we have evidence in humans that IGF-1 deficiency can also induce angiogenesis and VEGF activation in the absence of circulating IGF-1 (Laron & Weinberger 2003). You have shown that tumours have an increased number of IGF-1 receptors. Are certain genes responsible for this? If so, should we not then strive to recognize these genes with certain markers, so we can identify those patients in whom the tumours may develop increased numbers of IGF-1 receptors?

LeRoith: What you are suggesting is that there might be something like a polymorphism or some change in the receptor promoter, as opposed to something that is regulating its gene expression.

Werner: We have evidence that in certain pathologies there is a dose dependency effect between IGF-1R levels and the degree of cell proliferation. For example, a number of studies have shown that in overgrowth syndromes, such as Beckwith-Wiedemann, there is a trisomy of the IGF-1 receptor locus. As a result of the trisomy there is a threefold increase in the levels of expression of the receptor, which may lead to the overgrowth phenotype typical of these disorders. There are no reports of IGF-1 receptor trisomy in human cancer. However, in malignantly transformed cells receptor expression may be several-fold increased as a result of impaired regulation of the IGF-1R gene by mutated tumour suppressors or oncogenes. In this case there is a huge increase in receptor expression which may contribute to the neoplastic phenotype.

De Meyts: Have you dismissed IGF-2 too soon as a potential tumorigenic ligand? It is normally down-regulated in most normal tissues after birth in rodents, but not in humans where the circulating concentration is several-fold that of IGF-1, and in fact a number of tumours in humans can produce so much IGF-2 that the patients actually develop intractable hypoglycaemia. Also, in a number of tumours there is loss of imprinting of IGF-2. I wouldn't dismiss the role of autocrine IGF-2 loops in tumour progression once tumorigenesis has started.

Pollak: This might represent a case where chronic local high levels of ligand can even cause down-regulation of the receptor number, but nevertheless there is a very important amount of phosphorylation and signalling. This is why it may be dangerous to assume that the only tumours for which IGF1 receptors are relevant are those where it is overexpressed. This may be the source of some of the complexities in interpreting the levels in well differentiated versus poorly differentiated breast cancers. One model would have it that poorly differentiated breast cancers may express a lot of IGF-2, with chronic stimulation and a short autocrine loop which would down-regulate the IGF-1 receptor number. The next round of studies on tumour pathology in terms of receptor levels will have to look at receptor phosphorylation, because a small number of receptors, all of which are phosphorylated, might be more directly related to behaviour than just a large number of vacant receptors.

LeRoith: On that point, a question that we are tackling at the moment is the number of receptors needed for proliferation, which may be a question of overexpression, and how many are needed for apoptosis. If only a few are needed for apoptosis, then this supports the point—if you have less apoptosis you will have more tumour.

De Meyts: For the insulin receptor we have an instructive example, the T cell lymphoma (LB) discovered by David Naor in Israel with colleagues in Argentina. This cell line is completely devoid of IGF-1R. It has only 300 GH receptors and 1500 insulin receptors, and these appear to be the two that drive the growth of a very malignant tumour (Ish-Shalom et al 1997, Ursø et al 2003). This is a very small number of receptors, even compared with a normal cell.

LeRoith: Val Macaulay, you did a literature search once summarizing IGF-1 receptor expression in tumours. What is your impression of the overexpression of the receptors in various tumours?

Macaulay: People talk about IGFR overexpression in a lot of different tumours, but when you assess the data what they are often looking at is cell lines. We didn't find many tumour types where a careful assessment had been made of the tumour and the equivalent normal tissue, which is the most relevant comparison. Comparing cell lines is fairly meaningless. As you said, the data in breast cancer are conflicting (e.g. Papa et al 1993, Turner et al 1997). In prostate cancer we have evidence for IGF-1R overexpression (Hellawell et al 2002, recently confirmed by Grzmil et al 2004), although these results conflict with other reports (Tennant et al 1996, Chott et al 1999, Zhang et al 1999). Other tumours for which there is good evidence for IGF-1R overexpression include colon cancer (Hakam et al 1999), pancreatic cancer (Bergmann et al 1995), and melanoma (Kanter-Lewensohn et al 2002).

LeRoith: Is this from patients?

Macaulay: This is clinical material from patients compared with normal tissue.

LeRoith: So it is still a fairly open question in terms of what is happening in the patients themselves.

Holly: Elaborating on Pierre De Meyt's point about writing off IGF-2, you have expressed a bias against binding proteins so perhaps I will express my bias against the rodent models! They are vastly different from humans, because IGF-2 is virtually switched off at weaning in rodents, and therefore you are tinkering with IGF-1 against a background of virtually no IGF-2 in the circulation. In humans, there is a vast reservoir of IGF-2 as a background against the small variations in IGF-1. It is a very different scenario.

LeRoith: That is what makes the mouse model much cleaner! What is this very high level of IGF-2 in humans doing normally, and what is it doing in cancer situations? Do you need a local IGF-2 to propagate those tumours, or could this reservoir of this very high level in the circulation be involved. There are a lot of questions still open for discussion. But I accept the criticism of the mouse model.

Clark: To keep the IGF-2 theme going, there is a nice experiment of nature, the IGF-1 knockout in man (Woods et al 1996). These children have non-detectable IGF-1 levels, but high levels of IGF-2 yet they grow very poorly. This suggests that the growth promoting activity of IGF-2 in humans is absolutely miniscule.

LeRoith: And as yet they haven't developed tumours.

Clark: No, but they have over 1000 ng/ml of IGF-2. We don't understand IGF-2 at all.

References

Belfiore A, Frittitta L, Costantino A et al 1996 Insulin receptors in breast cancer. Ann NY Acad Sci 784:173–188

Bergmann U, Funatomi H, Yokoyama M, Beger HG, Korc M 1995 Insulin-like growth-factor-I overexpression in human pancreatic-cancer—evidence for autocrine and paracrine roles. Cancer Res 55:2007–2011

Cai D, Dhe-Paganon S, Melendez PA, Lee J, Schoelson SE 2003 Two new substrates in insulin signaling, IRS5/DOK4 and IRS6/DOK5. J Biol Chem 278:25323–25330

Chott A, Sun Z, Morganstern D et al 1999 Tyrosine kinases expressed in vivo by human prostate cancer bone marrow metastases and loss of the type 1 insulin-like growth factor receptor. Am J Pathol 155:1271–1279

Favre C, Gerard A, Clauzier E, Pontarotti P, Olive D, Nunes JA 2003 DOK4 and DOK5: new Dok-related genes expressed in human T cells. Genes Immun 4:40–45

Grimm J, Sachs M, Britsch S et al 2001 Novel p62dok family members, dok-4 and dok-5, are substrates of the c-Ret receptor tyrosine kinase and mediate neuronal differentiation. J Cell Biol 154:345–354

Grzmil M, Hemmerlein B, Thelen P, Schweyer S, Burfeind P 2004 Blockade of the type 1 IGF receptor in human prostate cancer cells inhibits proliferation and invasion, up-regulates IGF binding protein-3, and suppresses MMP-2 expression. J Pathol 202:50–59

Hakam A, Yeatman TJ, Lu L et al 1999 Expression of insulin-like growth factor-1 receptor in human colorectal cancer. Hum Pathol 30:1128–1133

Hellawell GO, Turner GD, Davies DR, Poulsom R, Brewster SF, Macaulay VM 2002 Expression of the type 1 insulin-like growth factor receptor is up-regulated in primary prostate cancer and commonly persists in metastatic disease. Cancer Res 62:2942–2950

Hu J, Liu J, Ghirlando R, Sattiel AR, Hubbard SR 2003 Structural basis for the recruitment of the adaptor protein APS to the activated insulin receptor. Mol Cell 12:1379–1389

Ish-Shalom D, Christoffersen CT, Vorwerk P et al 1997 Mitogenic properties of insulin and insulin analogues mediated by the insulin receptor. Diabetologia 40:S25–S31

Kanter-Lewensohn L, Dricu A, Girnita L, Wejde J, Larsson O 2002 Expression of insulin-like growth factor-1 receptor (IGF-1R) and p27Kip1 in melanocytic tumors: a potential regulatory role of IGF-1 pathway in distribution of p27Kip1 between different cyclins. Growth Factors 17:193–202

Laron Z, Weinberger D 2003 Diabetes and its vascular complications in primary IGFI deficiency (Laron Syndrome). Horm Res 60(suppl 2):43

Papa V, Gliozzo B, Clark GM et al 1993 Insulin-like growth factor-I receptors are overexpressed and predict a low risk in human breast cancer. Cancer Res 53:3736–3740

Saltiel AR, Pessin JE 2002 Insulin signalling pathways in time and space. Trends Cell Biol 12: 65–71

Schnarr B, Strunz K, Ohsam J, Benner A, Wacker J, Mayer D 2000 Down-regulation of insulin-like growth factor-I receptor and insulin receptor substrate-1 expression in advanced human breast cancer. Int J Cancer 89:506–513

Tennant MK, Thrasher JB, Twomey PA, Drivdahl RH, Birnbaum RS, Plymate SR 1996 Protein and messenger ribonucleic acid (mRNA) for the type 1 insulin-like growth factor (IGF) receptor is decreased and IGF-II mRNA is increased in human prostate carcinoma compared to benign prostate epithelium. J Clin Endocrinol Metab 81:3774–3782

Turner BC, Haffty BG, Narayanan L et al 1997 Insulin-like growth factor-I receptor overexpression mediates cellular radioresistance and local breast cancer recurrence after lumpectomy and radiation. Cancer Res 57:3079–3083

Ursø B, Ilondo MM, Holst PA et al 2003 IRS-4 mediated mitogenic signalling by insulin and growth hormone in LB cells, a murine T-cell lymphoma devoid of IGF-I receptors. Cell Signal 15:385–394

Werner H, Karnieli E, Rauscher FJ, LeRoith D 1996 Wild-type and mutant p53 differentially regulate transcription of the insulin-like growth factor I receptor gene. Proc Natl Acad Sci USA 93:8318–8323

Woods KA, Camacho-Hubner C, Savage MO, Clark AJ 1996 Intrauterine growth retardation and postnatal growth failure associated with deletion of the insulin-like growth factor I gene. N Engl J Med 335:1363–1367

Zhang L, Kashanchi F, Zhan Q et al 1996 Regulation of insulin-like growth factor II P3 promotor by p53: a potential mechanism for tumorigenesis. Cancer Res 56:1367–1373

Zhang P, Wang-Rodriguez J, Bailey D 1999 Insulin-like growth factor receptor expression in prostate cancer. Am J Clin Pathol 112:130

Physiology of the IGF system

Jeff Holly

University Division of Surgery, Bristol Royal Infirmary, Bristol BS2 8HW, UK

Abstract. The insulin-like growth factors (IGFs) comprise a complex regulation system with two growth factors, cell-surface receptors, 6 specific high affinity IGF binding proteins (IGFBP1–6), IGFBP-proteases, as well as other IGFBP-interacting molecules. Although the IGFs and their signalling receptor closely resemble the peptide hormone (after which they were named) and its cell receptor; their *modus operandi* is very different from that of traditional peptide hormones. The IGFs are not stored within cells of a specific tissue but are present at very high levels throughout the body. They circulate at total concentrations approximately 1000 times higher than that of most peptide hormones and although tissue levels are somewhat lower, they are still present in vast excess compared to that required for maximal cellular stimulation. These high levels are maintained due to their association with the IGFBPs, which dramatically slow their clearance. The IGFBPs bind the IGFs with greater affinity than their cell surface receptors, enabling them to tightly control tissue activity. The IGFBP proteases modify the IGFBPs, lowering the affinity with which they bind IGFs. In the tissues the IGFs are important regulators of cell survival, growth, metabolism and differentiated function; the complex system confers specificity on these actions.

2004 Biology of IGF-1: its interaction with insulin in health and malignant states. Wiley, Chichester (Novartis Foundation Symposium 262) p 19–35

General physiology

The insulin-like growth factors (IGF-1 and 2) were discovered in the late 1950s as skeletal growth factors produced in the liver that appeared to mediate the effects of the pituitary on whole-body somatic growth (Daughaday & Salmon 1999). It was only when these growth factors were chemically characterized many years later, and with the realization of their close structural homology to proinsulin, that they were given their present names. By that time it had been shown that in addition to production in the liver, both IGF-1 and IGF-2 were produced in most, if not all, tissues. The liver has however been confirmed as by far the main source of the large amount of IGF found in the circulation and it became increasingly apparent that pituitary growth hormone (GH) was not the only regulator but that they were also very strongly nutritionally dependent. Nutrition has many interacting effects upon the IGF system, including direct effects of certain nutrients upon hepatic expression and indirect effects via insulin and via changes in hepatic GH receptors (Ketelslegers et al 1995). The IGFs play an important role in regulating somatic growth according to nutritional conditions. It has also become apparent that this forms part of a very fundamental control, ensuring that the development of the organism proceeds appropriately to the nutritional supply. This control system has been conserved throughout evolution from yeast through to higher mammals. Genetic studies in *Caenorhabditis elegans*, *Drosophila* and rodents have established a conserved insulin-like system that links growth and development with nutrient supply. A plentiful food supply results in rapid growth and development and early acquisition of reproductive status. The organism can then reproduce so that the next generation can take advantage of the good food supply. This is also associated with a shorter lifespan, favoured on an evolutionary basis to make way for the next generation (Carter et al 2002). In contrast when nutrients are in short supply the activity of the insulin-like system is suppressed, growth and development are slowed, or even halted, and acquisition of a reproductive status is put off for as long as possible, waiting for the food supply to improve. This is associated with a lengthening of the lifespan. Increased activity of the insulin-like axis may increase cell turnover, accelerating ageing, whereas less activity may reduce cell turnover, slow ageing and hence lengthen lifespan. There is increasing interest in the factors responsible for human longevity, but the extrapolation from the genetic models to humans is extremely complex. In flies, worms and even in rodents lifespan is tightly linked to reproductive competence; when the organism is no longer efficient to reproduce it is in competition for food with the next generation and rapid death is favoured for the continuation of the species. Throughout the development of mammals, however, there became a stage when there was an evolutionary advantage for maintaining the older generation beyond its reproductive lifespan, presumably to pass on its acquired wisdom to the next generation. The physiology of ageing in this post-reproductive stage is less well understood and the experimental models employing lower species are of limited value. The limitations on human lifespan in the post-reproductive, aged population are generally chronic conditions such as cardiovascular disease and cancer; these are very different from the limitations on lifespan in nematodes, flies and even rodents. The relevance of the IGF system to longevity of humans is a subject of increasing research activity.

There is now considerable evidence indicating that within human populations there is a strong association between circulating IGF-1 concentrations and the risk of developing a number of cancers. A relatively high IGF-1 concentration in an individual is associated with an increased risk of developing colorectal, breast or prostate cancer. This implies that the IGF system may not only mediate the fundamental links between nutrition, growth, development and lifespan; but could also mediate the link between nutrition and the cancers that have become widespread in western societies. It has long been known that calorie restriction is effective at reducing cancer incidence and increasing evidence indicates that this is largely mediated via effects on the IGF system (Kari et al 1999). In relation to human populations the evidence that a relatively high circulating concentration of IGF-1 may increase the risk of cancer has to be balanced by the other potential consequences of interindividual differences in these concentrations. There is emerging evidence implying that a relatively low circulating IGF-1 concentration may be associated with increased risk of cardiovascular disease and cognitive decline, and predispose to osteoporosis. Any proposed manipulation of the IGF system in the elderly population, such as the administration of GH to counter age-related muscle and bone frailty would have to be undertaken against a careful consideration of the overall balance of consequences. An additional major factor that should also be considered is that the associations between IGF levels and cancer incidence imply an effect of IGF-1 early in life when these cancers are probably initiated. In the elderly population the risk of initiating new cancers is not the major concern: a much bigger concern would be the impact upon existing pre-clinical neoplasias. Many population screening and large-scale autopsy studies have established that in the elderly there is a very high prevalence of small neoplasias in tissues such as the breast, prostate and colorectum. The prevalence of these neoplasias is much higher than the incidence of the corresponding cancer within the population, presumably because most of the neoplasias detected at autopsy are slow, indolent lesions that would not develop into a clinical cancer before the individual dies of other causes. These data suggest that most individuals would probably be harbouring at least one sub-clinical neoplasia by the age of 70 years. The main concern in administering GH, or other manipulations to raise IGF-1 levels, to counter the effects of ageing, would then not be the risk of initiating new cancers, but what effect this would have on the sub-clinical cancers that would normally not present before the individual dies of a cardiovascular incident.

Modus operandi

The two growth factors IGF-1 and IGF-2 are single polypeptides that share a high degree of homology with proinsulin. Their actions on cells are mediated by a classical transmembrane tyrosine kinase cell surface receptor. Like the ligands, the IGF-1 receptor is remarkably similar to the insulin receptor, particularly in the tyrosine kinase domain, and they share considerable overlap in their intracellular signalling capability (Kim & Accili 2002). These receptors each exist as dimers within the cell surface and they are so similar that in cells where both are expressed there is substantial heterodimerization forming hybrid IGF-1/insulin receptors. These hybrids appear to act more like IGF-1 receptors *in vitro*, but their physiological role *in vivo* is poorly understood. There is also an IGF-2 receptor which is a single large transmembrane receptor that is completely unrelated to the IGF-1 and insulin receptors. The IGF-2 receptor does not appear to act as a traditional signalling receptor in response to ligand occupancy. In relation to IGF function it is thought to act as a clearance receptor for IGF-2, since disruption of gene expression in mice resulted in elevated IGF-2 levels and overgrowth. These receptors, are however, clearly multifunctional. Their most well characterized role is as mannose 6-phosphate receptors involved in the targeting of lysosomal enzymes to the lysosomes within the cell. They, however, also bind latent transforming growth factor (TGF)β and enable its activation on the cell surface, and they bind retinoids and urokinase-receptors. The potential functional consequences of interactions between IGF-2 and all the other possible ligands of the IGF-2 receptor are far from clear (Ghosh et al 2003).

Although the IGFs and their signalling receptors are remarkably similar to insulin, how they operate as a communication system within the body has evolved to be very different in mammals. The expression of insulin is very restricted, principally just to the β cells in the pancreas. It is stored in secretory granules within the cells of the pancreatic islets and secreted via the regulated pathway from these cells in response to stimuli. In contrast the IGFs are expressed widely in tissues throughout the body. In addition, like most other peptide growth factors and cytokines, the IGFs are not stored within secretory granules within cells, but they are secreted as they are produced, via the constitutive secretory pathway. Furthermore, when insulin is secreted from the pancreas it then enters the circulation and passes around the body until it encounters a cell receptor in a target tissue. In contrast, when the IGFs are secreted they then associate with soluble high-affinity binding proteins, the IGF binding proteins (IGFBPs). The IGFBPs bind the IGFs and considerably slow their clearance; enabling very high concentrations of IGFs to build up. In the circulation two of the IGFBPs, IGFBP-3 and IGFBP-5, are bound to a further large glycoprotein, the acid labile subunit (ALS) that is present in excess. This ternary complex formation slows clearance even more such that in adult humans the total IGF-1 and IGF-2 concentration in the circulation is around 100 nanomolar. This is around 1000 times higher than insulin and most peptide hormones. At the cellular level, optimal regulation of the IGF-1 receptor is achieved with just 1–2 nM concentrations, indicating that there is a vast excess in the circulation. In the tissues IGF concentrations are around a third of that in the circulation, but this is still a large excess over that needed for cell regulation. Therefore, while IGFs are not stored within cells, there appears to be a large extracellular store maintained in complexes with IGFBPs. With insulin the activity throughout the body is largely determined by the rate of secretion from the pancreas; in contrast, with the IGFs the constitutive secretion within any tissue is just one component of the total amount of IGF that the cells are exposed to. The IGFs are bound to the IGFBPs with higher affinity than to the IGF-1 receptor, so most of the IGF in the body is potentially not available for receptor activation. Activity in a tissue is therefore not necessarily determined by secretion rate of IGFs nor by total IGF concentration. It is also not safe to assume that IGF has to be released from a binding protein and it is then just the free IGF in solution that is active. There is considerable evidence that IGFBPs can not only sequester IGFs away from cell receptors and restrict activity, but also that they can enhance activity at the cellular level via a variety of mechanisms (Firth & Baxter 2002).

There are six high affinity binding proteins (IGFBP1–6) that are unrelated to the cell surface receptors. The IGFBPs are structurally closely related to each other, although they are each distinct gene products and they all have very distinct functional properties (Firth & Baxter 2002). In terms of physiology there is still very limited understanding of the exact role of each of the IGFBPs. In humans IGFBP-3 clearly acts as the main circulating carrier protein, but it is also expressed extensively in many tissues and obviously has many additional local functions. One of these proteins, IGFBP-1, is more restricted in its sites of expression; IGFBP-1 present in the circulation is predominantly derived from the liver where its expression is under the dynamic control of insulin which suppresses its production. In the circulation IGFBP-1 levels undergo a circadian variation due to this dynamic insulin regulation. This appears to provide an additional acute control to ensure that IGF activity is appropriate to nutritional conditions.

With the large quantities of IGFs associated with IGFBPs with greater affinity than the cell receptor, it is clear that there must be mechanisms for making this IGF available for actions in the tissues. In the circulation the majority of IGF is associated with IGFBP-3 and the ALS. The ALS binds to a C-terminal region of IGFBP-3 that also binds to proteoglycans present on cell surfaces and in the extracellular matrix (ECM). It is therefore possible that proteoglycans on the surface of the capillary endothelium compete for binding to IGFBP-3 and displace the ALS generating a binary complex from the ternary complex. The binary complex would then be more able to cross the endothelium and transport the IGF into the tissue. There is, however, another mechanism for controlling delivery of IGF from the circulatory reservoir. A circulating protease that acts specifically upon IGFBP-3 has been described in many different conditions. This protease results in limited cleavage of IGFBP-3. The cleaved IGFBP-3 still retains IGF in the ternary complex, but it is bound with a lower affinity. Even a small decrease in affinity could result in a shift in the complex equilibrium that must exist *in vivo* with the IGF re-equilibrating to other IGFBPs that are present, these are generally not cleaved by the same protease. These other IGFBPs only form binary complexes and therefore have greater ability to transport the IGFs out into target tissues. There have been many studies documenting increases in

IGFBP-3 proteolysis in the circulation in pregnancy and many other conditions, especially catabolic states (Maile & Holly 1999). In addition to the IGFBP-3 protease, it has become clear that each of the IGFBPs appears to be subject to specific proteolysis. In humans, proteases capable of cleaving IGFBP-3 appear to be ubiquitously present both in the circulation and in extravascular fluids. In the normal healthy individual there is little detectable IGFBP-3 protease activity in serum due to the presence of inhibitors which protect the IGFBP-3 from proteolysis. Increases in proteolysis that are observed in different conditions appear to be due to a decrease in these inhibitors, rather than an increase in levels of proteases (Maile et al 1998). Outside of the circulation in the tissues this system appears to operate quite differently. The protease inhibitors appear to be restricted to the circulation, whereas the same proteases that are present in the circulation are also present in extravascular interstitial fluids. Consequently IGFBP-3 protease activity is unopposed and proteolysis of IGFBP-3 is more extensive in the tissues, presumably making the IGF more available for cell receptors. This system in the tissues is disturbed in inflammatory conditions, where an increase in capillary permeability enables the circulating protease inhibitors access to the extravascular space and IGFBP-3 proteolysis is then suppressed (Maile et al 1998).

All of the IGF present in the body is effectively present in IGFBP complexes and there is clearly a very complex system with six IGFBPs, each of which is present in a number of functionally distinct forms due to various post-translational modifications. There are proteases and accompanying inhibitors for each of the individual IGFBPs, the most fully characterized being the PAPP-A system for cleaving IGFBP-4 (Chen et al 2002). It has also become clear that each of the IGFBPs interacts with high affinity with many other proteins, particularly in the ECM and on the cell surface. The pattern of expression of all of these interacting components varies between tissues and within a tissue varies with developmental stage and pathology. This sophisticated complexity of components for controlling IGF availability and actions provides an insight into how some specificity could be conferred on the system. Since their original description as cell growth factors, it was realised that they were also responsible for metabolic insulin-like activity and they have subsequently been shown to be pluripotential cell regulators. In addition to regulating growth and metabolism, they are very potent cell survival factors and can regulate cell motility, differentiation and most, if not all, differentiated cell functions. These peptides are therefore ubiquitously present in vast excess and can potentially regulate every cell function. The sophisticated interplay of multiple components appears to provide a means of conferring specificity such that their actions can be very finely controlled in a tissue specific manner.

As both IGF-1 and IGF-2 appear to act via the same cell surface, IGF-1 receptor, the distinction in their physiology has raised some puzzling questions. The distinction between the two IGFs is most clear in early development. IGF-2 plays a very important role in fetal and early neonatal growth and development. *In utero* IGF-2 has an important role in placental function and in the control of nutrient partitioning (Gluckman & Pinal 2003). Both IGF-2 and the IGF-2 receptor are imprinted genes. This imprinting appears to have evolved to balance the genetic conflict between parents. The paternal imprinted genes enhance nutrient extraction from the mother and growth of the fetus to ensure the survival and development of the father's offspring. This is enabled by paternal imprinting of the IGF-2 gene. In contrast, the mother needs to constrain the fetal development and balance nutrient extraction to ensure her own survival and reproductive competence for future potential fetuses, with potentially different fathers. This is enabled by maternal imprinting of the IGF-2 receptor gene (Reik et al 2003). As the pituitary develops and takes control of the endocrine system, pituitary GH drives systemic IGF-1 production which then plays a more dominant role in growth and development. In rodents there is a clear switch, at weaning the expression of IGF-2 has virtually ceased and there is an obvious end to the major role that IGF-2 plays. In higher mammals this switch does not occur and in humans IGF-2 is the most prevalent IGF throughout life. In adult humans there are around fourfold higher levels of IGF-2 in the circulation compared to IGF-1 and it remains unclear why or what is the role of this IGF-2. In the rodent there is virtually no IGF-2 in the adult circulation and therefore these experimental models are not informative regarding the role of IGF-2 in the adult human. This species difference also considerably limits the use of these experimental models for examining interventions targeting the IGF system for treating conditions in adult humans.

References

Carter CS, Ramsey MM, Sonntag WE 2002 A critical analysis if the role of growth hormone and IGF-1 in aging and lifespan. Trends Genet 18:295–301

Chen BK, Overgaard MT, Bale LK et al 2002 Molecular regulation of the IGF-binding protein-4 protease system in human fibroblasts: identification of a novel inducible inhibitor. Endocrinology 143:1199–1205

Daughaday WH, Salmon WD 1999 The origins and development of the somatomedin hypothesis. In: Rosenfeld R and Roberts (eds) Contemporary endocrinology: the IGF system. Humana Press Inc, Totowa, NJ, p 1–15

Firth SM, Baxter RC 2002 Cellular actions of the insulin-like growth factor binding proteins. Endocr Rev 23:824–854

Ghosh P, Dahms NM, Kornfield S 2003 Mannose 6-phosphate receptors: new twists in the tale. Nat Rev Mol Cell Biol 4:202–212

Gluckman PD, Pinal SC 2003 Regulation of fetal growth by the somatotrophic axis. J Nutr 133(suppl 2):S1741–S1746

Kari FW, Dunn SE, French JE, Barrett JC 1999 Roles for insulin-like growth factor-1 in mediating the anti-carcinogenic effects of caloric restriction. J Nutr Health Aging 3:92–101

Ketelslegers JM, Maiter D, Maes M, Underwood LE, Thissen JP 1995 Nutritional regulation of insulin-like growth factor-I. Metabolism 44(suppl 4):50–57

Kim JJ, Accili D 2002 Signalling through IGF-I and insulin receptors: where is the specificity? Growth Horm IGF Res 12:84–90

Maile LA, Holly JM 1999 Insulin-like growth factor binding protein (IGFBP) proteolysis: occurrence, identification, role and regulation. Growth Horm IGF Res 9:85–95

Maile LA, Xu S, Cwyfan-Hughes SC, Fernihough JK, Pell JM, Holly JM 1998 Active and inhibitory components of the insulin-like growth factor binding protein-3 protease system in adult serum, intersitial, and synovial fluid. Endocrinology 139:4772–4781

Reik W, Constancia M, Fowden A et al 2003 Regulation of supply and demand for maternal nutrients in mammals by imprinted genes. J Physiol 547:35–44

DISCUSSION

Lønning: I have a question concerning the increase we see in protease activity in inflammation, critical illnesses and advanced cancer. If I heard you correctly, you are suggesting that one of the explanations could simply be clipped IGFBP-3 leaking out from the tissue into the circulation. Is that correct? If the vessels in the tumour and in inflammation have a higher permeability, it could be the clipped protein that leaks back.

Holly: That is the explanation for seeing a large proportion of clipped IGFBP-3 in the circulation in normal healthy individuals. Where you can't find activity in the circulation it is presumably being clipped as soon as it gets out of the circulation and then what is washing back is in the clipped form. This happens in normal physiology. When you become catabolic or have advanced cancer, you get an increase in the protease in the circulation, so you actually get clipping occurring in the circulation as well as still occurring outside the circulation. The two processes are going on together. There is always the cleavage outside the circulation, and some of this is washing back. Then you get alterations in the clipping that is actually occurring in pathologies.

Lønning: To play the devil's advocate, we know that the vessels in the tumour tissue have a different fenestration compared to normal vessels. Could what you see be due to higher leakage of clipped proteins, which are being clipped in the tumour tissue?

Holly: We can do a number of different assays on the serum samples from these patients and show that there is increased activity in the circulation. We were originally very excited to find that there was an increase in proteolysis of IGFBP-3 in the circulation in patients with cancer. But then we went on to show that in normal tissues all the IGFBP-3 is already clipped, so what would happen in a tumour is a more difficult scenario to understand. There are interesting differences. In the normal tissue there is a limited cleavage. In the tumours you get other proteases such as cathepsins and the tumour starts to acidify, and there is a different pattern of cleavage. The consequences of this still need to be worked out in terms of different fragments. As soon as you acidify you release the IGF from the binding proteins anyway, so there is a different interpretation of the clipping again.

LeRoith: If I understand correctly from the data you presented on disease states, it is because of this inhibitor in interstitial tissue that you have intact binding protein and IGF-1 in the disease state. Are you suggesting that IGFBP-3 is preventing IGF-1 from acting, or enabling it to act?

Holly: In the arthritic joint there is an increase in capillary permeability and inhibitors are going into tissue. IGFBP-3 is no longer all clipped and in the low affinity state. More of it is maintained in a high-affinity state so less IGF-1 will be available for sustaining tissue integrity or whatever metabolic actions that it has.

LeRoith: So it is preventing IGF-1 action in target tissue.

Holly: In arthritis we have gone on to inject steroids into joints, and have shown that when there is a decrease in capillary permeability the protease activity goes up and all the IGFBP-3 is clipped.

Laron: We know that with increasing age the circulating level of IGF-1 as well as GH decrease. At the same time the incidence of malignancy goes up. What do we know about *in vivo* levels of free IGF-1? If indeed IGF-1 plays a role, there should be an increase or at least a stabilization of free IGF-1 with age.

Holly: I don't believe in free IGF. Roger Ekins put forward the free hormone hypothesis, breaking down complex systems into two compartments, a free fraction of hormone which is active and a bound fraction which is inactive (Ekins 1992). But over the last decade many of us have shown that with IGF and binding proteins in many cell systems, the bound is more active than the free. Breaking it down into two compartments is naïve. The situation outside the circulation is very different. Measuring free IGF in the circulation is like measuring something that has just fallen off the bus, because the small binding proteins are the shuttle service, and outside the circulation the mix of binding proteins and proteases is very different, therefore the equilibrium will be different. Free is the result of everything being in equilibrium. You can work out mathematically how much should be free and it agrees very well with the best technical measures. So the free level in the circulation is completely uninterpretable.

Laron: But how do you reconcile the basic finding that with age there is less IGF-1 and more malignancy. Does this mean that less IGF-1 is more dangerous than high levels?

Holly: There is the same sort of paradox in breast cancer. It is oestrogen driven, and oestrogen levels decrease at a time when you get more breast cancer. Androgen levels also decrease at a time when you get more prostate cancer. The age related decline in IGF-1 and GH may be protective to prevent you getting more cancer.

LeRoith: There are probably oncogenic hits that are causing the cancer, and IGF-1 in that system can turn the prevalence of tumours into incidence. In other words, it might stimulate underlying tumours to be doing something. It may be that this reduction in IGF-1/GH is protective. There is an animal model suggesting that the GH receptor antagonist knockout causes the animals to live longer. It is possible that we should allow GH/IGF-1 to decrease — perhaps this is good for us.

Holly: The decrease was presumably designed for a reason.

Lønning: The parallel with oestrogens is a good one. There is an increase in breast cancer incidence with age, and then suddenly around the menopause there is a plateau for a couple of years and then it starts to increase again. There is now experimental evidence *in vitro* to suggest that tumour cells may adapt to a reduction in the oestrogen concentration. This is probably through up-regulation by the MAP kinase and other systems.

Pollak: Often at this kind of meeting, the paradox that Zvi Laron raised is discussed. If all of this has any validity, why is there more cancer in the older people, who have lower IGF-1 levels? From an oncological perspective the question is important, but there is a lot of evidence that the rate of cancer in old people is determined when those people are young. Your fate in terms of having cancer at age 75 may be sealed at age 40. There are determinants of late cancer that operate early in life. We know that people stay true to their centile of IGF more or less throughout life. If you are in the top part of the population of IGF levels at age 60, you probably also were in the top centiles at age 15, 20 and 25. You may have had a different kind of history of your somatic cell divisions early in life which led to an increased accumulation of genetic damage because of a slight increased survival probability of damaged cells. The paradox you posed is an important one, but I think that there are at least two answers. One is that the late life cancers may be at least in part be determined by early life IGF experience, and the second part is the one that was already mentioned in the discussion, which is that although in general old people have a lower IGF-1 level than young people, among the old people there is a spread in the IGF-1 levels. What some of the epidemiology is telling us is that the people who have the slower rates of decline may be the ones who have more cancer.

Rosenfeld: You stated as an assumption that people will maintain their percentiles of IGF throughout life. In truth, this has never been adequately demonstrated. It is an assumption we make and there is logic to it, but there are no solid data supporting it. The issue of the age-associated changes in IGF-1 needs to be put in perspective. What makes this decline so striking is the adolescent increase in IGF-1. It is important to note that this is to a large extent a uniquely human phenomenon. We are the only species with an adolescent growth spurt. Even primates don't have skeletal adolescent growth spurts. This probably reflects the pubertal increase in GH secretion, which then remains the major controller of IGF-1 levels during ageing. To make your hypothesis stand, that it is what occurs in adolescence or young adult life that is predictor of adult cancer risk, the correlation between GH secretion, IGF secretion and maintenance of IGF-1 levels throughout the lifespan will need to be determined. In this regard, one important part of the underlying physiology is that we understand so little about the transcriptional regulation of IGF-1. We know that it is GH dependent postnatally, but we don't know what controls it prenatally. Since IGF-1 levels may be surrogates for so many other physiological phenomena besides GH secretion, such as obesity and nutrition, until we understand what controls IGF-1 levels throughout the lifespan we will have difficulty intervening to regulate these levels.

Holly: We have done a recent study on 770 men aged 60–70, where we have 6 monthly measures of growth throughout their childhood. Their IGF-1 levels measured at age 60 have been plotted against peak height velocity a measure of when mid-puberty occurred. Those that developed earlier have a nice dose dependent effect on their IGF-1 measured some 60 years later. This implies that IGF-1 through life does track to a certain extent. This is compatible with the hypothesis that the IGF-1 activity is tracking and reflecting what happened early in life. We also published data suggesting that childhood nutrition affects the risk of cancer in later life.

Carpentier: Here we speak about IGF-1 or the IGF-1 receptor, but each time we focus on only one component. I think we should consider the two elements. We should see whether if you have a high level of IGF-1 you will decrease the level of receptor. But if there is not such an effect then you will probably have things going wrong. We always need to take into account both elements and not just focus on one.

Kaaks: I am puzzled by what Jeff Holly said about pubertal IGF levels. The vast majority of cross-sectional studies have shown no association whatsoever between final adult height attained and IGF levels. The correlations are usually no more than 0.10 if they exist at all. This seems to argue against a major tracking effect. If one is willing to accept that final height is a marker of IGF level or exposure to IGF in the pubertal period, you would expect this association to persist later in life as well.

Holly: Your final height is dependent on the rate at which you are growing and for how long you grow. There are lots of good correlations with height and IGF-1 at individual stages throughout childhood. We know that if you increase or decrease IGF-1 it affects the rate of growth. Where you end up is determined by the length of the adolescent period. If you develop early and cease growing early you can have grown faster but end up with shorter final height. The IGF-1 level gives you a measure of the rate at which you are growing, but also the final height is determined by the tempo and length of time you grow for. The correlations with longitudinal growth are there throughout childhood and disappear in adulthood.

Kaaks: So you are arguing that peak height velocity is a better marker for cumulative exposure to IGF in the pubertal period, or just at a given point in time at which the peak height velocity is expressed?

Holly: Peak height velocity tells you what is going in at the most rapid period of change. It's like a car accident: the faster you are going the bigger the crash.

Lønning: There were some epidemiological studies back in Norway on young girls who went through puberty during the wartime period during 1940–45 when there were food restrictions (Nilsen & Vatten 2001). In general, they have slightly lower height compared with those who had their growth spurts just before the war or afterwards. They also seem to have a somewhat lower incidence of breast cancer.

Rosenfeld: My understanding of the epidemiological data is different. I thought they did support a correlation between adult height and IGF-1 levels, and also between adult height and certain cancers.

Kaaks: Cancers for sure. But with IGF-1 many of our data and many other studies that we have looked at indicate that there is no correlation with height.

Pollak: Part of the answer to this paradox is that adult height is poorly correlated with IGF-1. In part, this is because when adult height is measured in old enough people, there are other variables that have to do with loss of height that complicate the situation in older people. The correlation of adult cancers to IGF-1 is stronger than the correlation of height to IGF-1. In Scandinavia, when they look at height to cancer risk relationships, there is a reproducible although very weak relationship that is found when groups as large as 10 000 people are studied. This is because the adult height is a poor surrogate for IGF-1 levels, whereas adolescent height or height at age 20 would be more closely correlated with the IGF-1 level.

Rosenfeld: Even better would be height pre-pubertally, say at age 10 or 12. This is because a critical determinant of adult height will be the timing of epiphyseal fusion.

Holly: We have published that of all the childhood anthropometry, prepubertal leg length measurements are the strongest correlate with risk of getting the epithelial cancers throughout the rest of life.

Thomas: In the earlier part of your paper you pointed out how all the model systems contribute to our understanding of what the signalling components are doing in terms of longevity and nutritional sensing. Are there any homologues of these binding proteins in *Drosophila* or *Caenorhabditis elegans*?

Holly: In *C. elegans* it is quite complicated: there are now 38 ligands (Duret et al 1998). There are certainly binding proteins in insects.

De Meyts: There is an insulin binding protein in insects that does not have an orthologue in humans or other species so far (Andersen et al 2000), but I don't know of any IGF-1 binding proteins.

Holly: It is not my field, but Zee Upton told me that insects do have IGF binding proteins.

Thomas: I was going to make a suggestion. If we do have such an orthologue, we could think about setting up a genetic screen.

Holly: Ron Rosenfeld has reviewed that the proteins are part of a superfamily, and lots of these genes go back a long way. Whether these always had a role as binding proteins is unclear.

Laron: There is a new hormone which links nutrition, GH and feeding—ghrelin. There are many papers published on this hormone. Is anything known that connects ghrelin with cancer?

Kaaks: Not as far as I know. These may be difficult studies to do because of the large variation between fasting and non-fasting states. One would have to do thorough controls.

LeRoith: In obese patients there is no fasting state.

Laron: It would be of interest to do these studies, because ghrelin is secreted in the stomach. Is anything known about ghrelin concentrations in stomach cancer?

Pollak: No. The epidemiology is always at least a few weeks if not a few years behind the research! You are defining a future area of research. I think it is on the radar screens of many people to look at these things in a population context, but there is always a time delay. I suspect those papers will come out in a few years.

Clark: On the ghrelin story, Merck, Pfizer and Genentech have made small ligands against the ghrelin receptor. This was done before we knew about endogenous ghrelin. These small molecule GH secretagogues were taken into development, and in formal toxicology studies large doses were given in long-term studies. There was no evidence that they induced tumours in animals, and long-term clinical studies were performed in humans (Murphy et al 2001). In terms of whether the ghrelin system is the link between IGF-1 and oncology, the data from the small molecules don't suggest that there is any vast toxicology there.

Jenkins: In vitro we have looked at the effects of ghrelin on cancer cells. It seems to have a biphasic response. At high doses it inhibits both breast and colon cancer cells, but at more physiological doses (10^{-10} M) it seems to have a slight independent stimulatory effect on cell growth. This is independent of IGF-1.

Grimberg: Another hormone that might be important to look at is leptin. Leptin has been shown to induce the expression of IGF-1 receptor in the growth plates (Maor et al 2002), and leptin is produced by fat cells.

Holly: I think some people have already done this.

Kaaks: We have done a few studies looking at the association between leptin and cancer. I find the results very difficult to interpret because leptin has so many functions, on the regulation of appetite and energy balance, cellular fatty acid metabolism, pituitary gonadotropin secretion and steroidogenesis. A second problem is that I don't see a direct link with signalling pathways in the cells that are well established to be involved in cancer development. There is such a link for IGF-1 and insulin, if you look at the Ras/Raf/MAP kinase or the PI3K/Akt pathways, which are both directly related to the tyrosine kinase receptors, including the receptors of insulin and IGF-1. I don't see any such link emerging for leptin. Leptin correlates strongly with obesity. Because of this you'd expect to see an association with some cancers that are obesity-related. It may be simply a marker of adiposity and no more than that.

Rosenfeld: To me it seems to boil down to the fact that in humans we have not identified anything other than GH that is a strong transcriptional regulator of IGF-1. For any action that we think affects IGF-1 levels such as nutrition or obesity, unless we can find some other way it manipulates IGF-1 other than through GH, we are at a loss. If there is any effect of leptin or ghrelin, it is all going to be through GH secretion. Is anyone aware of anything else that physiologically transcriptionally regulates IGF-1?

Jenkins: IGF-1 must be transcriptionally regulated other than by GH. In a physiological situation, if you have total GH deficiency with a complete absence of your pituitary, circulating IGF-1 levels are usually still at the low end of the normal range or just below this. This is telling us that there is something other than GH that is regulating IGF-1 levels. There may be constitutive production from other tissues such as muscle.

Rosenfeld: Prepubertally, if you totally eliminate GH secretion or action, IGF-1 levels are virtually unmeasurable. There are factors post-pubertally that regulate basal IGF-1 secretion.

Holly: Certainly at the age when people get cancer, a lot of the GH-deficient subjects have normal IGF-1 levels. It is less GH-driven and more driven by something else at the ages where people get cancer.

LeRoith: In liver, for example, we know that GH is a strong stimulant. The only way to show this is to hypox the animal. You are really suggesting that there is some other hormonal contribution there, although we know that GH stimulates powerfully. This is regulated by nutrition. The other tissues in the body are also regulated by other factors, perhaps even more strongly than GH.

Rosenfeld: I don't disagree. Those pathways need to be identified.

LeRoith: Some of them must contribute to the circulating level as well, even in the absence of GH.

Roberts: We are assuming that all the regulation of IGF-1 gene expression is transcriptional. This is probably not the case. It is clear from a lot of recent array studies that the extent of translational control is significantly more than we appreciate. There is work that Derek LeRoith and I did some years ago which showed that in certain circumstances you can have very strong translational regulation of IGF-1 because it is a gene that has very complicated 5′ and 3′

untranslated regions, which are important regulators of translational efficiency. We may be missing some potential transcriptional regulators, but there may be other things out there that we are not going to see in terms of mRNA levels.

LeRoith: Ron Rosenfeld's point is that we don't understand any of that after 20 years.

De Meyts: As a prominent politician said recently, the fact that they have not been found doesn't mean that they don't exist!

Holly: The situation is far more complicated than just transcriptional or translational control. The protein levels are controlled as much, if not more, by clearance than by IGF-1 production.

Pollak: What is the consensus on prolactin as a regulator of IGF synthesis in humans?

Clark: In patients with Laron syndrome the prolactin receptor is normal and there are high levels of GH which does bind to the prolactin receptor. These patients have very low IGF-1 levels so the evidence from humans is that prolactin receptor doesn't regulate IGF-1. It probably regulates IGF-2, on the other hand.

Laron: If I am not mistaken, there are certain malignancies that are increased in pregnancy, but has this anything to do with sex hormones or with placental lactogen? What do we know about the signal transmission of placental lactogen and its post receptor effects? Is it similar to normal GH-1?

Rosenfeld: Placental lactogen and prolactin both stimulate the Jak/STAT system and phosphorylate STAT5B, a major transcriptional regulator of IGF-1. But as Ross Clark said, physiologically in humans they don't appear to be important stimulators of IGF-1.

Laron: I read somewhere that there is increased production of prolactin in prostate cancer.

Pollak: There are a lot of papers out about prolactin receptors on prostate cancer tissue. It is not my work and I am not prepared to defend it, but I am interested that for at least a decade papers have been published showing prolactin receptors, GHRH and other hypothalamic or pituitary receptors present on neoplastic tissue. The relevance of these observations has never really been established.

LeRoith: I can comment on one of them. Andrew Schally from Tulane University has done a lot of work on GHRH receptors and lung cancer, and has given antagonists. He suggests that it inhibits IGF-2 production by the tumours, and this is how it may work as a tumour inhibitor. He has then given this with bombesin inhibitors and combined the two. This has actually inhibited the tumour growth even more. The relevance may not be through IGF-1 but through some other system, like in this case IGF-2, through the GHRH receptor. I am not sure how this works.

Thomas: One of the IGF-2 transcripts is controlled at the translational level by the TOR pathway. Nutrients are necessary and sufficient to drive this pathway. By nutrition you could drive IGF-2.

Ohlsson: 10 years ago we published a report showing that IGF-2 expression in human liver drops dramatically after the age of 30 (Ohlsson et al 1994).

Kaaks: One prospective cohort study on prolactin levels in prostate cancer found no association (Stattin et al 2001).

Lønning: The studies on prolactin are in patients who have already been diagnosed with cancer cannot be counted on. They relate to stress hormone levels and all these issues. I also have a comment with respect to pregnancy and cancer risk. There is a very slight increase in the risk of breast cancer in pregnancy and the first year after. But it is very low, and also it should be borne in mind that pregnancy doesn't just involve one hormone. It is a totally homeostatic change so it is very difficult to identify the factors involved. There is no doubt that this is related to a more rapid growth of cancers that were already present and not induction of new tumours.

Carbone: I have a question regarding the *NEJM* paper correlating obesity with increased cancer risk (Calle et al 2003). One issue that isn't addressed in that paper is the fact that lung cancer was specifically not elevated in overweight individuals, yet *in vitro* models of lung cancer are very sensitive to IGF-1 stimulation. Do you think that this is just an artefact of the predominantly environmental causality of lung cancer?

Kaaks: There is no simple direct relationship between BMI as an index of obesity and IGF-1. We have shown in one large cross-sectional study a non-linear relationship where there is a peak around a BMI of 25–26 and which goes down afterwards (Lukanova et al 2002). We have repeated this on a large cross-sectional study of 1800 women from the EPIC cohort and we see the same thing. One shouldn't simplify this reasoning too much. It seems that up to a certain level, maybe through higher insulin levels, when people become more obese they may become more sensitive to the GH-stimulated synthesis of IGF-1, but after a certain point there could be a dominant-negative feedback of the free IGF on the GH axis. This is the kind of interpretation we have given to this observation. It matches the observation that BMI above 30 is associated with lower IGF-1 levels. Anorexia is also associated with lower than normal IGF-1 levels. There must be a maximum in the middle.

Holly: In relation to lung cancer, isn't there a confounding issue of relationships between BMI and smoking?

Lønning: Yes. First of all, in lung cancer there is a very strong exogenous carcinogen that is causing the bulk of lung cancers. There is also a negative association between smoking and BMI. In general, heavy smokers have a lower BMI, so it goes in exactly the opposite direction.

Yee: At the beginning of your talk you focused on protease regulation and binding proteins. Is there any evidence that the body regulates BP proteases to influence IGF action?

Holly: There is not the evidence. The proteases and inhibitors haven't been identified; all the measures are still fairly crude.

Rosenfeld: At the extremes, such as in anorexia, you can see some increased proteases.

Holly: Yes, there are huge increases. But in the normal physiological range the changes are more subtle.

References

Andersen AS, Hansen PH, Schäffer L et al 2000 A new secreted insect protein belonging to the immunoglobulin superfamily binds insulin and related peptides and inhibits their activities. J Biol Chem 275:16948–16953

Calle EE, Rodriguez C, Walker-Thurmond K, Thun MJ 2003 Overweight, obesity, and mortality from cancer in a prospectively studied cohort of U.S. adults. N Engl J Med 348:1625–1638

Duret L, Guex N, Peitsch MC et al 1998 New insulin-like proteins with atypical disulfide bond pattern characterized in *Caenorhabditis elegans* by comparative sequence analysis and homology modelling. Genome Res 8:348–353

Ekins R 1992 The free hormone hypothesis and measurement of free hormones. Clin Chem 38:1289–1293

Lukanova A, Soderberg S, Stattin P et al 2002 Nonlinear relationship of insulin-like growth factor (IGF)-I and IGF-I/IGF-binding protein-3 ratio with indices of adiposity and plasma insulin concentrations (Sweden). Cancer Causes Control 13:509–516

Maor G, Rochwerger M, Segev Y, Phillip M 2002 Leptin acts as a growth factor on the chondrocytes of skeletal growth centers. J Bone Miner Res 17:1034–1043

Murphy MG, Weiss S, McClung M et al 2001 Effect of alendronate and MK-677 (a growth hormone secretagogue), individually and in combination, on markers of bone turnover and bone mineral density in postmenopausal osteoporotic women. J Clin Endocrinol Metab 86:1116–1125

Nilsen TI, Vatten LJ 2001 Adult height and risk of breast cancer: a possible effect of early nutrition. Br J Cancer 85:959–961

Ohlsson R, Hedborg F, Holmgren L, Walsh C, Ekström T 1994 Overlapping expression of IGF2 and H19 expression during human development: biallelic expression of IGF2 correlates with a lack of H19 expression. Development 120:361–368

Stattin P, Rinaldi S, Stenman UH et al 2001 Plasma prolactin and prostate cancer risk: a prospective study. Int J Cancer 92:463–465

Molecular basis of insulin action

Yehiel Zick

Department of Molecular Cell Biology, The Weizmann Institute of Science, Rehovot, 76100, Israel

Abstract. Insulin signalling at target tissues results in a large array of biological responses. These events are essential for normal growth and development, and for normal homeostasis of glucose, fat and protein metabolism. Elucidating the intracellular events following activation of the insulin receptor and the interactions between the insulin and IGF-1 signalling systems has been the main focus of a large number of investigators, and for excellent reasons. Improved understanding of the signalling pathways involved in insulin action and the impact of IGF-1 on these processes could lead to a better understanding of the pathophysiology of insulin resistance associated with obesity and type 2 diabetes and the identification of key molecules that could lead to newer and more effective therapeutic agents for treating these common disorders that are already an uprising epidemic of the 21st century. This chapter will summarize our current understanding of the molecular basis of insulin action, beginning with outlining key elements that constitute the insulin signalling pathways. Then, impairments in insulin signalling pathways and new paradigms regarding the molecular basis of insulin and IGF-1 resistance will be analysed.

2004 Biology of IGF-1: its interaction with insulin in health and malignant states. Wiley, Chichester (Novartis Foundation Symposium 262) p 36–55

Insulin signalling

Insulin is the major anabolic hormone. Its action is essential for growth, development, homeostasis of glucose, fat, and protein metabolism, and the proper function of pancreatic β cells (LeRoith & Zick 2001). At the molecular level, insulin binding to its transmembrane receptor (IR) stimulates the intrinsic Tyr kinase activity of the receptor (IRK) which then phosphorylates selected Tyr residues of target proteins. IR substrates include the three isoforms of Shc, IRS proteins (IRS1–6), $p60^{dok}$, Cbl, APS and Gab-1 (LeRoith & Zick 2001, Zick 2001, Khan & Pessin 2002, Saltiel & Pessin 2002).

The Tyr-phosphorylated IR substrates function as signalling scaffolds, providing a docking interface for proteins with Src-homology 2 (SH2) domains. Some of the SH2 proteins are enzymes, including the P-Tyr phosphatase SHP2 (SH-PTP2) and the cytoplasmic Tyr kinase Fyn. Other SH2 proteins, such as the p85 regulatory subunit of PI3K, Grb2 or APS function as adaptor proteins for downstream effectors that further propagate the metabolic and growth-promoting effects of insulin.

IRS proteins are considered as the major IR substrates. They contain a conserved pleckstrin homology (PH) domain, located at their N-terminus, that serves to anchor the IRS proteins to membrane phosphoinositides and helps to localize the IRS proteins in close proximity to the receptor (Voliovitch et al 1995; Fig. 1). The PH domain of IRS proteins is flanked by a P-Tyr binding (PTB) domain. The PTB

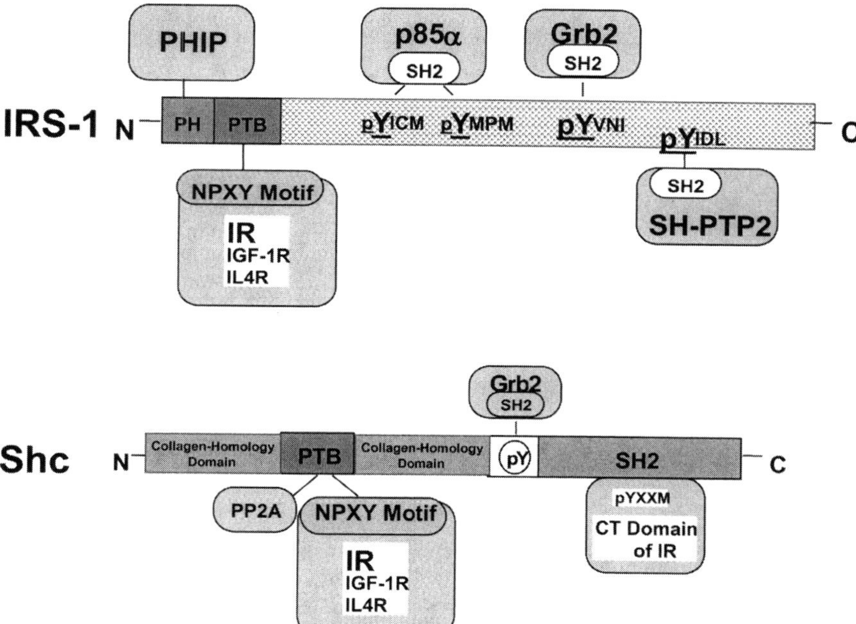

FIG. 1. Structural features of Shc and IRS proteins. IRS proteins have a conserved pleckstrin homology (PH) domain, located at their amino terminus, that serves to anchor the IRS proteins to membrane phosphoinositides and helps to localize the IRS proteins in close proximity to the insulin receptor. The PH domain also promotes protein–protein interactions with proteins such as PHIP. The PH domain is flanked by a P-Tyr binding (PTB) domain. The PTB domain functions as a binding site to the NPXY motif of the juxtamembrane (JM) region of the insulin and other receptors such as the IGF-1 and interleukin (IL)-4 receptor. The C-terminal region of IRS proteins contains multiple Tyr phosphorylation motifs that serve as docking sites for SH2 domain-containing proteins such as the p85a regulatory subunit of PI3K, Grb2, Nck, Crk, Fyn and SHP-2. Shc proteins have a PTB domain at their N-terminus, a collagen-homology domain (CH1), and a C-terminal SH2 domain. Shc can interact with the JM domain of IR through its PTB domain, while its SH2 domain binds the Tyr-phosphorylated CT domain of IR. Tyr-phosphorylated Shc serves as docking site for downstream effectors having SH2 domains such as Grb2. The Ser/Thr phosphatase PP2A can also bind to the PTB domain of Shc and inhibit its interaction with IR.

domain functions as a binding site to the NPXY motif of the juxtamembrane (JM) region of IR, IGF-1R and other receptors (Wolf et al 1995). The C-terminal region of IRS proteins is poorly conserved. It contains multiple Tyr phosphorylation motifs that serve as docking sites for SH2 domain-containing proteins including the p85a regulatory subunit of PI3K, Grb2, Nck, Crk, Fyn, SHP2 and others, which mediate various aspects of insulin action (LeRoith & Zick 2001, Zick 2001, Khan & Pessin 2002, Saltiel & Pessin 2002).

IRS1, similarly to the other IRS proteins, contains over 70 potential Ser/Thr phosphorylation sites with homologies to casein kinase II, PKB, PKC, MAP kinases, CDC2, and cAMP- and cGMP-dependent protein kinase consensus phosphorylation sites (Sun et al 1991). Indeed, several kinases that can phosphorylate IRS1 have been identified. These include casein kinase II, glycogen synthase kinase 3, MAP kinase, and even a lipid kinase, the PI3K (reviewed in Zick 2001). In non-treated cells, IRS1 is strongly phosphorylated on Ser residues and weakly phosphorylated on Tyr residues. Following insulin stimulation, Tyr and Ser phosphorylation of IRS1 is increased. Ser phosphorylation of IRS1 reduces its ability to undergo Tyr-phosphorylation and serves to shut off insulin signalling (Zick 2001, see below).

Insulin signalling propagates through three major pathways: the PI3K, the MAP kinase, and the Cbl/CAP pathways (Fig. 2). While these pathways share several signalling elements that intricately affect one another, each of these pathways has some unique characteristics. The MAPK pathway can be considered as a general signalling pathway which is activated by a number of growth factor receptors including insulin, all leading to enhanced cell growth, while the PI3K and the Cbl/CAP pathways, triggered by insulin, generate biological responses that are more unique to insulin action. Recruitment of the

FIG. 2. The insulin signalling network. The activated insulin receptor kinase (IRK) phosphorylates substrate proteins such as Shc, Gab1, Cbl, APS and the family of IRS proteins on selective Tyr residues that serve as docking sites for downstream effector molecules. This trigger three major kinase signaling cascades, the MAP kinase, the PI3K and the Cbl/TC10 pathway. Recruitment of Grb2 and mSos to Tyr-phosphorylated Shc activates the MAPK signalling cascade, while association of PI3K with the IRS proteins, results in production of PIP_3 that activates PDK1 and its downstream effector kinases PKB, mTOR, p70S6 kinase, and the atypical isoforms of PKC (PKC ζ/λ). The pathway leading to insulin-dependent activation of JNK and p38 is less well understood. Phosphorylation of Cbl mediates glucose transport in a PI3K-independent manner through activation of TC10 and its interaction with the exocyst complex and CIP4/2 (Cdc42-interacting protein 4/2). Insulin also promotes the recruitment of Myo1c, which contains a motor domain, to GLUT4 vesicles, thus facilitating glucose transport. Collectively, these signalling pathways mediate the metabolic and growth-promoting functions of insulin including the translocation of vesicles containing GLUT4 glucose transporters to the plasma membrane; stimulation of glycogen and protein synthesis; and initiation of specific gene transcription, while inhibiting the transcription of gluconeogenic genes (see text for details).

proteins Grb2 and Sos to Tyr-phosphorylated Shc activates the MAP kinase cascade and leads to enhanced gene transcription (Johnson & Lapadat 2002), while association of PI3K with the IRS proteins results in production of phosphatidylinositol-3,4,5-phosphate (PIPS) that activates PDK1 (PIP_3-dependent kinase 1) and its downstream effector kinases PKB (protein Ser/Thr kinase B, also named Akt); mTOR, p70S6 kinase, and the atypical isoforms of PKC (PKCζ/λ), all leading to enhanced glucose transport, glycogen and protein synthesis (Cantley 2002). Tyr phosphorylation of Cbl by IRK mediates glucose transport in a PI3K-independent manner through activation of the GTP-binding

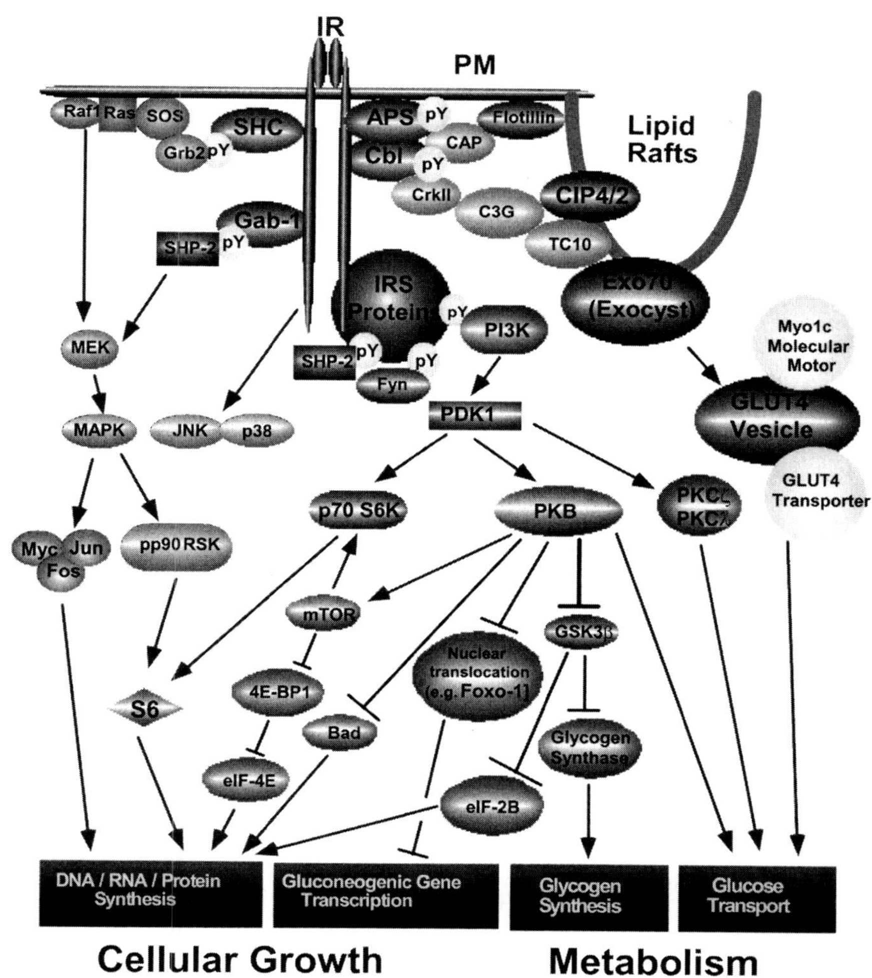

protein TC10 and its interaction with the exocyst complex and CIP4/2 (Cdc42-interacting protein 4/2) (Chiang et al 2001, Inoue et al 2003). Insulin also promotes the recruitment of Myo1c, which contains a motor domain, to GLUT4 vesicles, thus facilitating glucose transport (Bose et al 2002). Collectively, these signalling pathways mediate the metabolic and growth-promoting functions of insulin including the translocation of vesicles containing GLUT4 glucose transporters to the plasma membrane, the stimulation of glycogen and protein synthesis, and the regulation of β cell function and initiation of specific gene transcription, while inhibiting the transcription of gluconeogenic genes.

Inhibition of insulin receptor signalling

The duration and extent of insulin signalling is regulated at several levels. Some of the control mechanisms are set into motion immediately following insulin stimulation. They act to terminate insulin's effects through activation of lipid or protein phosphatases and through the induction of Ser/Thr kinases that phosphorylate and uncouple various elements along the insulin signalling pathways. Other negative control mechanisms, which operate on a longer timescale involve a reduction in the cellular content of the insulin receptor, its substrates, and other signalling elements.

Insulin receptor internalization and degradation

Internalization of the insulin receptor is a multi-step process. Following surface redistribution, the receptor–insulin complex progressively concentrates in clathrin-coated pits, which represent the internalization gates. The internalized receptor undergoes sorting, which determines whether it will be subjected to degradation in lysosomes or whether it will recycle back to the plane of the membrane (Carpentier & McClain 1995). Stimulation of the IRK is a prerequisite for surface redistribution of receptor–insulin complexes, but the nature of the protein substrates being involved remains unclear. We have shown that IRK internalization occurs independent of its ability to phosphorylate IRS proteins (Boura-Halfon et al 2003), whereas impaired internalization of IR is associated with impaired phosphorylation of Shc (Biener et al 1996).

We have further demonstrated that the cellular environment regulates IR internalization. In particular, IR internalization is affected by the nature of the extracellular matrix (ECM) proteins onto which the cells adhere. Interaction of different ECM proteins with cell surface integrins results in different cytoskeletal organizations that affect the rate of IR endocytosis (Boura-Halfon et al 2003). It appears that specific polymerized actin structures, in the form of filamentous actin tracks, are required to maintain proper IR internalization. Accordingly, IR internalization is impaired upon disruption of actin filaments, or when cells adhere to matrices such as galectin 8 (Levy et al 2003), in which actin is organized in cortical elements, exhibiting poorly developed filamentous structures (Boura-Halfon et al 2003).

Role of protein and lipid phosphatases

Insulin signalling is negatively regulated by phosphatidylinositol-3-phosphatases such as PTEN (Simpson et al 2001) and SHIP2 (Hori et al 2002). Accordingly, disruption of the genes of theses lipid phosphatases yields mice with increased insulin sensitivity (Clement et al 2001). Protein tyrosine phosphatases (PTPs) also have a prominent role in the control of IR signalling. PTPs dephosphorylate the IR and its substrates and thus serve to terminate IR signalling. Several PTPs have been implicated in the negative regulation of insulin action. These include PTPIB and its close homologue TCPTP. For example, mice lacking PTP1B have increased insulin sensitivity and resistance to obesity induced by a high-fat diet (Elchebly et al 1999), while loss of TCPTP enhances IR activation (Galic et al 2003).

Ser phosphorylation as a physiological regulatory mean to terminate insulin signalling

Control mechanisms are integral part of any signalling network. Control can be achieved by autoregulation, whereby downstream enzymes inhibit upstream elements (homologous desensitization). Alternatively, signals from apparently unrelated receptor pathways can inhibit the signal (heterologous desensitization). The insulin receptor, IRS and Shc proteins, which are key players in propagating insulin signalling, are subjected to such network control. Recent studies from our laboratory have focused on Ser/Thr phosphorylation of IRS proteins as a key feedback control mechanism that uncouples the IRS proteins from their upstream and downstream effectors and terminates signal transduction in response to insulin (Paz et al 1997, Liu et al 2001, Zick 2001).

We have shown that insulin-stimulated Ser/Thr phosphorylation of IRS proteins has a dual function in serving either as a positive or a negative modulator of insulin signalling (Fig. 3). Phosphorylation of Ser residues within the PTB domain of IRS1 by insulin-stimulated PKB, protects IRS proteins from the rapid action of PTPs, and enables the IRS proteins to maintain their Tyr-phosphorylated active conformation, thus implicating PKB as a positive regulator of IRS-1 functions (Paz et al 1999). By contrast, Ser/Thr phosphorylation of IRS proteins by other insulin-stimulated Ser/Thr kinases, such as PKCξ (Liu et al 2001) serves as a physiological negative feedback control

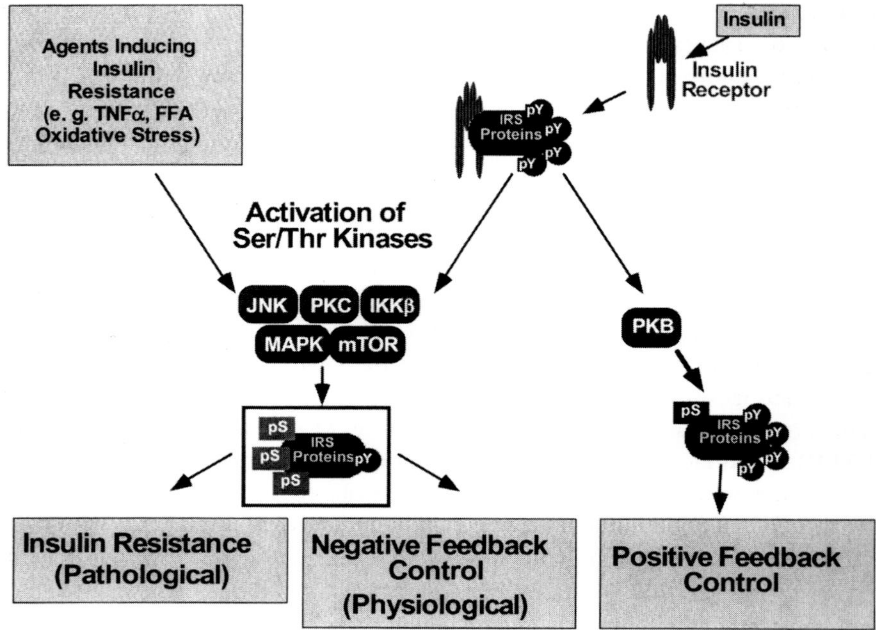

FIG. 3. Ser/Thr-phosphorylated the IRS proteins as modulators of insulin action and insulin resistance. Ser/Thr phosphorylation of IRS protein has a dual role, either to enhance or to terminate insulin's signal. Ser residues of the PTB domain of IRS-1, located within consensus PKB phosphorylation sites, presumably function as positive effectors of insulin signalling by protecting IRS proteins from the action of PTPs. Hence, PKB propagates insulin signalling by phosphorylating downstream effectors, and by phosphorylating IRS proteins, thus generating a positive feedback loop for insulin action. Insulin also activates other Ser/Thr kinases including mTOR, JNK, PKCζ and IKKβ, that mediate phosphorylation of IRS proteins. Phosphorylation of these Ser sites is part of a negative feedback control mechanism, induced by insulin, that results in the termination of insulin signal. Agents that induce insulin resistance, such as FFAs and TNFα, take advantage of this negative-feedback control mechanism by activating either the same or other Ser/Thr kinases that phosphorylate the IRS proteins, inhibit their function, terminate insulin action and induce insulin resistance.

mechanism that inhibits further Tyr phosphorylation of IRS proteins. Ser/Thr phosphorylation can induce the dissociation of IRS proteins from the insulin receptor (Paz et al 1997, Liu et al 2001); hinder Tyr phosphorylation sites of IRS proteins (Mothe & Van Obberghen 1996); release the IRS proteins from intracellular complexes that maintain them in close proximity to the receptor (Tirosh et al 1999); induce IRS proteins degradation (Pederson et al 2001); or turn IRS proteins into inhibitors of the IRK (Hotamisligil et al 1996; Fig. 4). These multiple effects place the spotlight on Ser/Thr kinases that phosphorylate the IRS protein and the Ser sites that are getting phosphorylated.

The activity of insulin-stimulated IRS kinases is blocked by inhibitors of the PI3K pathway, implicating downstream effectors of PI3K as negative regulators of IRS protein function (Paz et al 1999, Liu et al 2001). One potential candidate is the mammalian target of rapamycin (mTOR), which enhances phosphorylation of Ser residues at the C-terminus of IRS1. This phosphorylation inhibits insulin-stimulated Tyr phosphorylation of IRS1 and its ability to bind PI3K (Li et al 1999). Another candidate is PKCξ. PKCξ mediates phosphorylation of IRS proteins (Liu et al 2001, Ravichandran et al 2001) that leads to the dissociation of the IR–IRS complexes (Liu et al 2001). This inhibits the ability of IRS proteins to undergo further insulin-stimulated Tyr phosphorylation and as a result, it terminates insulin signalling. IRS1 serves as a substrate for PKCξ *in vitro*, and endogenous IRS1 forms complexes with PKCξ in an insulin-dependent manner (Ravichandran et al 2001). These findings suggest that PKCξ can function as an insulin-stimulated IRS kinase, although downstream effectors of PKCξ could also fulfil this role. A potential candidate effector is IKKβ. IKKβ is a Ser/Thr kinase that is part of the IKK complex that phosphorylates the inhibitor of NF-κB, IκB. This results in the degradation of IκB, allowing for the nuclear translocation and activation of the transcription factor NF-κB (Karin 1999). IKKβ can bind PKCξ both *in vitro* and *in vivo*, serves as an *in vitro* substrate for PKCξ, and is activated by a functional PKCξ (Lallena et al 1999). IKKβ is activated by insulin in Fao rat hepatoma cells. Furthermore, insulin-stimulated Ser phosphorylation of IRS1 is inhibited by salicylates, implicating IKKβ as an insulin-stimulated IRS kinase (Y. F. Liu and Y. Zick, unpublished data). This conclusion is supported by recent evidence indicating that IRS1 is a direct substrate for IKKβ that phosphorylates IRS1 on Ser 312 (the human homologue of mouse Ser 307) following cellular stress (Gao et al 2002). Because Ser307 is adjacent to the PTB domain of IRS1, its phosphorylation might disrupt the interaction between the juxtamembrane domain of the IR and the PTB domain IRS1, and in such a way inhibit insulin-stimulated Tyr phosphorylation of IRS1.

JNK, a member of the MAP kinase family of protein kinases, is activated by insulin by an as yet unknown mechanism. Recent studies have shown that JNK associates with IRS1 and phosphorylates it at Ser307 in an insulin-dependent manner (Lee et al 2003). Insulin stimulation of JNK activity requires PI3K and Grb2 signalling, suggesting that JNK activation is mediated by a number of signalling pathways. Direct binding of JNK to IRS1 is not required for JNK activation by insulin. However, direct interactions between JNK and IRS1 are required for Ser 307 phosphorylation (Lee et al 2003).

PKB, mTOR, PKCξ and IKKβ are downstream effectors of PI3K along the insulin signalling pathway. This suggests that their action should be orchestrated to allow phosphorylation by PKB and sustained activation of IRS1, prior to the activation of mTOR, JNK or PKCξ, the actions of which are expected to terminate

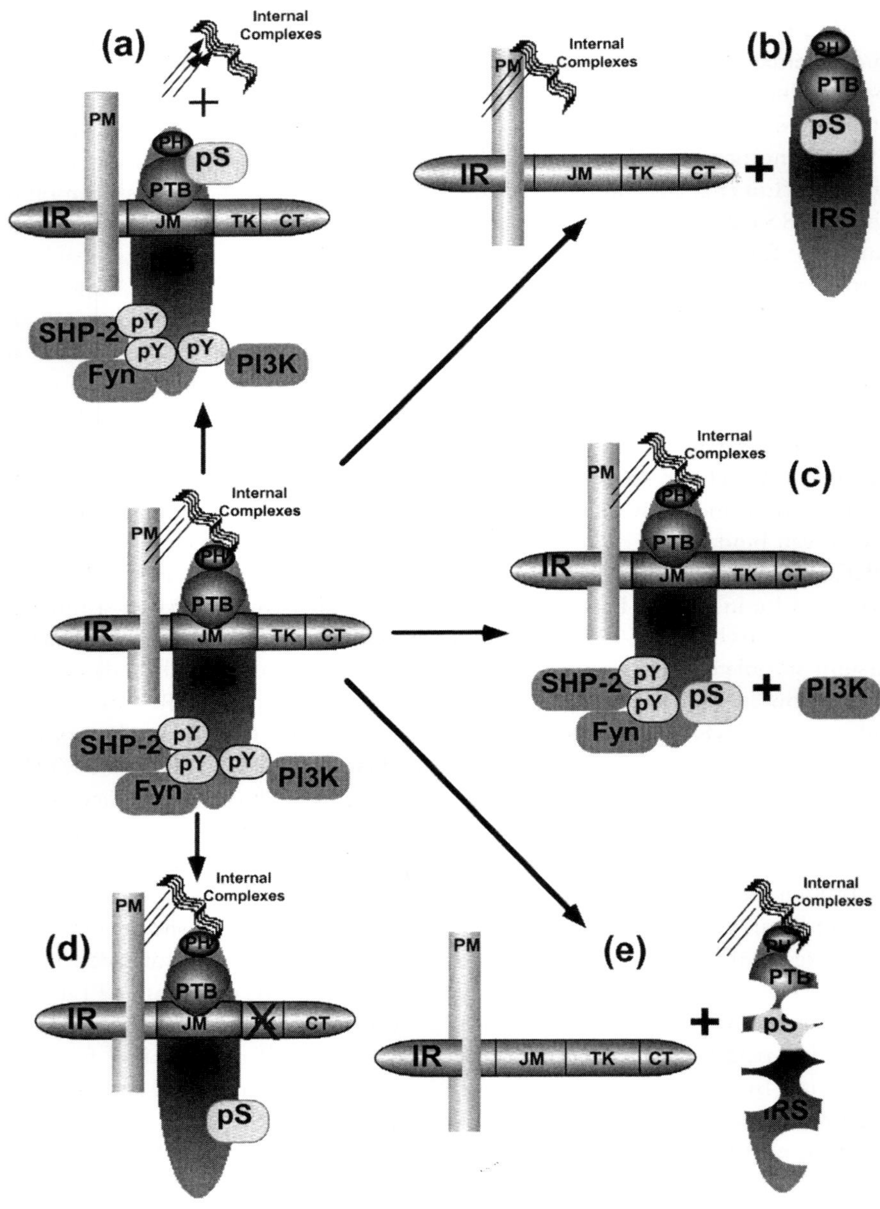
(a)
Internal
Complexes
PM
PH
pS
PTB
IR
JM
TK
CT
SHP-2
pY
pY
pY
Fyn
PI3K
(b)
PM
Internal
Complexes
IR
JM
TK
CT
PH
PTB
pS
IRS
(c)
Internal
Complexes
PM
PH
PTB
IR
JM
TK
CT
SHP-2
pY
pY
pS
Fyn
PI3K
Internal
Complexes
PM
PH
PTB
IR
JM
TK
CT
SHP-2
pY
pY
pY
Fyn
PI3K
(d)
Internal
Complexes
PM
PH
PTB
IR
JM
CT
pS
(e)
PM
IR
JM
TK
CT
Internal
Complexes
PTB
pS
IRS

insulin signal transduction. Of note, the negative-feedback control mechanism induced by PKCξ (or mTOR) includes a self-attenuation mode, whereby PI3K-mediated activation of mTOR and PKCξ inhibits IRS1 function, thereby inhibiting further activation of mTOR and PKCξ themselves (Liu et al 2001, Zick 2001).

IRS proteins also serve as substrates for the IGF-1 receptor (LeRoith & Zick 2001). The structural similarity between the IR and IGFR further suggests that elevated Ser/Thr phosphorylation of IRS proteins might as well interfere with IGFR interactions with IRS proteins, and inhibit IGFR signalling. This raises the possibility that a similar feedback control mechanism is part of the IGF-1 signalling pathway, and brings up the question as to which Ser kinases, triggered by IGF-1, might act as negative modulators of IGFR function.

Ser phosphorylation of IRS proteins and insulin resistance

Insulin resistance is a common pathological state in which target cells fail to respond to ordinary levels of circulating insulin (Kahn & Flier 2000). Individuals with insulin resistance are predisposed to developing type 2 diabetes, a 21st century epidemic. Insulin resistance is frequently associated with a number of other health disorders including obesity, hypertension, chronic infection, and cardiovascular diseases, making it the focus of interest of a large number of studies (Kahn & Flier 2000). Recent studies by us and others indicate that Ser/Thr phosphorylation of IRS proteins that uncouples them from their upstream and downstream effectors in response to insulin under physiological conditions, could also be the underlying mode of action of inducers of insulin resistance (Zick 2001). Emerging data suggest that agents such as tumour necrosis factor (TNF)α, free fatty acids (FFAs) and cellular stress that inhibit insulin signalling and induce insulin resistance activate Ser/Thr kinases that phosphorylate the IRS proteins and inhibit their function. Thus, while the underlying molecular pathophysiology of insulin resistance is still not well understood, Ser phosphorylation of IRS proteins represents an important new mechanistic theme (Zick 2001) that should be considered along with other potential mechanisms for

FIG. 4. The impact of Ser/Thr phosphorylation on IRS proteins function. Ser/Thr phosphorylation of IRS proteins inhibits insulin-stimulated Tyr phosphorylation of the IRS proteins because: (a) it releases the IRS proteins from intracellular insoluble multiprotein complexes that include cytoskeletal elements that maintain the IRS proteins in close proximity to the receptor; (b) it induces the dissociation of IRS proteins from the JM domain of IR; (c) it inhibits the ability of downstream effectors such as PI3K to dock and bind to specific Tyr residues at the C-terminal tail of the IRS proteins; (d) it turns IRS proteins into inhibitors of IRK; and (e) it induces the degradation of the IRS proteins.

the induction of insulin resistance such increased activity of lipid- or protein-Tyr phosphatases (Kahn & Flier 2000).

Because Ser/Thr phosphorylation of IRS proteins is stimulated by insulin treatment and by inducers of insulin resistance, it suggests that the same Ser kinases might be utilized to phosphorylate the IRS proteins under both physiological and pathological conditions (Fig. 3). This conclusion is based, for example, upon the fact that TNFα can induce activation of sphingomyelinase and production of ceramide, which stimulates PKCξ and its downstream target IKKβ. Indeed, the inhibitory effects of TNFα on insulin-stimulated Tyr phosphorylation of IRS proteins are mimicked by sphingomyelinase and ceramide analogues (Kanety et al 1996, Paz et al 1997). Alternatively, TNFα can induce complex formation between PKCξ, p62 and RIP proteins that serve as adaptors of the TNF receptor and link PKCξ to TNFα signalling (Sanz et al 1999).

IKKβ is an additional IRS kinase, the activity of which is stimulated by FFA, pro-inflammatory cytokines and other inducers of insulin resistance. Activation or overexpression of IKKβ attenuates insulin signalling, whereas IKKβ inhibition by high doses of salicylates or by a reduction in IKKβ gene dose reverses obesity- and diet-induced insulin resistance in animal models (Yuan et al 2001) and improves glucose metabolism in type 2 diabetic subjects (Hundal et al 2002). The mechanism by which FFA might activate IKKβ presumably involves an increase in FFA-derived metabolites, such as diacylglycerol and ceramide, which are potent activators of PKCθ and PKCξ, both known to activate IKKβ. At the molecular level, inhibition of IKKβ prevents Ser/Thr phosphorylation of IRS proteins induced by a high-fat diet, TNFα, or phosphatase inhibitors, whereas it improves insulin-stimulated Tyr phosphorylation of IRS proteins. Hence, IKKβ might serve as a point of convergence, where Ser kinases downstream of insulin signalling and Ser kinases activated by pro-inflammatory cytokines activate IKKβ to inhibit insulin signalling both under physiological and pathological conditions.

JNK is activated by pro-inflammatory cytokines such as TNFα, and its activity is abnormally elevated in obesity. Conversely, an absence of JNK1 results in decreased adiposity, significantly improved insulin sensitivity and enhanced insulin receptor signalling capacity in two different models of mouse obesity (Hirosumi et al 2002). The inhibitory effects of JNK on insulin signalling can be attributed, at least partially, to its function as an IRS kinase (Aguirre et al 2000) that phosphorylates Ser307, to uncouple IRS-1 from the insulin receptor.

'Novel' PKC isoforms, such as PKCθ, were implicated as mediators of FFA-induced insulin-resistance in skeletal muscle, in a process that involves phosphorylation of IRS-1 at Ser307 (Yu et al 2002). In contrast, 'conventional' members of the PKC family such as PKCα, which are activated by phorbol esters or endothelin-1, utilize members of the MAPK pathway to phosphorylate IRS-1 at

Ser612 (located in a consensus MAPK phosphorylation site) and at additional sites in its C-terminal tail (DeFea & Roth 1997). Other potential IRS kinases include glycogen synthase kinase-3 (GSK3) (Eldar-Finkelman & Krebs 1997), casein kinase II (Tanasijevic et al 1993) and a novel kinase that phosphorylates IRS1 at Ser 789 (Qiao et al 2002). The S789 kinase is presumably activated under conditions of insulin resistance because increased phosphorylation of this site is observed in livers of insulin-resistant rodent models (Qiao et al 2002).

Future perspectives

Current findings implicate IRS proteins as major targets for insulin-induced, phosphorylation-based negative feedback control mechanisms that uncouple the insulin receptor from its downstream effectors and terminate insulin signalling under physiological conditions. The kinases involved are still under investigation, with current focus on PKCξ, IKKβ, JNK and mTOR as potential candidates. A variety of agents and conditions that induce insulin resistance such as TNFα, FFAs and stress inducers also activate IRS kinases. At present, different PKC isoforms, IKKβ, MAPK, JNK and mTOR appear as potential candidates but additional kinases are likely to emerge. Since each of the potential IRS kinases has a unique substrate specificity, the question remains as to which Ser sites are being modified by each kinase and what are the consequences of such phosphorylation. Present studies indicate that negative regulatory sites are found both in close proximity to the PTB domain (e.g. Ser307) and at the C-terminal end of IRS1 (e.g. Ser612), and it still remains to be determined whether phosphorylation of Ser residues distributed along the IRS molecule contributes to a given functional change (e.g. enhanced dissociation of IR/IRS complexes) or whether phosphorylation of Ser residues clustered within a confined region results in a unique functional consequence. Another question still unresolved is whether the same or different signalling pathways are being utilized by insulin or agents that induce resistance to regulate the activity of IRS kinases. While the same kinases (PKCξ, JNK, IKKβ) can be activated by insulin, FFAs and TNFα, there is no evidence that these kinases are being activated along the same pathways. Indeed, at least under certain circumstances, kinases localized along different pathways are activated by insulin and TNFα to induce phosphorylation of the inhibitory Ser307 site. Given the large number of stimuli, pathways, kinases and potential sites involved, it appears that Ser/Thr phosphorylation of IRS proteins represents a combinatorial consequence of several kinases, activated by different pathways, acting in concert to phosphorylate multiple sites. Still, in spite of the complexity and dynamic of the system, unravelling IRS kinases and their biological role is expected to provide a novel viewpoint of the molecular basis for insulin resistance. This should enable a rationale for drug design to selectively inhibit the activity of relevant kinases and generate a novel class of therapeutic agents for the treatment of insulin resistance and type 2 diabetes.

Finally, it should be noted that Ser phosphorylation of IRS proteins also has essential bearings on IGF-1 signalling. Unlike insulin, IGF-1 is a major inducer of tumorigenesis. Therefore, agents that selectively inhibit the growth-promoting activity of IGF-1 might be potential targets as anticancer drugs. Ser/Thr kinases that phosphorylate IRS proteins are potential targets because they can induce the dissociation of IRS–IGFR complexes and thus inhibit the biological activity of IGF-1. By revealing the kinases that negatively regulate IRS protein functions and the specific residues modified by these enzymes, we might be in a position to offer new means to selectively potentiate these kinase activities and thus inhibit the growth-promoting activity of the IGFR, which is associated with tumour cell growth. Conversely, development of selective means to inhibit IRS kinases might offer new strategies to potentiate IGF-1 action as a survival factor in the brain and other tissues and thus inhibit its sensitivity to the action of neurodegenerative agents such as TNFα

References

Aguirre V, Uchida T, Yenush L, Davis R, White MF 2000 The c-Jun NH(2)-terminal kinase promotes insulin resistance during association with insulin receptor substrate-1 and phosphorylation of Ser(307). J Biol Chem 275:9047–9054

Biener Y, Feinstein R, Mayak M, Kaburagi Y, Kadowaki T, Zick Y 1996 Annexin II is a novel player in insulin signal transduction. Possible association between annexin II phosphorylation and insulin receptor internalization. J Biol Chem 271:29489–29496

Bose A, Guilherme A, Robida SI et al 2002 Glucose transporter recycling in response to insulin is facilitated by myosin Myo1c. Nature 420:821–824

Boura-Halfon S, Voliovitch H, Feinstein R, Paz K, Zick Y 2003 Extracellular matrix proteins modulate endocytosis of the insulin receptor. J Biol Chem 278:16397–16404

Cantley LC 2002 The phosphoinositide 3-kinase pathway. Science 296:1655–1657

Carpentier JL, McClain D 1995 Insulin receptor kinase activation releases a constraint maintaining the receptor on microvilli. J Biol Chem 270:5001–5006

Chiang SH, Baumann CA, Kanzaki M et al 2001 Insulin-stimulated GLUT4 translocation requires the CAP-dependent activation of TC10. Nature 410:944–948

Clement S, Krause U, Desmedt F et al 2001 The lipid phosphatase SHIP2 controls insulin sensitivity. Nature 409:92–97

DeFea K, Roth RA 1997 Modulation of insulin receptor substrate-1 tyrosine phosphorylation and function by mitogen-activated protein kinase. J Biol Chem 272:31400–31406

Elchebly M, Payette P, Michaliszyn E et al 1999 Increased insulin sensitivity and obesity resistance in mice lacking the protein tyrosine phosphatase-1B gene. Science 283:1544–1548

Eldar-Finkelman H, Krebs EG 1997 Phosphorylation of insulin receptor substrate 1 by glycogen synthase kinase 3 impairs insulin action. Proc Natl Acad Sci USA 94:9660–9664

Galic S, Klingler-Hoffmann M, Fodero-Tavoletti MT et al 2003 Regulation of insulin receptor signaling by the protein tyrosine phosphatase TCPTP. Mol Cell Biol 23:2096–2108

Gao Z, Hwang D, Bataille F et al 2002 Serine phosphorylation of insulin receptor substrate 1 (IRS-1) by inhibitor κB kinase (IKK) complex. J Biol Chem 277:48115–48121

Hirosumi J, Tuncman G, Chang L et al 2002 A central role for JNK in obesity and insulin resistance. Nature 420:333–336

Hori H, Sasaoka T, Ishihara H et al 2002 Association of S112-containing inositol phosphatase 2 with the insulin resistance of diabetic db/db mice. Diabetes 51:2387–2394

Hotamisligil GS, Peraldi P, Budavari A et al 1996 IRS-1-mediated inhibition of insulin receptor tyrosine kinase activity in TNF-alpha- and obesity-induced insulin resistance. Science 271:665–668

Hundal RS, Petersen KF, Mayerson AB et al 2002 Mechanism by which high-dose aspirin improves glucose metabolism in type 2 diabetes. J Clin Invest 109:1321–1326

Inoue M, Chang L, Hwang J, Chiang SH, Saltiel AR 2003 The exocyst complex is required for targeting of Glut4 to the plasma membrane by insulin. Nature 422:629–633

Johnson GL, Lapadat R 2002 Mitogen-activated protein kinase pathways mediated by ERK, JNK, and p38 protein kinases. Science 298:1911–1912

Kahn BB, Flier JS 2000 Obesity and insulin resistance. J Clin Invest 106:473–481

Kanety H, Hemi R, Papa MZ, Karasik A 1996 Sphingomyelinase and ceramide suppress insulin-induced tyrosine phosphorylation of the insulin receptor substrate-1. J Biol Chem 271:9895–9897

Karin M 1999 The beginning of the end: IkappaB kinase (IKK) and NF-kappaB activation. J Biol Chem 274:27339–273342

Khan AH, Pessin JE 2002 Insulin regulation of glucose uptake: a complex interplay of intracellular signalling pathways. Diabetologia 45:1475–1483

Lallena M-J, Diaz-Meco MT, Bren G, Paya CV, Moscat J 1999 Activation of IkappaB kinase beta by protein kinase C isoforms. Mol Cell Biol 19:2180–2188

Lee YH, Giraud J, Davis RJ, White MF 2003 cJUN N-terminal kinase (JNK) mediates feedback inhibition of the insulin signaling cascade. J Biol Chem 278:2896–2902

LeRoith D, Zick Y 2001 Recent advances in our understanding of insulin action and insulin resistance. Diabetes Care 24:588–597

Levy Y, Ronen D, Bershadsky AD, Zick Y 2003 Sustained induction of ERK, PKB and p70S6K regulates cell spreading and formation of F-actin microspikes upon ligation of integrins by galectin-8, a mammalian lectin. J Biol Chem 278:14533–14542

Li J, DeFea K, Roth RA 1999 Modulation of insulin receptor substrate-1 tyrosine phosphorylation by an Akt/phosphatidylinositol 3-kinase pathway. J Biol Chem 274: 9351–9356

Liu YF, Paz K, Herschkovitz A et al 2001 Insulin stimulates PKCzeta-mediated phosphorylation of insulin receptor substrate-1 (IRS-1). A self-attenuated mechanism to negatively regulate the function of IRS proteins. J Biol Chem 276:14459–14465

Mothe I, Van Obberghen E 1996 Phosphorylation of insulin receptor substrate-1 on multiple serine residues, 612, 632, 662, and 731, modulates insulin action. J Biol Chem 271: 11222–11227

Paz K, Hemi R LeRoith D et al 1997 A molecular basis for insulin resistance: elevated serine/threonine phosphorylation of IRS-1 and IRS-2 inhibits their binding to the juxtamembrane region of the insulin receptor and impairs their ability to undergo insulin-induced tyrosine phosphorylation. J Biol Chem 272:29911–29918

Paz K, Yan-Fang L, Shorer H et al 1999 Phosphorylation of insulin receptor substrate-1 (IRS-1) by PKB positively regulates IRS-1 function. J Biol Chem 274:28816–28822

Pederson TM, Kramer DL, Rondinone CM 2001 Serine/threonine phosphorylation of IRS-1 triggers its degradation: possible regulation by tyrosine phosphorylation. Diabetes 50:24–31

Qiao LY, Zhande R, Jetton TL, Zhou G, Sun XJ 2002 *In vivo* phosphorylation of insulin receptor substrate 1 at serine 789 by a novel serine kinase in insulin-resistant rodents. J Biol Chem 277:26530–26539

Ravichandran LV, Esposito DL, Chen J, Quon MJ 2001 PKC-zeta phosphorylates IRS-1 and impairs its ability to activate PI 3-kinase in response to insulin. J Biol Chem 276:3543–3549
Saltiel AR, Pessin JE 2002 Insulin signaling pathways in time and space. Trends Cell Biol 12: 65–71
Sanz L, Sanchez P, Lallena MJ, Diaz-Meco MT, Moscat J 1999 The interaction of p62 with RIP links the atypical PKCs to NF-kappaB activation. EMBO J 18:3044–3053
Simpson L, Li J, Liaw D et al 2001 PTEN expression causes feedback upregulation of insulin receptor substrate 2. Mol Cell Biol 21:3947–3958
Sun XJ, Rothenberg P, Kahn CR et al 1991 Structure of the insulin receptor substrate IRS-1 defines a unique signal transduction protein. Nature 352:73–77
Tanasijevic MJ, Myers MG Jr, Thoma RS, Crimmins DL, White MF, Sacks DB 1993 Phosphorylation of the insulin receptor substrate IRS-1 by casein kinase II. J Biol Chem 268:18157–18166
Tirosh A, Potashnik R, Potashnik R, Bashan N 1999 Oxidative stress disrupts insulin-induced cellular redistribution of insulin receptor substrate-1 and phosphatidylinositol 3-kinase in 3T3-L1 adipocytes. A putative cellular mechanism for impaired protein kinase B activation and GLUT4 translocation. J Biol Chem 274:10595–10602
Voliovitch H, Schindler D, Hadari YR, Taylor SI, Accili D, Zick Y 1995 The pleckstrin-homology (PH) domain of insulin receptor substrate-1 (IRS0-1) is required for proper interaction of IRS-1 with the insulin receptor. J Biol Chem 270:18083–18087
Wolf G, Trub T, Ottinger E et al 1995 PTB Domains of IRS-1 and Shc have distinct but overlapping binding specificities. J Biol Chem 270:27407–27410
Yu C, Chen Y, Cline GW et al 2002 Mechanism by which fatty acids inhibit insulin activation of IRS-1 associated phosphatidylinositol 3-kinase activity in muscle. J Biol Chem 277:50230–50236
Yuan M, Konstantopoulos N, Lee J et al 2001 Reversal of obesity and diet induced insulin resistance with salicylates or targeted disruption of IKK beta. Science 293:1673–1677
Zick Y 2001 Insulin resistance: a phosphorylation-based uncoupling of insulin signaling. Trends Cell Biol 11:437–441

DISCUSSION

LeRoith: There are two things that come to mind when we discuss this subject. One is work by Boris Draznin who showed that PI3K is blocked under insulin-resistant conditions; this allows the MAP kinase pathway to be more active (Montagnani et al 2002). So when IGF-1, PDGF and pathways come along, there is much more mitogenic activity in endothelial cell lines. This could be explained by some of what you have suggested: that you are blocking PI3K and you are allowing other pathways such as Shc to be enhanced. He has shown this in endothelial cells and vascular cells. This is interesting.

Zick: There are some reports in the literature that insulin can stimulate kinases that induce the phosporylation of Shc (Sasaoka et al 2000). Perhaps a similar pathway could operate along the Shc pathway. We can have association with IRS proteins or the Shc pathway.

LeRoith: So there are other ways to get MAP kinase activated. The paradigm may fit into what he has been showing with the vascular cells. The second point I wanted to open up for discussion is that when patients were given rhIGF-1 and they had severe insulin resistance, they responded very well to IGF-1 treatment. Is this working in the muscle to stimulate uptake of glucose, which IGF-1Rs can support? If on the one hand you have insulin resistance and perhaps chronically an IRS1 abnormality in muscle, how would one conceive of the IGF-1R stimulating glucose uptake? The pathway should go IRS, TC10 and eventually lead to glucose transporter translocation. This would speak a little bit against the IRSs being common to both, at least in muscle. It may be that there are different IRS molecules involved? Am I correct that rhIGF-1 worked well in those circumstances?

Clark: Yes. It is interesting that the pathways are divergent enough that if you are insulin resistant, you are not necessarily IGF resistant. There are patients with insulin receptor mutations which completely abrogate insulin signalling, but some of those patients still respond to IGF-1 (Nakae et al 1998). Alan Moses' experience was that some patients responded to IGF and some didn't. I think it is worth going back to those rare patients and looking at them to figure out the mutations, because some of them weren't insulin receptor mutations — they were patients with insulin resistance that looked like a Type A patient but didn't have a receptor mutation but rather a signalling mutation (Moses et al 1995). Overall, the experience with IGF-1 at Genentech in several hundred patients was that their responsiveness to IGF-1 and insulin don't go hand in hand.

LeRoith: One possibility is that your paradigm for the insulin receptor doesn't work for the IGF-1 receptor. Prof Zick and I are collaborating on this project. It would be nice if we could show that the paradigm didn't work for the IGF-1R but it did for the insulin receptor. It could help us on this Holy Grail trail.

Holly: There is a complex triangle. We did some work with Dave Dunger in type I diabetics looking at the effects of IGF-1 on insulin sensitivity. There was clearly a component that was due to the IGF-1 feeding back on the pituitary and suppressing GH. We did a study giving somatostatin, so we blocked pituitary output of GH, gave pulses of GH and then looked to see whether IGF-1 still had an effect on insulin sensitivity. This study appeared to show that every pulse of GH was followed by a wave of insulin resistance. The IGF-1 then had an effect only on that insulin resistance caused by the GH. The IGF-1 was imparting insulin sensitivity in that post-GH phase. I was trying to figure out in my mind how your feedback effects could factor into that kind of situation.

Zick: That is what Derek LeRoith has already alluded to. There is a divergence between the insulin receptor signalling and IGF-1R signalling. There are now at least six IRS proteins, and we already know that between IRS1 and IRS2 there are differences in the location of the serine sites and there are differences in responsiveness of the different IRS proteins. This could add another layer of complexity to the story: which IRS proteins are coupled to which receptor at any given time, and which are getting phosphorylated?

LeRoith: Furthermore, we know that pancreas, liver and muscle use different IRS proteins. Some of that effect could be dissociating because a different IRS is more important for the insulin function in that tissue. It is complicated.

Holly: Giving IGF-1 to diabetics, you'd assume that there are not functional IGF receptors on the liver or the adipocytes. It is mainly in the muscle, therefore, that you are looking at the triangle between GH, insulin and IGF-1.

LeRoith: To return to GH, its effects are complicated. In our animal model we showed that there is first muscle resistance and then liver resistance. Either way, this effect could be through the SOCS proteins initially. By reducing GH you allow for release of whatever GH was inhibiting. This is one mechanism in the type I diabetic patients. The problem in the type II patients is that it is hard to invoke GH because they have GH that is elevated, normal or reduced. So, in uncontrolled type I diabetics with high GH, that is one mechanism to explain the resistance, but a lot of people felt and some of the studies suggested that it was muscle glucose uptake sensitivity that improved with rhIGF-I administration, which may be a direct effect of IGF-1 on muscle.

Holly: Our study in the type I patients suggested that IGF-1 was independent of GH, but it was linked to the GH–insulin resistance.

Thomas: Has anyone ever taken a mouse that has been on a high fat diet, injected it with insulin in the tail vein, and looked at the pathway in peripheral tissues? We have done this with PKB, for example, and see resistance of activation in this pathway. Has anyone gone back and done the same experiment with IGF-1?

Clark: We did a lot of studies comparing IGF-1 and insulin in different animal models. It is much harder to see IGF resistance than to see insulin resistance (Clark et al 1997).

LeRoith: I am not sure that this study has been done.

Thomas: I am just curious as to whether one would see a differential effect at that level. If you did, you could dissect the system.

Roberts: In your model, your idea is that PKB phosphorylation is positive feedback, and anything inducing serine/threonine phosphorylation is negative. A number of recent studies have shown that specifically for the IGF-1R and IR-A/IGF-2 binding version of the insulin receptor that with those two receptors, but not the IR-B receptor, you can induce nuclear translocation of IRS1 and IRS2. IRS2 doesn't go to exactly the same place in the nucleus as IRS1. If we accept this, then it could be the difference between insulin and IGF signalling. If you take all this into account, it could turn part of your model upside down, at least for IGF signalling. It also may explain some of the differences between IGF and insulin signalling.

Laron: You didn't mention the effects of the knockouts of the various IRSs. How did these models clarify the above issues?

Zick: There are a many studies relating to IRS1 and IRS2 knockouts. They end up having different phenotypes. The IRS1 knockout is not so much diabetic. It is small in size, suggesting that the main defect is a defect in growth. You can push the system further, for example by giving them a high fat diet. Then they may become slightly diabetic, depending on whose results you look at. The consensus is that IRS1 null mice are smaller but are not extremely diabetic. The situation is different in IRS2 nulls, which are overtly diabetic. The major defect is failure of development of the beta cells of the pancreas. This suggests that the effects of IRS2 are more related to the fundamental effects of insulin with respect to β cell function and induction of diabetes.

Laron: Wouldn't you then say from the results of these animal models that they demonstrate a dissociation between the pathway at IGF-1 and insulin?

Zick: It is very clear, at least to me, that the various IRS proteins do not mediate exactly the same functions. Just in terms of simplicity, we place them together as IRS1–4 for the sake of discussion. If you go deeper into the mechanisms, they differ in structure, function and tissue distribution. Their knockouts show different phenotypes. On top of everything, they interact differently with the insulin receptor, and the IGF-1R. These IRS proteins also interact with other receptors, including several of the interleukins and integrins. We are talking about a complicated network, and I just tried to shed light on a narrow corner of the whole picture.

Carpentier: You say that your mutant IRS protein is not dephosphorylated as well as the normal receptor. In this case, IRS1 is not dephosphorylated. But is the receptor itself phosphorylated?

Zick: That's an interesting question that people haven't really paid attention to. If we go back 20 years when we looked initially at tyrosine phosphorylation of the insulin receptor and the IGF-1R, it was clear that at a basal level both receptors are able to be phosphorylated on serine residues. Furthermore, if you trigger these receptors with insulin or IGF-1, first and foremost there is increased serine phosphorylation of the receptors. Obviously, you also get tyrosine phosphorylation that everyone studies, but the serine phosphorylation has been ignored. There are some 150 serine/threonine phosphorylation sites in the insulin or IGF-1 receptors. Numerous studies were done as far back as the late 1980s with various kinases showing that they can phosphorylate the receptor. For example, one study in the late 1980s showed that cAMP-dependent protein kinase can phosphorylate insulin receptors even at a 1:1 molar ratio, but there was no physiological consequence to that phosphorylation (Roth & Beaudoin 1987). This was the big problem. Most studies, either mutating serine sites or overexpressing kinases that induce insulin or IGF-1 receptor phosphorylation (on serine residues), did not show any clear biological consequence. This is the reason why this whole field somehow got marginalized. However, recently Shoelson and colleagues looked at the effects of free fatty acids on the induction of insulin resistance. They can then treat these cells with salicylates to inhibit IKK and improve insulin action. They claim that the effects are on the IRS protein serine phosphorylation, but part of the effect is on the insulin receptors themselves (Yuan et al 2001).

Carpentier: In your case, do you see inhibition of the dephosphorylation of the insulin receptor?

Zick: We don't know this. The beauty of the system here is that we are looking at isolated juxtamembrane domains of the receptor to avoid this problem. We wanted to avoid the issue of which is more serine-phosphorylated (the receptor or the IRS proteins), so we expressed the isolated juxtamembrane domains of the insulin receptors and IFG1-Rs, and in such a way we could avoid the issue of what happens to the receptors. We just concentrated on what happens to the IRS proteins interacting with the isolated juxtamembrane domains.

Thomas: One point where I became lost is that you showed that the phosphorylation of PKB in that domain was a positive effector, whereas in the negative feedback loop it was PKCλ that was coming in. Yet you were mutating all those sites. Under those conditions which is dominant?

Zick: Initially, we had mutations that were generated at PKB phosphorylation sites, and only then we added mutations at potential PKC phosphorylation sites. It seems that phosphorylation of the inhibitory (PKC) sites dominates the phosphorylation of the stimulatory (PKB) sites. To us, this suggests that PKB should phosphorylate first and maybe produce a positive effect, and then the negative effects should come later. We shouldn't forget that the inhibitory kinase that is involved is PKCζ. We know from the studies of Farese and colleagues that these kinases are also important for *bona fide* insulin action and glucose transport. If you knock them down you affect glucose transport. They should first act on whatever targets to do their beneficial effects. Later on, they should come back for their negative feedback effect to dissociate the IRS proteins from the receptors and inhibit IR–IRS interactions. But their role is not purely as negative regulators. They first have their own biological effects and only then they come back and do their job as negative regulators of IR–IRS interactions.

Thomas: Do you know how the PKB site works? What is the phosphorylation site?

Zick: Once we phosphorylate the PKB sites we prevent tyrosine dephosphorylation. What happens at the 60 min time point is that we see a reduction in tryosine phosphorylation, so clearly phosphatases were acting there to dephosphorylate the IRS proteins. We can, for example, mimic the effects of PKB simply by adding vanadate. Once we inhibit tyrosine phosphatase we don't need this protective effect of PKB. We assume PKB acts by preventing phosphatases from getting access to IRS proteins.

References

Clark RG, Thomas GB, Mortensen DL et al 1997 Growth hormone secretagogues stimulate the hypothalamic–pituitary–adrenal axis and are diabetogenic in the Zucker diabetic fatty rat. Endocrinology 138:4316–4323

Montagnani M, Golovchenko I, Kim I et al 2002 Inhibition of phosphatidylinositol 3-kinase enhances mitogenic actions of insulin in endothelial cells. J Biol Chem 18:1794–1799

Moses AC, Morrow LA, O Brien M, Moller DE, Flier JS 1995 Insulin-like growth factor I (rhIGF-I) as a therapeutic agent for hyperinsulinemic insulin-resistant diabetes mellitus. Diabetes Res Clin Pract Suppl:S185–194

Nakae J, Kato M, Murashita M, Shinohara N, Tajima T, Fujieda K 1998 Long-term effect of recombinant human insulin-like growth factor I on metabolic and growth control in a patient with leprechaunism. J Clin Endocrinol Metab 83:542–549

Roth RA, Beaudoin J 1987 Phosphorylation of purified insulin receptor by cAMP kinase. Diabetes 36:123–126

Sasaoka T, Kobayashi M 2000 The functional significance of Shc in insulin signaling as a substrate of the insulin receptor. Endocr J 47:373–381

Yuan M, Konstantopoulos N, Lee J et al 2001 Reversal of obesity and diet-induced insulin resistance with salicylates or targeted disruption of IKKβ. Science 293:1673–1677 (Erratum in Science 295:277)

IGF-1 and insulin as growth hormones

Zvi Laron

Endocrinology and Diabetes Research Unit, Schneider Children's Medical Center, WHO Collaborating Center for the Study of Diabetes in Youth, Petah Tikva and Sackler School of Medicine, Tel Aviv University, Tel Aviv, Israel

Abstract. IGF-1 generated in the liver is the anabolic effector and linear growth promoting hormone of the pituitary growth hormone (GH). This is evidenced by dwarfism in states of congenital IGF-1 deficiency, *Igf1* gene mutation/deletions or knockouts, and in Laron syndrome (LS), due to GH receptor gene mutations/deletions or IGF-1 receptor blocking. In a positive way, daily IGF-1 administration to stunted patients with LS or hGH gene deletion accelerates linear growth velocity. IGF-1 acts on the proliferative cells of the epiphyseal cartilage. IGF-1 also induces organ and tissue growth; its absence causing organomicria. Insulin shares a common ancestry with IGF-1 and with 45% amino acid homology, as well as very close relationships in the structure of its receptors and post-receptor cascade, also acts as a growth hormone. It has protein anabolic activity and stimulates IGF-1 synthesis. Pancreas agenesis causes short babies, and obese children with hyperinsulinism, with or without pituitary GH, have an accelerated growth rate and skeletal maturation; so do babies with macrosomia. Whether the insulin growth effect is direct, or mediated by IGF-1 or leptin is controversial.

2004 Biology of IGF-1: its interaction with insulin in health and malignant states. Wiley, Chichester (Novartis Foundation Symposium 262) p 56–83

The genes for insulin-like growth factor 1 (IGF-1) and insulin are homologous and are thought to have arisen from a common ancestor. However, the *IGF1* gene resides on chromosome 12 (Brissenden et al 1984) and that of insulin on chromosome 11 (Bennett et al 1995). Both share 45% amino acid homology but the C-peptide region of IGF-1 bears no homology with the proinsulin C-peptide, and is not cleaved from the molecule as occurs in proinsulin processing (Rinderknecht & Humbel 1978). The IGF-1 receptor is closely related to the insulin receptor and binds IGF-1 with high affinity and insulin with low affinity (LeRoith et al 1996). Despite their physiological interactions and synergistic anabolic effects, the growth promoting effects of the two hormones differ in their intensity (Zapf et al 1999).

Action of IGF-1 on ephiphyseal growth cartilage

Whether IGF-1 has a direct effect on linear growth, or whether a preparatory or synergistic action with pituitary growth hormone (GH) is needed, is controversial

(Daughaday 1993, Zapf et al 1999, Laron 2001). The unsettled question is whether IGF-1 can activate the cartilage cells in the germinal layer (the prechondrocytes) (Green et al 1985) or concomitant GH activity on these cells is needed (Lindahl et al 1986, 1987, Nilsson 1995). Using murine mandibular condyle cultures as a model, Maor et al (1993) demonstrated that paracrine IGF-1 is present in the chondroprogenitor zone in the mandibular condyles of 2 day old mice, and that the distribution of the IGF-1 receptors was parallel to that of IGF-1 production in the chondroprogenitor zone.

In vivo growth effects of IGF-1

In GH-deficient hypophysectomized rats, IGF-1 restored longitudinal growth and weight gain in a dose-dependent manner similar to GH (Schoenle et al 1982). The same was found when treating Snell dwarf mice (Pit 1 mutation causing GH, TSH, and PRL deficiency) with IGF-1 (Van Buul-Offers et al 1986, 2000).

Experimental gene knockouts

Igf1 gene deficient mice have reduced size at birth and severe postnatal growth retardation (Baker et al 1993), so do the mice in which the growth hormone receptor binding protein gene was disrupted (the Laron mouse) and which are unable to generate IGF-1 (Zhou et al 1997). It is of interest that Bikle et al (2001), using histomorphometric methods on bones of mice rendered IGF-1 deficient, reported that the bones, although smaller, appeared more compact. Mice lacking the IGF-1 receptor also have intrauterine growth retardation (Powell-Braxton et al 1993). The birth weight of *Igf1* null mice is 60% of normal; that of *Igf1* receptor nulls is 45%. By 2 months of age, the size of *Igf1* knockout mice is 30% of normal. It seems that in mice, prenatally IGF-1 mediates growth independently of GH; postnatally GH is needed for hepatic IGF-1 synthesis (Lupu et al 2001). By combining the *Igf-1* mutation with a null *Ghr* mutation, Lupu et al (2001) have analysed the relative contributions of IGF-1 and GH to bone formation. They concluded that the actions of GH to promote osteogenesis depend on the presence of IGF-1. In addition to growth, *Igf1* gene mutants or knockouts have delayed embryonic and postnatal bone maturation as well as bone matrix mineralization (Zhang et al 2002).

Igf1 transgenic mice

A line of transgenic mice expressing *Igf1* under the control of the mouse metallothionien 1 promoter grew large but only on a temporary basis (Behringer et al 1990).

IGF-1 binding proteins (IGFBPs)

IGFBP1, IGFBP2 and IGFBP6 act as growth inhibitors of an IGF-dependent proliferation of growth plate chondrocytes in rats, whereas IGFBP3 can inhibit IGF-independent and IGF-dependent cell proliferation (Kiepe et al 2002). Furthermore, coadministration of IGFBP1 with IGF-1 to GH-deficient Snell mice (Pit 1 deficiency) inhibited the IGF1 effect on body growth (Van Buul-Offers et al 2000). Overexpression of IGFBP1 in transgenic mice results in growth retardation (Rajkumar et al 1995).

Peak bone mineral density (bone mass)

Mice lacking IGF-1 (*Igf1* knockouts) exhibited impairment in bone accretion (Mohan et al 2003).

IGF-1 effect on growth in human

Prenatal

Babies born with hereditary or congenital IGF-1 deficiency due to GH receptor deletions or mutations (Laron syndrome=primary GH insensitivity; Laron 1993) or deletion of exons of the *IGF1* gene (Wood et al 1996) are born short (Table 1). Some are of low normal body length, denoting variability of either

TABLE 1 Birth length and weight of 11 babies with Laron syndrome from the Israeli cohort

Patient no.	*Sex*	*Gestational age*	*Delivery*	*Birth length (cm)*	*Birth weight (g)*
1	F	Full term	Normal	46[a]	3400
2	F	Full term	Normal	49	3200
3	M	Full term	Normal	47	3740
4	M	Full term	Normal	50	3050
5	F	Full term	Normal	46[a]	2900
6	M	Full term	Normal	45[a]	3000
7	M	Full term	Normal	49	3000
8	F	Full term	Normal	46[a]	3100
9	M	Full term	Normal	46[a]	3250
10	F	Full term	Normal	47	3200
11	M	Full term	Normal	44[a]	3200

[a]Two SDs below the mean birth weight for respective ethnic community.

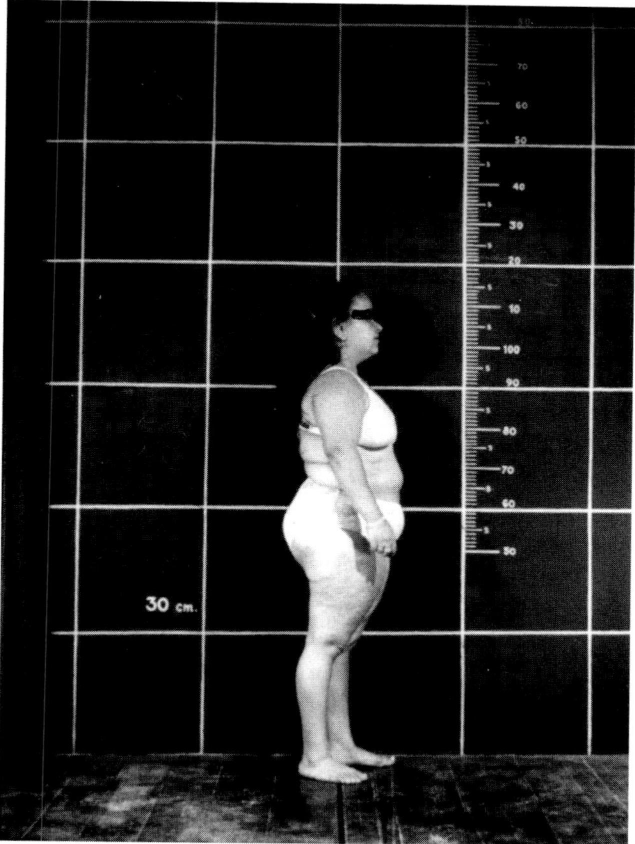

FIG. 1. Dwarfism (height 115 cm) of a 26 year old female patient with Laron syndrome. Note obesity.

parental height or intrauterine conditions. This phenotype is similar to that described in congenital absence of hGH (Laron & Pertzelan 1969, Gluckman et al 1992).

There are scattered reports of prenatal and postnatal growth deficiencies in children with intrauterine growth retardation and chromosomal abnormalities, such as 15q26.1qter associated with monozygosity for the IGF-1 receptor (Roback et al 1991), or a girl with Silver–Russell syndrome and multiple dysmorphic abnormalities (Tamura et al 1993). It is suspected but not proven that a certain percentage of children with intrauterine growth retardation (IUGR) and postnatal growth deficits have defects in the IGF-1 gene receptor (Nakae et al 2001).

Growth promoting effect by administration of biosynthetic IGF-1 to children with IGF-1 deficiency

There are three states with IGF-1 deficiency in which IGF-1 treatment has been administered:

Laron syndrome (LS; primary GH insensitivity, resistance); isolated growth hormone deficiency due to *GH1* gene deletion and antibody formation to GH; and *IGF1* exon deletion (one patient). The largest and longest experience has been with LS.

LS is a form of dwarfism caused by molecular defects (deletions or mutations) of the GH receptor or post-receptor pathways, causing primary IGF-1 deficiency (Laron 1995, 1999a). Untreated patients reach an adult height of 116–142 cm in males and 108–136 cm in females (Laron 1999a) (Fig. 1). The only effective treatment is biosynthetic IGF-1, available since 1986 (Niwa et al 1986). Unfortunately the restricted amount of drug for clinical trials permitted treatment of only a small number of patients.

The biosynthetic IGF-1 used by different clinics is, with the exception of Israel and Japan who used the same preparation, of different manufacture but with an identical structure. The only difference is that whereas our group uses one subcutaneous injection per day administered before breakfast to avoid the hypoglycaemic effect of IGF-1, the other groups administer two injections of IGF-1 per day (Laron 1999b).

Short-term and transitory effects are water and electrolyte retention and calciuria (Laron & Klinger 1994, Klinger & Laron 1994). Administration of IGF-1 for months or years persistently suppressed GH, and serum insulin, preventing hypoglycaemia, and stabilizing blood glucose levels, provided that meals were regular (Laron et al 1993a). This was also confirmed by Walker et al (1992). Sensitive markers of IGF-1 activity during treatment are a rise in serum alkaline phosphatase, procollagen 1 (PICP) and procollagen 3 (PIIINP) (Klinger et al 1996), serum phosphate and GFR (Klinger & Laron 1994). IGF-1 administration also raised sex hormone binding protein (Gafny et al 1994) and decreased serum lipoprotein(a) (Laron et al 1997), and to a lesser degree, cholesterol (Laron & Klinger 1994).

IGF-1 administration also affects its specific binding proteins participating in its own regulation of available free hormone. During the first weeks of administration IGF-1 suppresses the IGFBPs (Laron et al 1992a) including IGFBP3 (Laron et al 1992b) but longer administration leads to the generation of the IGFBP3 (Kaneti et al 1993) and of its acid labile fraction (Kaneti et al 1997). This finding has practical importance as it prolongs the biological half-life of the administered IGF-1 during long-term treatment (Laron et al 1999), and requires in most patients a progressive reduction of the IGF-1 dose in order to prevent over-dosage and adverse effects.

TABLE 2 Linear growth response of children with Laron syndrome treated by IGF-1

			At start				*Growth velocity (cm/yr)*			
Author	*Year*	*n*	*Age (yr) range*	*BA (yr)*	*Ht SDS M*	*IGF-1 dose µg/kg/d*	*0 before*	*1st year*	*2nd year*	*3rd year*
Ranke et al[a]	1995	31	3.7–19	1.8–13.3	−6.5	40–120 b.i.d.	3.9±1.8	(n=26) 8.5±2.1	(n=18) 6.4±2.2	
Backeljauw & Underwood[a]	1996	5	2–11	0.3–6.8	−5.6	80–120 b.i.d.	4.0	(n=5) 9.3	(n=5) 6.2	(n=1) 6.2
Klinger & Laron[b]	1995	9	0.5–14	0.2–11	−5.6	150–200 once	4.7±1.3	(n=9) 8.2±0.8	(n=6) 6±1.3	(n=5) 4.8±1.3*
Guevarra-Aguirre[a]	1997	15	3.1–17	4.5–9.3		120 b.i.d.	3.4±1.4	(n=15) 8.8±11	(n=15) 6.4±1.1	(n=6) 5.7±1.4
		8				80 b.i.d.	3.0±1.8	(n=8) 9.1±2.2	(n=8) 5.6±2.1	

*The younger children had a growth velocity of 5.5 and 6.5 cm/yr.
BA = bone age; SDS M = standard deviation score below the median for sex and age.
[a]Two injections per day (s.c.); [b]one daily injection (s.c.).

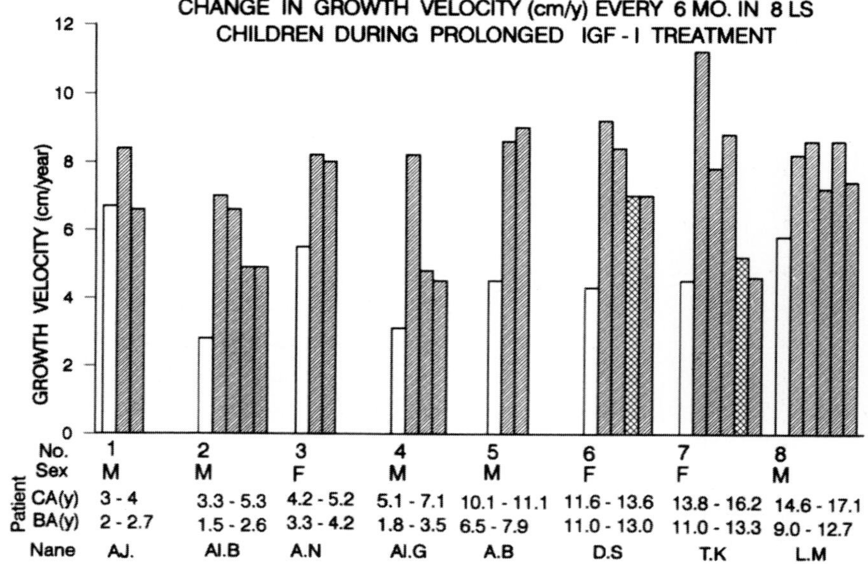

FIG. 2. Change of growth velocity during long-term IGF-1 treatment of eight children with Laron syndrome. White column: pretreatment growth velocity.

One of the major effects of IGF-1 is acceleration of linear growth. Due to limitations in the availability of the drug there are only few reports on long-term treatment of children with LS. There are four reports on 2 or 3 years treatment (Klinger & Laron 1995, Ranke et al 1995, Backeljauw & Underwood 1996, Guevara-Aguirre et al 1997) one for 4 years (Enberg et al 2000), one for 5 years (Backeljauw & Underwood 1996), and one on 7 year treatment (Krzisnik & Battelino 1997). In the first year of treatment the growth velocity was higher than in subsequent years (Table 2, Fig. 2). It seems that once-daily IGF-1 administration (Klinger & Laron 1995) is as effective in promoting growth as twice-daily IGF-1 administration (Ranke et al 1995, Backeljauw & Underwood 1996, Guevara-Aguirre et al 1997, Backeljauw et al 2001) (Figs 3 and 4). On the other hand, twice-daily injections or not decreasing the IGF-1 dose with time (Klinger & Laron 1995) caused more adverse effects (Klinger & Laron 1995, Laron 1999b; Table 3). With continuous treatment there was also a progressive growth of the extremities (hands, feet, chin and nose). Despite the effective stimulation of linear growth, the growth velocity is not as intense as that of GH in GH deficiency (Laron & Klinger 2000, Backeljauw et al 2001) (Figs 5 and 6). During IGF-1 treatment we also registered a fast catch-up of the head circumference even at ages 10–14 (Laron

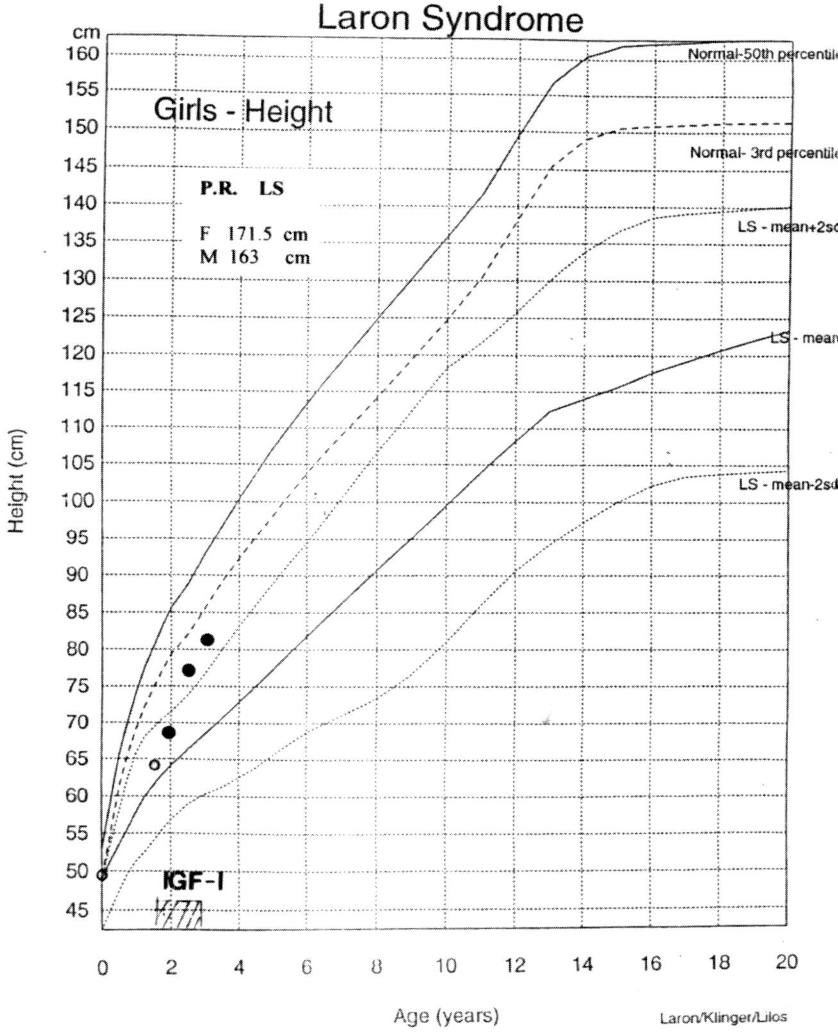

FIG. 3. Enhancement of growth by IGF-1 treatment of a female infant with Laron syndrome. Drawn on Laron syndrome growth chart (Laron et al 1993b).

et al 1992c; Fig. 7) denoting brain growth, and some reduction in adipose tissue as measured by skinfold thickness. Recently we found the IGF-1 treatment of patients with LS to have a significant stimulatory effect on erythropoesis (Sivan et al 2003). Whether this effect is mediated by erythropoietin is under investigation.

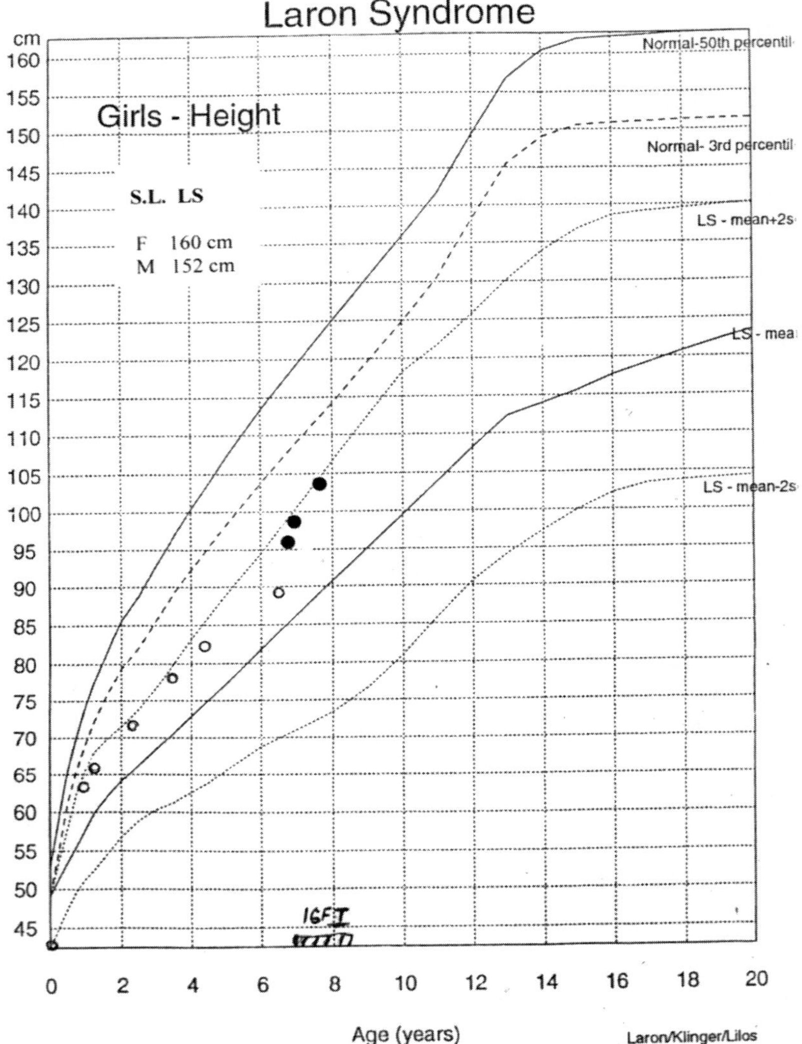

FIG. 4. Growth acceleration by initiation of IGF-1 treatment of a prepubertal girl with Laron syndrome. Drawn on Laron syndrome growth chart (Laron et al 1993b).

Backeljauw et al (2001) treated three children who developed hGH antibodies with IGF-1. The response was that only one of the children achieved normal height. One patient with a defect in the *IGF1* gene has been described by Woods et al (1996) did not respond to hGH and only partially to IGF-1 (Camacho-Hubner et al 1999).

TABLE 3 Adverse effects reported during IGF–1 treatment of children with Laron syndrome

	Ranke et al (1995) n=*31*	*Backeljauw & Underwood (1996)* n=*5*	*Klinger & Laron (1995)* n=*9*	*Guevarra-Aguirre et al (1997)* n=*22*
Headaches (early)	21	2	–	?
Nausea, vomiting	?	–	–	3
Hypoglycaemia	13	+ early	1 (transitory)	6
Papilloedema (transitory)	1	2	–	–
Bell's palsy	1	–	–	–
Lipohypertrophy	7	–	–	–
Enlargement of lymphoid tissue	3	4	1	?
Thickening of nose	5	2	2	?
Local reaction (transitory)	?	?	2	3
Transient tachycardia	?	?	2	16
Increased hyperandrogenicity	?	?	2	?

The causes of reduced growth response to IGF-1, compared to that of GH in states of GH deficiency, remains to be clarified. It may be due to inappropriate dosage administration, not really comparable data, or indeed the concomitant need of GH to obtain a maximal growth effect. In contrast to the growth response of the long bones and organs, the brain growth response seen with IGF-1 compares well with that of hGH (Laron et al 1992c).

Insulin and growth

Clinical observations that insulin deficiency or oversecretion affect growth in opposed directions is not new (Laron 1981, 1982). Advances in technology and genetics have added knowledge on the physiology of insulin, its interaction with IGF-1 and effects on growth.

Experimental evidence on the need of insulin for early growth

Inactivation of the two insulin genes *Ins1* and *Ins2* in mice resulted in slight impairment of embryonic growth (Duvillie et al 1997). Mice lacking the insulin

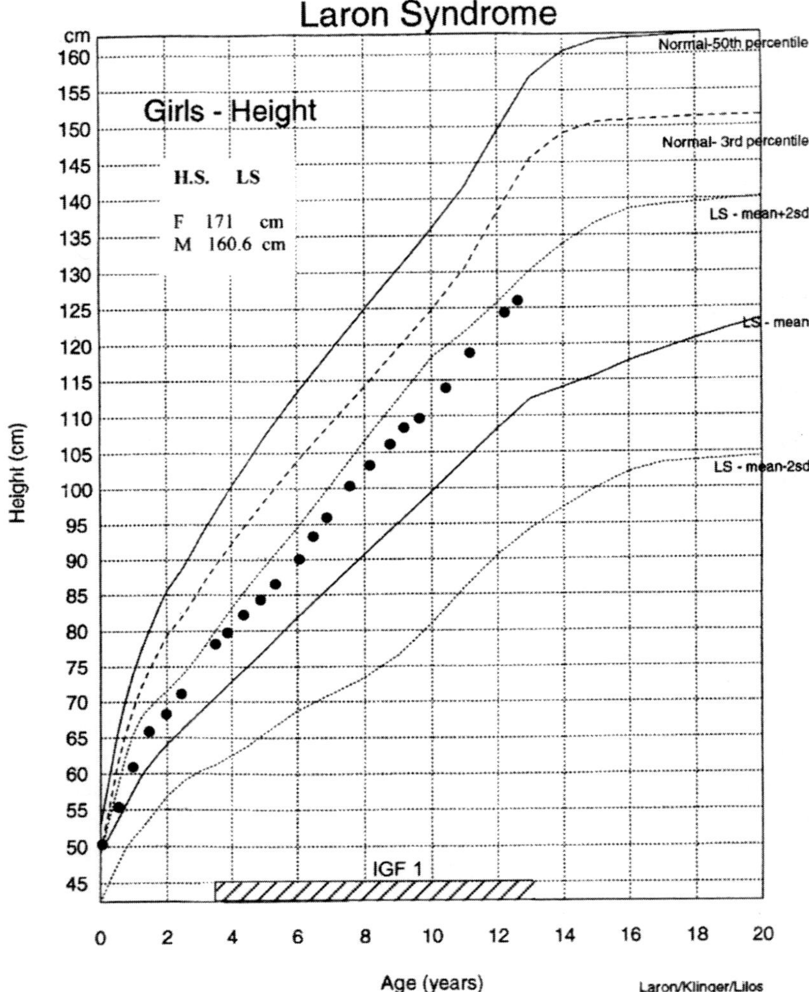

FIG. 5. The long-term growth response to IGF-1 once daily of a girl with Laron syndrome and a molecular defect in the transmembrance domain of the GH receptor (Silbergeld et al 1997). Note that she improved height, maintaining a normal growth velocity forage, but lacking a full catch up to normal stature.

receptor are born with slight growth retardation (Louvi et al 1997). These animals die shortly after birth by ketoacidosis.

In vitro studies using mice condylar cartilage, demonstrated that addition of insulin to the culture caused a marked (+96%) increase in DNA synthesis and a

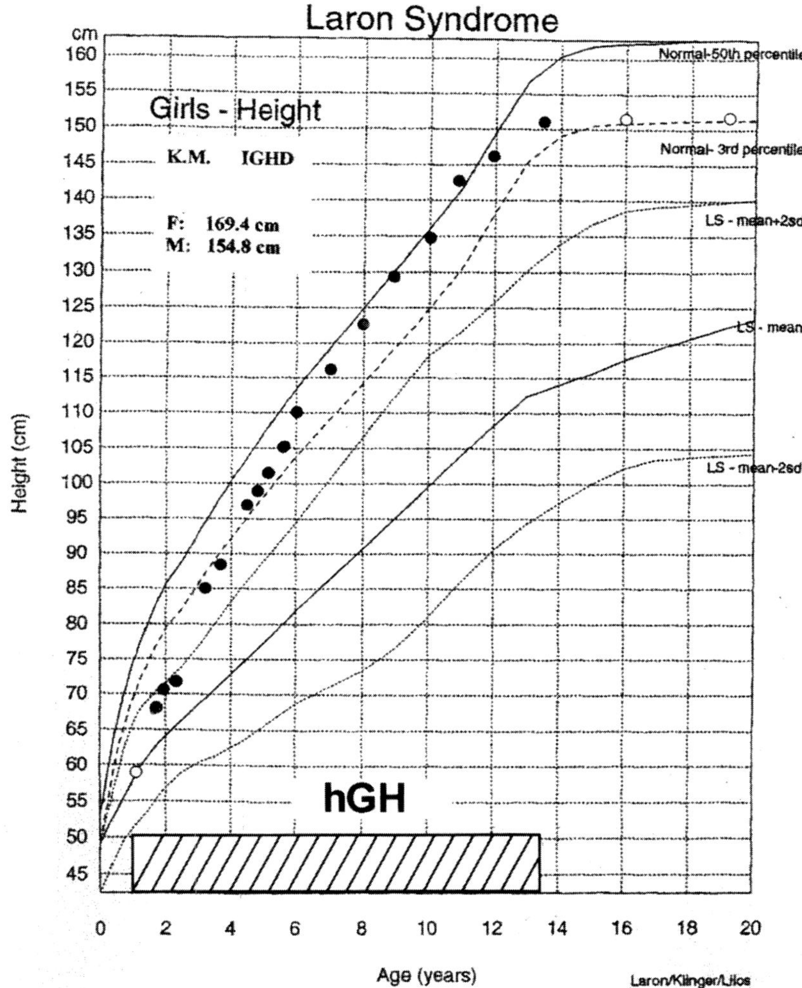

FIG. 6. Growth response to human growth hormone (hGH) injection (0.1 U/kg/d s.c. once daily) to a girl with isolated GH deficiency due to *hGH1* gene deletion. Empty circles: height before and after stopping therapy. Drawn for comparison on Laron syndrome growth charts (Laron et al 1993b).

60% increase in the size of the culture explants. Insulin also enhanced the differentiation of the progenitor cartilage cells, and their proliferation (Maor et al 1993). Insulin also stimulates skeletal growth *in vivo*. Salter & Best (1953) injected long-acting insulin to hypophysectomized rats 14 days after operation and found evidence of skeletal growth in sections of the tibia.

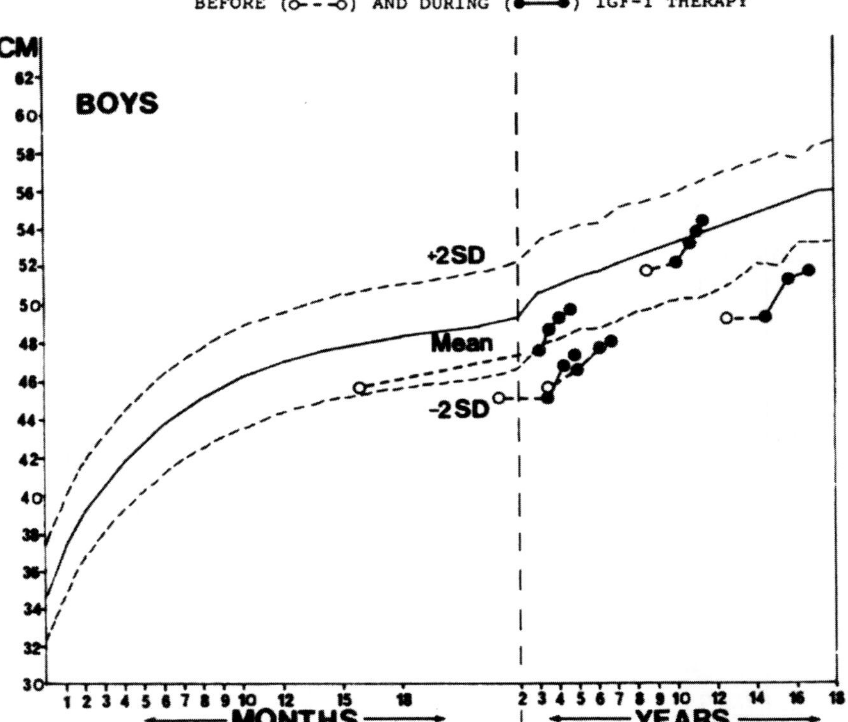

FIG. 7. Fast catch up growth of head circumference to IGF-1 treatment in boys with Laron syndrome.

Perfusion of livers of hypophysectomized rats with insulin demonstrated that the insulin increased somatomedin (IGF-1) activity in the perfusate (Daughaday et al 1976).

Insulin as a fetal growth factor in humans

Null mutations of the insulin gene transcription factor PDX1 cause pancreas agenesis, and result in severe IUGR (Stoffers et al 1997), as occurs in infants with congenital diabetes (Dodge & Laurence 1977). Newborns with insulin receptor (IR) mutations are severely growth retarded (Takahashi et al 1997). In contrast fetuses exposed to high insulin concentrations *in utero* are big, such as in maternal diabetes (Tyrala 1996), Beckwith-Wiedemann syndrome (DeBaun et al 2000), erythroblastosis fetalis (Barrett & Oliver 1968) and nesidioblastosis (Reinecke-Luthge et al 2000). Thus in contrast to mice insulin, human insulin is an important early growth factor.

Postnatal influence of insulin on growth

Hypoinsulinism

In clinical conditions such as metabolically uncontrolled diabetes mellitus (Laron et al 1977), constitutional short stature and lean body mass (Karp et al 1973) and hypocaloric states due to reduced food consumption (as occurs in chronic disease, coeliac disease, weight reducing, dieting, anorexia nervosa, all of which are accompanied by hypoinsulinaemia) there is a slowing of the growth velocity (Laron 1981) and short stature (Figs 8 and 9). These states are also causing secondary GH resistance and a reduction in IGF-1 secretion.

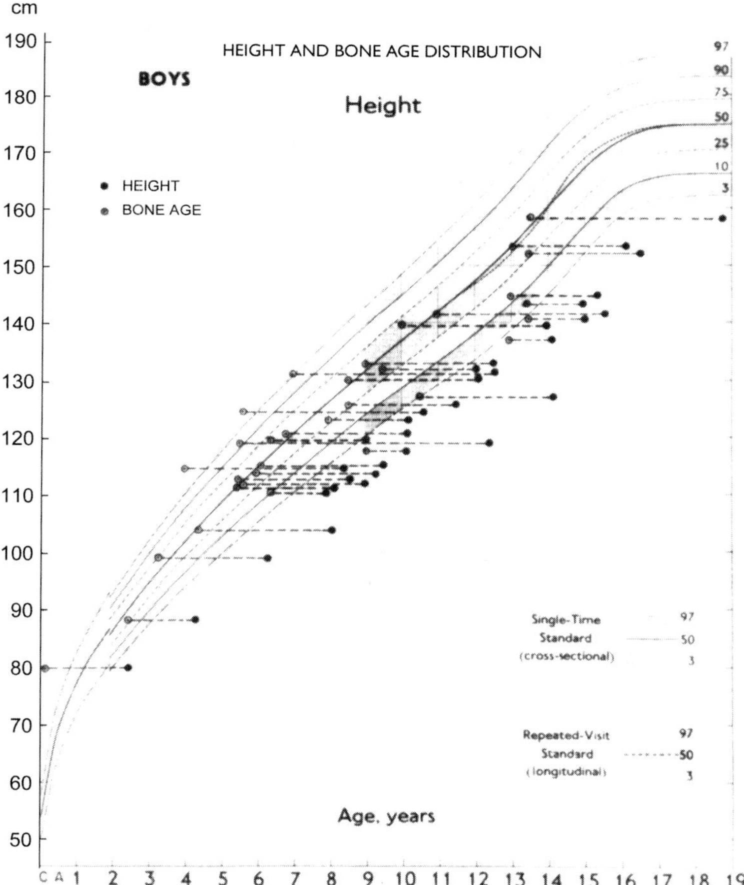

FIG. 8. Short stature in 32 underweight boys with constitutional growth retardation. Note marked skeletal age retardation.

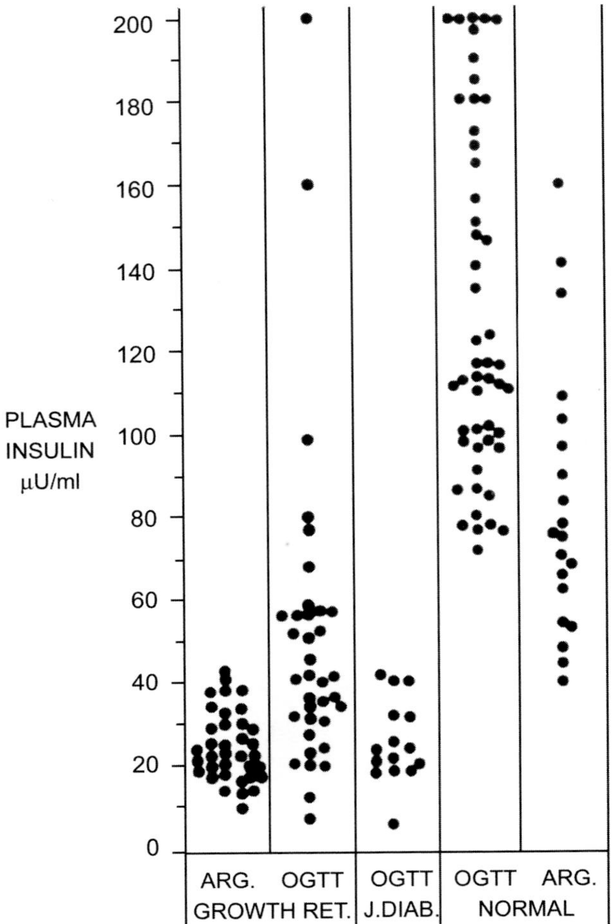

FIG. 9. Low insulin response to arginine or oral glucose stimulation in the boys shown in Fig. 8, compared to newly diagnosed Type 1 diabetic children and normal controls.

Hyperinsulinism

Obese children have high serum insulin (Sims & Danforth 1974) often accompanied by an enhanced rate of growth and tall stature for age (Laron et al 1978) (Fig 10).

Growth without growth hormone

The phenomenon of enhanced growth after extirpation of pituitary tumours in children has been an intriguing question for years both in animals (Baumann

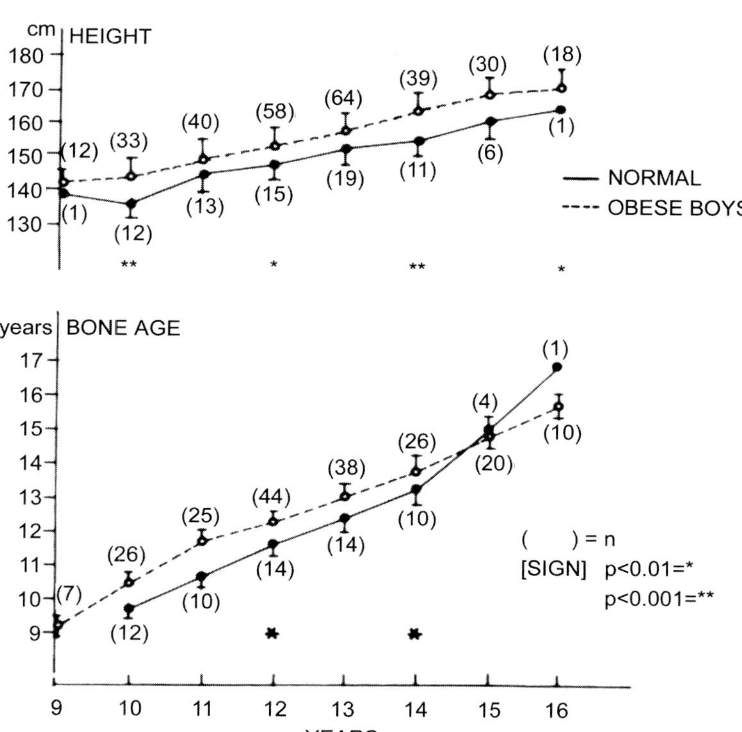

FIG. 10. The growth pattern and skeletal age of boys with simple obesity (Laron 1981).

1997) and in man (Laron et al 1975, Geffner 1996). In children it is mostly accompanied by hyperbulimia, weight gain and hyperinsulinaemia (Fig. 11). The levels of IGF-1 reported have been normal or increased (Laron 1981). Hyperinsulinaemia with or without elevated IGF-1 is one possible explanation. Bucher et al (1983), Dattani (2002) and Murashita et al (1999) proposed an undefined growth promoting agent (GPA) of 70 000 kDa. Recent experimental studies raise the possibility that leptin and insulin are the unknown growth factors in obesity (Maor et al 2002).

The identification of the IGF-1 and insulin post-receptor pathways should enable a better understanding of the role of these hormones on growth.

Insulin receptor substrates

Insulin receptor substrate (IRS) proteins act as post-receptor mediators of insulin, IGFs and cytokine signalling. The IRS family consists of five members. Absence of

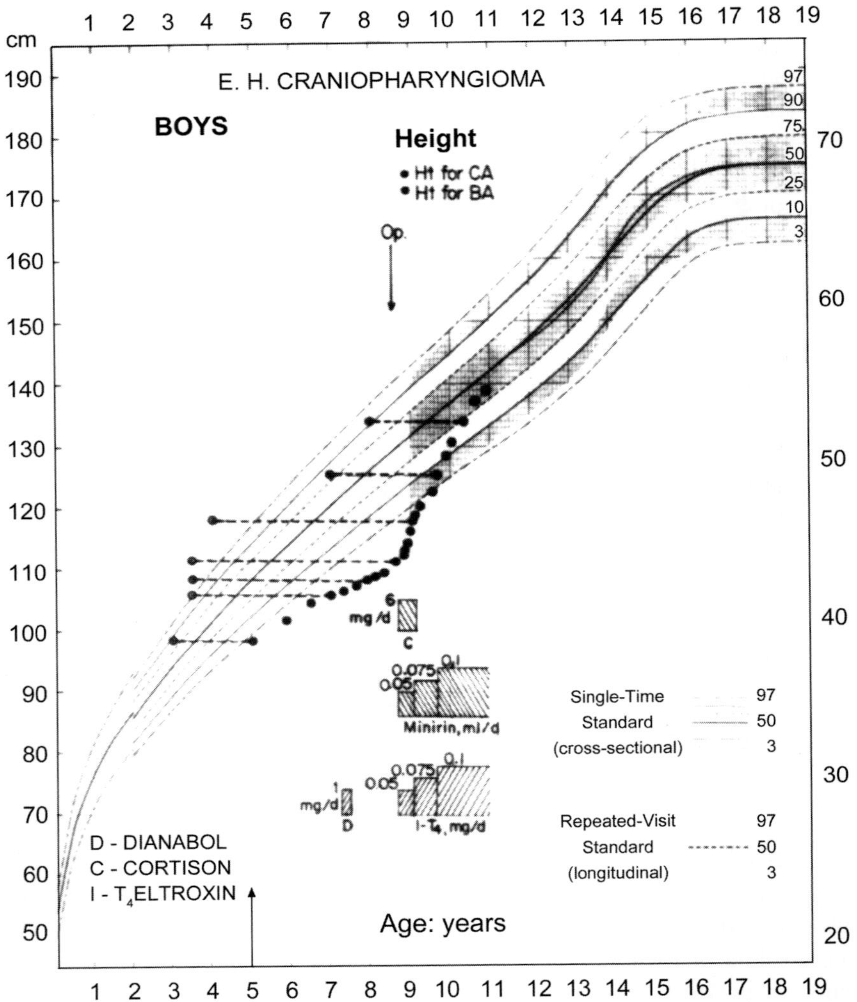

FIG. 11. The growth pattern of a boy with craniopharyngioma before and after extirpation of the tumour which included the pituitary gland. Note slowing of growth before operation and first catch up after operation accompanied by a marked weight increase and hyperinsulinaemia (not shown) and no demonstrable GH.

IRS1 in mice causes prenatal and postnatal growth retardation and insulin resistance (Tamemoto et al 1994). The pattern of growth retardation of IRS1-deficient mice is similar to that of IGF-1 deficient mice. Ablation of IRS4 results in modest growth retardation.

Conclusions

Clinical observations, radioimmunoassays, and molecular biological tools in genetics have advanced our knowledge on the physiological actions of IGF-1 and insulin (Rotwein et al 2002, Laron 2004a,b). Though related in structure, in their receptors and post-receptor pathways these two hormones affect linear growth with different intensities. Despite more knowledgeable about their actions we still lack detailed understanding on the synergistic and antagonistic pathways of IGF-1 and insulin.

Acknowledgements

The expert secretarial help of Mrs Gila Waichman and Mrs Kitty Tohar is acknowledged.

References

Backeljauw PF, Underwood LE 1996 Prolonged treatment with recombinant insulin-like growth factor-I in children with growth hormone insensitivity syndrome—a clinical Research Center study. GHIS Collaborative Group. J Clin Endocrinol Metab 81:3312–3317

Backeljauw PF, Underwood LE, and The GHIS Collaborative Group 2001 Therapy for 6.5–7.5 years with recombinant insulin-like growth factor I in children with growth hormone insensitivity syndrome: a clinical research center study. J Clin Endocrinol Metab 86:1504–1510

Baker J, Liu J-P, Robertson EJ, Efstratiadis A 1993 Role of insulin-like growth factors in embryonic and postnatal growth. Cell 75:73–82

Barrett CT, Oliver TK Jr 1968 Hypoglycemia and hyperinsulinism in infants with erythroblastosis fetalis. N Engl J Med 278:1260–1262

Baumann G 1997 Growth without a pituitary?—Lessons from the guinea pig. Endocrinology 138:3575–3576

Behringer RR, Lewin TM, Quaife CJ, Palmiter RD, Brinster RL, D'Ercole AJ 1990 Expression of insulin-like growth factor-I stimulates normal somatic growth in growth hormone-deficient transgenic mice. Endocrinology 127:1033–1040

Bennett ST, Lucassen AM, Gough SC et al 1995 Susceptibility to human type 1 diabetes at IDDM 2 is determined by tandem repeat variation at the insulin gene minisatellite locus. Nat Genet 9:284–292

Bikle D, Majumdar S, Laib A et al 2001 The skeletal structure of insulin-like growth factor I-deficient mice. J Bone Miner Res 16:2320–2329

Brissenden JE, Ullrich A, Francke U 1984 Human chromosomal mapping of genes for insulin-like growth factors I and II and epidermal growth factor. Nature 310:781–784

Bucher H, Zapf J, Torresani T, Prader A, Froesch ER, Illig R 1983 Insulin-like growth factor I and II, prolactin and insulin in 19 growth hormone-deficient children with excessive, normal, or decreased longitudinal growth after operation for craniopharyngioma. N Engl J Med 309:1142–1146

Camacho-Hubner C, Woods KA, Miraki-Moud F et al 1999 Effects of recombinant human insulin-like factor I (IGF-1) therapy on the growth hormone–IGF system of a patient with a partial IGF-I gene deletion. J Clin Endocrinol Metabol 84:1611–1616

Dattani MT 2002 GH deficiency might be associated with normal height in PROP1 deficiency. Clin Endocrinol 57:157–158

Daughaday WH 1993 Are there direct, non-IGF-I mediated effects of hGH? In: Laron Z, Parks JS (eds) Lessons from Laron Syndrome (LS) 1966–1992. Pediatr Adolesc Endocrinol 24:338–345

Daughaday WH, Phillips LS, Mueller MC 1976 The effects of insulin and growth hormone on the release of somatomedin by the isolated rat liver. Endocrinology 98:214–1219

DeBaun MR, King AA, White N 2000 Hypoglycemia in Beckwith–Wiedemann syndrome. Semin Perinatol 24:164–171

Dodge JA, Laurence KM 1977 Congenital absence of the pancreas and intrauterine growth retardation. Pediatrics 64:255–257

Duvillie B, Corconnier N, Deltour L et al 1997 Phenotypic alterations in insulin-deficient mutant mice. Proc Natl Acad Sci USA 94:5137–5140

Enberg B, Luthman H, Segnestam K, Ritzen EM, Sundstorm M, Norstedt G 2000 Characterization of novel missense mutations in the GH receptor gene causing severe growth retardation. Eur J Endocrinol 143:71–76

Gafny M, Silbergeld A, Klinger B, Wasserman M, Laron Z 1994 Comparative effects of GH, IGF-I and insulin on serum sex hormone binding globulin. Clin Endocrinol 41:169–175

Geffner ME 1996 The growth without growth hormone syndrome. Endocrinol Metab Clin North Am 25:649–663

Guevara-Aguirre J, Rosenbloom AL, Vasconez O et al 1997 Two year treatment of growth hormone (GH) receptor deficiency with recombinant insulin-like growth factor-I in 22 children: comparison of two dosage levels and to GH treated GH deficiency. J Clin Endocrinol Metab 82:629–633

Gluckman PD, Gunn AJ, Wray A et al 1992 Congenital idiopathic growth hormone deficiency is associated with prenatal and early postnatal growth failure. J Pediat 121:920–923

Green H, Morikawa M, Nixon T 1985 A dual effector theory of growth hormone action. Differentiation 29:195–198

Kaneti H, Karasik A, Klinger B, Silbergeld A, Laron Z 1993 Long-term treatment of Laron type dwarfs with insulin-like growth factor I increases serum insulin-like growth factor-binding protein 3 in the absence of growth hormone activity. Acta Endocrinol 128:144–149

Kaneti H, Silbergeld A, Klinger B, Karasik A, Baxter RC, Laron Z 1997 Long-term effects of insulin-like growth factor-I (IGF-I) on serum IGF-I, IGF-binding protein-3 and acid labile subunit in Laron syndrome patients with normal growth hormone binding protein. Eur J Endocrinol 137:626–630

Karp M, Laron Z, Doron M 1973 Insulin secretion in children with constitutional familial short stature. J Pediatr 83:241–246

Kiepe D, Ulinski T, Powell DR, Durham SK, Mehls O, Tonshoff B 2002 Differential effects of insulin-like growth factor binding proteins-1, -2, -3, and -6 on cultured growth plate chondrocytes. Kidney Int 62:1591–1600

Klinger B, Laron Z 1994 Renal function in Laron syndrome patients treated by insulin-like growth factor-I. Pediatr Nephrol 8:684–688

Klinger B, Laron Z 1995 Three year IGF-I treatment of children with Laron Syndrome. J Pediatr Endocrinol Metab 8:149–158

Klinger B, Jensen LT, Silbergeld A, Laron Z 1996 Insulin-like growth factor-I raises serum procollagen levels in children and adults with Laron syndrome. Clin Endocrinol 46:423–429

Klinger B, Anin S, Silbergeld A, Eshet R, Laron Z 1998 Development of hyperandrogenism during treatment with insulin-like growth factor-I (IGF-I) in female patients with Laron syndrome. Clin Endocrinol 48:81–87

Krzisnik C, Battelino T 1997 Five year treatment with IGF-I of a patient with Laron syndrome in Slovenia (a follow-up report). J Pediatr Endocrinol Metab 10: 443–447

Laron Z 1981 Insulin as a growth-promoting hormone. In: Collu R, Ducharme J, Guyda H (eds) Pediatric endocrinology. Raven Press, New York, p 149–165

Laron Z 1982 Somatomedin, insulin, growth hormone and growth: a review. Isr J Med Sci 18:823–829

Laron Z 1993 Laron syndrome: from description to therapy. Endocrinologist 3:21–28

Laron Z 1995 Prismatic cases: Laron Syndrome (primary growth hormone resistance). From patient to laboratory to patient. J Clin Endocrinol Metab 80:1526–1573

Laron Z 1999a Natural history of the classical form of primary growth hormone (GH) resistance (Laron syndrome). J Pediatr Endocrinol Metab 12:231–249

Laron Z 1999b Somatomedin-1 (recombinant insulin-like growth factor-I). Clinical pharmacology and potential treatment of endocrine and metabolic disorders. BioDrugs 11:55–70

Laron Z 2001 Insulin-like growth factor 1 (IGF-1): a growth hormone. J Clin Pathol Mol Pathol 54:311–316

Laron Z 2004a Laron syndrome (primary growth hormone resistance or insensitivity). The personal experience 1958–2003. J Clin Endocrinol Metab 89:1031–1044

Laron Z 2004b Biologic and clinical aspects of molecular defects along the growth hormone-insulin-like growth factor I axis. Chapter 9. In: Pescovitz OH, Eugster EA (eds). Pediatric endocrinology: mechanisms, manifestations, and management. Lippincott, Williams & Wilkins, Philadelphia, PA, USA, p 123–150

Laron Z, Pertzelan A 1969 Somatotrophin in antenatal and perinatal growth and development. Lancet 1:680–681

Laron Z, Klinger B 1994 IGF-I treatment of adult patients with Laron syndrome: preliminary results. Clin Endocrinol (Oxf) 41:631–638

Laron Z, Klinger B 2000 Comparison of the growth-promoting effects of insulin-like growth factor I and growth hormone in the early years of life. Acta Paediatr 88:38–41

Laron Z, Pertzelan A, Kiwity S, Livneh-Zirinsky M, Keret R 1976 Growth without growth hormone: Myth or fact? In: Convegno Internazionale di Endocrinologia Pediatrica, Bologna, June 1975, Pacini, Pisa, p 131–152

Laron Z, Volovitz V, Karp M 1977 Linear growth and insulin dose as indices of control in children with diabetes mellitus. In: Laron Z (ed) Medical aspects of balance of diabetes in juveniles. Pediatric and Adolescent Endocrinology. Vol. 2. S. Karger, Basel, p 60–69

Laron Z, Ben-Dan I, Shrem M, Dickerman Z, Lilos P 1978 Puberty in simple obese boys and girls. In: Cacciari E, Laron Z, Raiti S (eds) Obesity in childhood. Academic Press, London, p 29–40

Laron Z, Anin S, Klipper-Aubach Y, Klinger B 1992a Effects of insulin-like growth factor on linear growth, head circumference and body fat in patients with Laron-type dwarfism. Lancet 339:1258–1261

Laron Z, Klinger B, Blum WF, Silbergeld A, Ranke MB 1992b IGF binding protein 3 in patients with Laron type dwarfism: effect of exogenous rIGF-I. Clin Endocrinol (Oxf) 36:301–304

Laron Z, Suikkari AM, Klinger B et al 1992c Growth hormone and insulin-like growth factor regulate insulin-like growth factor binding protein-1 in Laron type dwarfism, growth hormone deficiency and constitutional short stature. Acta Endocrinol 127:351–358

Laron Z, Anin S, Klinger B 1993a Long-term IGF-I treatment of children with Laron syndrome. In: Laron Z, Parks JS (eds) Lessons from Laron syndrome (LS) 1966–1992. Pediatric and adolescent endocrinology, vol. 24, Karger, Basel–New York, p 226–236

Laron Z, Lilos P, Klinger B 1993b Growth curves for Laron syndrome. Arch Dis Child 68:768–770

Laron Z, Klinger B, Silbergeld A 1999 Serum insulin-like growth factor-I (IGF-I) levels during long-term IGF-I treatment of children and adults with primary GH resistance (Laron Syndrome). J Pediatr Endocrinol Metab 12:145–152

Laron Z, Wang XL, Silbergeld A, Wilcken DEL 1997 Growth hormone increases and insulin-like growth factor-I decreases circulating lipoprotein(a). Eur J Endocrinol 136:377–381

LeRoith D, Werner H, Beitner-Johnson D, Roberts CT Jr 1996 Molecular biology of the IGF-I receptor. In: Merimee T, Laron Z (eds) Growth hormone, IGF-I and growth. New views of old concepts. Modern Endocrinology and Diabetes. Vol 4. Freund Publishing House Ltd, London–Tel Aviv, p 73–99

Lindahl A, Isgaard J, Nilsson A, Isaksson OGP 1986 Growth hormone potentiates colony formation of epiphyseal chondrocytes in suspension culture. Endocrinology 118:1843–1848

Lindahl A, Isgaard J, Carlsson L, Isaksson OGP 1987 Differential effects of growth hormone and insulin-like growth factor I on colony formation of epiphyseal chondrocytes in suspension culture in rats of different ages. Endocrinology 121:1061–1069

Louvi A, Accili D, Efstratiadis A 1997 Growth-promoting interaction of IGF-II with the insulin receptor during mouse embryonic development. Dev Biol 189:33–48

Lupu F, Terwilliger JD, Lee K, Segre GV, Efstratiadis A 2001 Roles of growth hormone and insulin-like growth factor 1 in mouse postnatal growth. Dev Biol 229:141–162

Maor G, Silbermann M, von der Mark K, Heingard D, Laron Z 1993 Insulin enhances the growth of cartilage in organ and tissue cultures of mouse neonatal mandibular condyle. Calcif Tissue Int 52:291–299

Maor G, Rochwerger M, Segev Y, Phillip M 2002 Leptin acts as a growth factor on the chondrocytes of skeletal growth centers. J Bone Miner Res 17:1034–1043

Mohan S, Richman C, Guo R et al 2003 Insulin-like growth factor regulates peak bone mineral density in mice by both growth hormone-dependent and -independent mechanisms. Endocrinology 144:929–936

Murashita M, Tajima T, Nakae J, Shinohara N, Geffner ME, Fujieda K 1999 Near-normal linear growth in the setting of markedly reduced growth hormone and IGF-I. Horm Res 51:184–188

Nakae J, Kido Y, Accili D 2001 Distinct and overlapping functions of insulin and IGF-I receptors. Endocr Rev 22:818–835

Nilsson A 1995 Bone growth and metabolism in health and disease. In: Laron Z, Mastragostino S, Romano C, Boero S, Cohen A (eds) Limb lengthening: for whom, when and how? Freund Publishing House, London–Tel Aviv, p 79–91

Niwa M, Sato S, Saito Y et al 1986 Chemical synthesis, cloning and expression of genes for human somatomedin C (insulin like growth factor I) and 59Val somatomedin C. Ann NY Acad Sci 469:31–52

Powell-Braxton L, Hollingshead P, Warburton C et al 1993 IGF-I is required for normal embryonic growth in mice. Genes Dev 7:2609–2617

Rajkumar K, Barron D, Lewitt MS, Murphy LJ 1995 Growth retardation and hyperglycemia in insulin-like growth factor binding protein-1 transgenic mice. Endocrinology 136: 4029–4034

Ranke MB, Savage MD, Chatelain PG et al 1995 Insulin-like growth factor (IGF-I) improves height in growth hormone insensitivity: two years' results. Horm Res 44:253–264

Reinecke-Luthge A, Koschoreck F, Kloppel G 2000 The molecular basis of persistent hyperinsulinemic hypoglycemia of infancy and its pathologic substrates. Virchows Arch 436:1–5

Rinderknecht E, Humbel RE 1978 The amino acid sequence of human insulin like growth factor I and its structural homology, with proinsulin. J Biol Chem 253:2769–2776

Roback EW, Barakat AJ, Dev VG, Mbikay M, Chretien M, Butler MG 1991 An infant with deletion of the distal long arm of chromosome 15 (q26,1qter) and loss of insulin-like growth factor 1 receptor gene. Am J Med Genet 38:74–79

Rotwein P, Billiard J, Woelfle J 2002 Molecular physiology of IGF-I expression. J Pediatr Endocrinol Metab 15(suppl 5):1455–1458

Salter JM, Best CH 1953 Insulin as growth hormone. Br Med J 2:353–356

Schoenle E, Zapf J, Humbel RE, Froesch ER 1982 Insulin-like growth factor I stimulates growth in hypophysectomized rats. Nature 323:169–171

Silbergeld A, Dastot F, Klinger B et al 1997 Intronic mutation in the growth hormone (GH) receptor gene from a girl with Laron syndrome and extremely high serum GH binding protein: extended phenotypic study in a very large pedigree. J Pediatr Endocrinol Metab 10:265–274

Sims EAH, Danforth E Jr 1974 Role of insulin in obesity. Isr J Med Sci 10:1222–1229

Sivan B, Lilos P, Laron Z 2003 Effects of insulin-like growth factor -I deficiency and replacement therapy on the hematopoietic system in patients with Laron syndrome (primary growth hormone insensitivity). J Pediatr Endocrinol Metab 16:509–520

Stoffers DA, Zinkin NT, Stanojevic V, Clarke WL, Habener JF 1997 Pancreatic agenesis attributable to a single nucleotide deletion in the human IPF1 gene coding sequence. Nat Genet 15:106–110

Takahashi Y, Kadowaki H, Momomura K et al 1997 A homozygous kinase-defective mutation in the insulin receptor gene in a patient with leprechaunism. Diabetologia 40:412–420

Tamemoto H, Kadowaki T, Tobe K et al 1994 Insulin resistance and growth retardation in mice lacking insulin receptor substrate-1. Nature 372:182–186

Tamura T, Tohma T, Ohta T et al 1993 Ring chromosome 15 involving deletion of the insulin-like growth factor 1 receptor gene in a patient with features of Silver–Russell syndrome. Clin Dysmorphol 2:106–113

Tyrala EE 1996 The infant of the diabetic mother. Obstet Gynecol Clin North Am 23:221–241

Van Buul-Offers S, Veda I, van den Brande JL 1986 Biosynthetic somatomedin C (SM-C/IGF-I) increases the length and weight of Snell dwarf mice. Pediatr Res 20:825–827

Van Buul-Offers SC, van Kleffens M, Koster JG et al 2000 Human insulin-like growth factor (IGF) binding protein-1 inhibits IGF-I-stimulated body growth but stimulates growth of the kidney in Snell dwarf mice. Endocrinology 141:1493–1499

Walker JL, Van Wyk JJ, Underwood LE 1992 Stimulation of statural growth by recombinant insulin-like growth factor I in a child with growth hormone insensitivity syndrome (Laron type). J Pediatr 121:641–646

Woods KA, Camacho-Hubner C, Savage MO, Clark AJL 1996 Intrauterine growth retardation and postnatal growth failure associated with deletion of the insulin-like growth factor I gene. N Engl J Med 335:1363–1367

Zapf J, Froesch R, Schmid C 1999 Metabolic effects of IGF's. In: Rosenfeld R, Roberts Jr. C (eds) Contemporary endocrinology: the IGF system. Humana Press Inc, Totowa, NJ, p 577–616

Zhang M, Xuan S, Bouxsein ML et al 2002 Osteoblast-specific knockout of the insulin-like growth factor (IGF) receptor gene reveals an essential role of IGF signaling in bone matrix mineralization. J Biol Chem 277:44005–44012

Zhou Y, Xu BC, Maheshwari HG et al 1997 A mammalian model for Laron syndrome produced by targeted disruption of the mouse growth hormone receptor/binding protein gene (the Laron mouse). Proc Natl Acad Sci USA 94:13215–13220

DISCUSSION

De Meyts: I would like to clarify whether insulin is a growth factor in fetal growth in mice. This has been unequivocally answered by gene knockout studies, which you presented in a slightly confusing way. What you showed was actually the residue of growth, not the decrease in growth. If you knockout the IGF-1 receptor, the mice are born at 45% of normal size. If the IGF-1 receptor was mediating the effect of both IGF-1 and IGF-2 it shouldn't make any difference if you knock out that receptor plus the ligand. That is what you observe if you also knockout IGF-1. But if you knock out the IGF-1 receptor and IGF-2, the mice only have 30% of the normal size at birth. This is a difference of 15% that is not due to IGF-2 acting through the IGF-1 receptor but through another receptor. Efstratiadis and colleagues have tested whether that other receptor is the insulin receptor, and indeed if you knockout the IGF-1 receptor and the insulin receptor, they are born with 30% of normal size, similar to knocking out the IGF-1 receptor and IGF-2. This proves that IGF-2 is exerting part of its effect through the insulin receptor, about 15% of total fetal growth. Looking at the insulin receptor knockout mice, they were initially described to be of normal size. But if you study enough mice to reach significance, you can show they are actually 85–90% of the normal size. Why don't you see more size loss when you lose the role of insulin receptors mediating the effect of IGF-2? This is because there is a two-fold up-regulation of the IGF-1 receptor which partially compensates. If you knockout insulin — and there are two genes for insulin in mice — the mice are also 10–15% smaller. This decrease is only seen on the very last day of pregnancy, on day 18.5. This clearly shows that the insulin receptor does play some role in mediating the effects of IGF-2 on fetal growth, but insulin itself has a minor role in fetal growth and only at the very last stage of pregnancy. For review of this issue, see Efstratiadis (1998). Does this tell us anything about human pregnancy? We can't extrapolate to humans. Insulin receptor knockouts die within a few days in mice, and in humans there are two leprechaun patients with insulin receptor deletion that have lived several years, so it looks like the IGF-1 receptor in humans can at least for a while compensate for loss of metabolic effects of insulin. I don't know whether I've managed to clarify the issue!

LeRoith: It is clear, but on the other hand if we look at diabetic mothers and fetal macrosomia, the fetus there seems to have hyperinsulinaemia which was thought to be the cause of the macrosomia. But there is experimental evidence that insulin in fetal tissues can actually stimulate *IGF1* gene expression. This brings us back to the issue of gene expression under growth hormone effect. In liver, it is strongly controlled by nutrition and insulin. It may be that in fetal tissue that the hyperinsulinaemia that causes macrosomia is via the expression of IGF-1 working through its receptors. All of this could speak against insulin as being by itself a major growth factor, at least physiologically.

Holly: What about IGF-2? Zvi Laron was asking why these kids grow without IGF-1: why isn't IGF-2 the answer?

Laron: The role of IGF-2 isn't known. It could also play a role in the brain, where it is present. But there is a basic problem that in some respects, rodents do not behave like humans. The GH receptor knockout mice are not obese — they are lean — and we don't know the explanation for this at the moment. This contrasts with the human model, patients with LS, who are very obese.

Ohlsson: I would like to point out that the macro-organomegly associated with Beckwith–Wiedemann syndrome patients strongly correlates with tissues that are normally expressing high levels of *IGF2* in normal development (Hedborg et al 1994). There was one patient in particular that we were able to follow, and we could see that the organomegaly feature emerged only after week 17, not before. Interestingly, this is the stage when fetal insulin is being produced. When we looked at the pancreas of this patient, who unfortunately died of hypoglycaemia, there was a vast increase in the insulin-producing cells. We think that perhaps IGF-2 induced proliferation of the insulin-producing cells. Maybe there is also a link between having insulin collaborating with IGF-2, since this effect could only be seen once fetal insulin was being produced. Given that the effect was restricted to the endothelial tissues which are expressing high levels of IGF-2, we reasoned that there must be some kind of systemic–local factor involvement.

LeRoith: Why do you think the Laron dwarfs develop obesity?

Laron: I don't know. One explanation may be the insulin, which is high (Laron et al 1997). I don't know which is the cart and which is the horse, but they certainly have an abnormal fat metabolism.

Rosenfeld: They have no GH action. Interestingly, when they have IGF-1 replacement, there is not a decrease in obesity.

Laron: In GH-deficient adult patients who are treated with GH, there is a decrease in adipose tissue which is transitory, lasting for just a year. Then this stops (Laron & Klinger 1994). They don't become lean, and neither do our patients. I have a young patient who was treated for eight years. At the beginning she lost weight, and then this stopped. She is now very obese.

Rosenfeld: The implication, I think, is that in a GH-insensitive patient the adiposity reflects a defect in GH action independent of the IGF axis. This is because when you replace them with IGF, you do not correct the obesity.

LeRoith: There are certain mechanistic issues we have to look at. For example, GH is known to be lipolytic. This potentially could be the reason for fat loss. We also know that IGF-1 can cause differentiation of adipocytes. In our work in human mesenchymal stem cells it is IGF-1 and not insulin that pushes them through to the development of the adipocyte in differentiation. If you give GH to GH-deficient children, it could be that they lose their fat because of the lipolysis.

Laron: They too lose their fat only for a short time. Then the fat loss stops. I think that the mechanism is more complicated.

LeRoith: Now you are stimulating IGF-1 which could counteract that by causing differentiation of adipocytes and balance loss with differentiation. What is the IGF-1 level in the Laron dwarfs?

Laron: It is not measurable, or extremely low.

Rosenfeld: It is unmeasurable pre-pubertally, but in the adults it is measurable—about 25–30% of normal adult levels. Our experience in both Ecuador and Europe has been that pre-pubertal patients have unmeasurable levels, but post-pubertal levels are typically 50–70 ng/ml. Whereas the classical GH insensitive patients due to receptor mutation have truncal adiposity; the one case of the *IGF1* gene deletion and the one case of the *STAT5B* mutation are not obese. Presumably the GH pathways that don't involve the Jak/STAT *IGF1* gene transcription are the ones involved in lipolytic actions.

Holly: We always have to remember the triangle of insulin/GH/IGF-1. GH and IGF-1 appear to have important actions on insulin resistance, but the GH effect is mainly in the adipose tissue where the GH receptors are prevalent but there are no IGF-1 receptors. The IGF-1 effect is almost entirely in the muscle. It seems quite clear why Zvi Laron's patients are obese. It is because they haven't got the GH lipolysis action in the adipose tissue.

LeRoith: Something still has to drive the adipocytes to differentiate and then to increase their lipid storage.

Holly: It could be IGF-2. It does it experimentally as well as IGF-1.

Laron: GH treatment is advocated in Prader–Willi syndrome and other obese patients to reduce body fat. I don't think it works beyond an initial period, and it doesn't make these patients slim.

Pollak: I have a separate clinical question. I was intrigued by the mental deficiencies that you described and by the catch-up brain growth. I am curious: in the clinical management of these patients, has there been any psychometric improvement in the neurological deficits with treatment?

Laron: We investigated a group of LS patients after a 10 year interval. The verbal achievements were improved, the others were not (Galatzer et al 1993). The spectrum of defects is wide. We have a patient who is interned in a hospital for mental retardation, and at the other end of the spectrum there is a patient with a PhD. We have found that those who have the highest mental deficit have organic defects in the CNS detected by magnetic resonance imaging (MRI) (Kornreich et al 2002). Why one has more CNS damage than the other is as yet unclear. It is more than simply lack of IGF-1 action. There were different conclusions in the Ecuadorial group of patients (Kranzler et al 1998).

Rosenfeld: The other problem in looking at intellectual deficiencies in these patients is that many of them are subject to hypoglycaemia during the neonatal and infantile periods. For those who are retarded it is not clear how much this reflects the IGF brain growth effect and how much reflects hypoglycaemia.

Pollak: Another point came from these studies. You referred to the increase in IGF-1 in puberty. Earlier today we were asking about other regulators of IGF-1 expression besides GH. What do you understand as the explanation for the pubertal rise in IGF-1 levels?

Rosenfeld: There are a lot of difficult questions. To backtrack a little, we don't understand what it is at birth that triggers GH dependence of IGF-1. IGF-1 production *in utero* is largely GH-independent. Whatever triggers that off in the first few weeks of life is reflected in the very low IGF-1 levels of all studies of Laron dwarves. IGF-1 levels are virtually unmeasurable until puberty. Then, at puberty there clearly is a rise. IGF-1 levels remain measurable but low throughout adult life. Presumably, at least temporally this is related to the production of sex steroids. Normal physiology would suggest that most of the sex steroid effect is due to increased GH secretion that occurs at puberty, but there does appear to be some direct effect of sex steroids on IGF-1 levels. It is presumed that the non-GH-dependent production of IGF-1 that begins in puberty and continues throughout adult life is at least in part entrained if not dependent on sex steroids.

LeRoith: There were studies by Mark Sperling of Pittsburgh on the glucagon receptor and its function during birth (Ganguly et al 1983). He showed that prior to birth the cAMP connection to the glucagon receptor was present, but there was no proper connection. Post-birth they were then able to stimulate cAMP production with glucagon stimulation. If I could suggest an experiment, why not look at the STAT pathway prior to and post puberty to see whether the expression is there before but there is a lack of connection as a developmental alteration that could then be altered in development.

Pollak: Tamoxifen modestly reduces IGF-1 levels.

Rosenfeld: Is that through its effects on GH?

Pollak: It is a liver effect.

LeRoith: This observation goes back 30 years when we used to treat acromegalic patients with oestrogen and other sex steroids to block GH function. Now Ken Ho from Australia has shown that those compounds block the effect of GH at the liver through STAT effects (Leung et al 2003). So you may get increased secretion at puberty, but if you give enough of the sex steroid you can block the GH–STAT connection. I think he shows that it works through the SOCS feedback.

Kaaks: The same has been shown for hormone-replacement therapy and oral contraceptives. As long as they are taken by mouth and as long as they lead to fairly high concentrations of the steroids in the first pass through the liver after absorption this effect is seen. Patches don't have the same effect. There need to be supraphysiological levels of the steroids in the liver to see such things. The question is, if sex steroids play a role in IGF production, is this a pharmacological effect only, or does this relationship also have a regulatory role at normal, physiological levels of (endogenous) sex steroids?

LeRoith: Your studies show that tamoxifen reduces circulating IGF-1. Presumably this is the liver effect of blocking production.

Lønning: If you look at what happens when tamoxifen is given by the oral route, or if high-dose oestrogen is given in breast cancer therapy, there is a significant suppression of IGF-1 (Lønning et al 1992, Helle et al 2001). Oestrogen (diethyl stilbestrol given at 15 mg daily) is even more potent in this respect than tamoxifen. On the other hand, if we take regular hormone-replacement therapy as administered to post-menopausal women, and switch the same patients between parenteral, oral or patch administration, we just see marginal effects on the IGF system. Physiological replacement even by the oral route causes minor effects. However, with tamoxifen and high-dose oestrogen there is a profound effect at the liver level.

I have another question. Sex steroids up-regulate GH. At the same time, LS patients experience delayed puberty—it is not the other way round, that GH secretion triggers puberty. Why not?

LeRoith: So the question is, isn't GH–IGF normal stimulation at the time of puberty involved in pubertal growth?

Laron: These patients have a reduced pubertal growth spurt. Not only is puberty delayed, but also the extent of pubertal growth is reduced. We could show this especially in boys (Laron et al 1980).

LeRoith: So are their oestrogen and testosterone levels lower?

Laron: I don't have the figures in my head, but I would think, yes.

Lønning: It seemed from your results that the growth curve was delayed. The Laron patients continued to have a kind of late growth even beyond the age of 16, where pubertal growth stops in normal children. The reason why it stops is because oestrogen closes the epiphyseal lines in both sexes. This tells me that this process must be delayed in some way in Laron patients.

Laron: The girls are less delayed than the boys. If you take two biological markers, the age of menarche in girls is slightly delayed and the age of first nocturnal ejaculation in males can be delayed up to the age of 20 or more. This means that the bone age at that time is about 13.5 years.

Holly: Martin Savage showed many years ago that there is a close integration between GH, IGF-1 and insulin. (Savage et al 1992). There is a pubertal rise in fasting insulin, and at the same time there is a rise in GH and IGF-1. The pubertal rise in fasting insulin suppresses IGFBP1 and SHBG, revealing the IGF and unleashing the sex hormones (Holly et al 1989). In trying to understand what is going on with IGF-1 at puberty, have you looked at fasting insulin levels? Is there a pubertal increase in fasting insulin, and a suppression of IGFBP1 and SHBG?

Laron: Yes.

LeRoith: There is resistance at puberty, so there is a slight rise in insulin.

Rosenfeld: I don't think that pubertal rise in insulin resistance is seen, because they are GH resistant.

Holly: So they don't get the suppression of IGFBP1 or SHBG.

Rosenfeld: I don't know.

Kaaks: It has been shown that the insulin resistance during puberty is largely attributable to the GH-induced lipolysis which increases the free fatty acids in the circulation.

References

Efstratiadis A 1998 Genetics of mouse growth. Int J Dev Biol 42:955–976

Galatzer A, Anan O, Nagelberg N, Rubitzek J, Laron Z 1993 Cognitive and psychological functioning of young adults with Laron Syndrome. In: Laron Z, Parks JS (eds) Lessons from Laron Syndrome, 1966–1992. Paediatric and Adolescent Endocrinology. Vol 24. Karger, Basel, p 53–60

Ganguli S, Sinha MK, Sterman B, Harris P, Sperling MA 1983 Ontogeny of hepatic insulin and glucagon receptors and adenylate cyclase in rabbit. Am J Physiol 244:E624–631

Hedborg F, Holmgren L, Sandstedt B, Ohlsson R 1994 The cell type-specific IGF2 expression during early human development correlates to the pattern of overgrowth and neoplasia in the Beckwith–Wiedemann syndrome. Am J Pathol 145:802–817

Helle SI, Geisler J, Anker GB, Leirvaag B, Holly JM, Lonning PE 2001 Alterations in the insulin-like growth factor system during treatment with diethylstilboestrol in patients with metastatic breast cancer. Br J Cancer 85:147–151

Holly JM, Smith CP, Dunger DB et al 1989 Relationship between the pubertal fall in sex hormone binding globulin and insulin-like growth factor binding protein-I. A synchronized approach to pubertal development? Clin Endocrinol (Oxf) 31:277–284

Kornreich L, Horev G, Schwarz M, Karmazyn B, Laron Z 2002 Craniofacial and brain abnormalities in Laron syndrome (primary growth hormone insensitivity). Eur J Endocrinol 146:499–503

Kranzler JH, Rosenbloom AL, Martinez V, Guevara-Aguirre J 1998 Normal intelligence with severe insulin-like growth factor I deficiency due to growth hormone receptor deficiency: a controlled study in a genetically homogeneous population. J Clin Endocrinol Metab 83:1953–1958

Laron Z, Klinger B 1994 IGF-I treatment of adult patients with Laron syndrome: preliminary results. Clin Endocrinol (Oxf) 41:631–638

Laron Z, Sarel R, Pertzelan A 1980 Puberty in Laron type dwarfism. Eur J Pediatr 134:79–83

Laron Z, Avitzur Y, Klinger B 1997 Insulin resistance in Laron Syndrome (primary insulin-like growth factor I deficiency) and effect of IGF-I replacement therapy. J Pediatr Endocrinol Metab 10(suppl):105–115

Leung KC, Doyle N, Ballesteros M et al 2003 Estrogen inhibits GH signaling by suppressing GH-induced JAK2 phosphorylation, an effect mediated by SOCS-2. Proc Natl Acad Sci USA 100:1016–1021

Lonning PE, Hall K, Aakvaag A, Lien EA 1992 Influence of tamoxifen on plasma levels of insulin-like growth factor I and insulin-like growth factor binding protein I in breast cancer patients. Cancer Res 52:4719–4723

Savage MO, Smith CP, Dunger DB, Gale EA, Holly JM, Preece MA 1992 Insulin and growth factors adaptation to normal puberty. Horm Res 37(suppl 3):70–73

Insulin-like growth factors and neoplasia

Michael N. Pollak

Department of Oncology, McGill University and Lady Davis Research Institute, 3999 Rue Côte Sainte Catherine, Montréal, Québec, H3T 1E2, Canada

Abstract. Prospective studies suggest that individuals with circulating levels of insulin-like growth factor 1 (IGF-1) at the high end of the normal range are at increased risk for several common cancers. Further data implicate IGF-1 and hyperinsulinism as candidate mediators of the effects of body size on cancer risk and prognosis. Ongoing research seeks to confirm these findings, to clarify the underlying physiology, and to assess their relevance to patterns of cancer incidence. *In vivo* models have not only provided data consistent with the epidemiological observations, but also suggest that IGF-1 signalling stimulates growth of established cancers. This has led to the development of novel IGF-1 receptor targeting therapies which have impressive antineoplastic activity in experimental systems.

2004 Biology of IGF-1: its interaction with insulin in health and malignant states. Wiley, Chichester (Novartis Foundation Symposium 262) p 84–107

Signalling systems based on proteins homologous to those involved in IGF-1 signalling arose early in evolution as regulators of cellular proliferation in relation to nutrient availability (Longo & Finch 2003). In mammals, insulin and IGF-1 receptors play key roles in regulating cellular proliferation and apoptosis, energy utilization, body size, longevity and a variety of more specialized organ-specific functions (Baserga et al 2003, Giudice 2002, Jones & Clemmons 1995, Nakae et al 2001).

Recent laboratory and epidemiological research has led to interest in the relationship of insulin and IGF signalling to neoplasia (Baserga et al 2003, Holly 1998, Burroughs et al 1999) and to the related issue of ageing at the cellular and whole-organism levels (Tatar et al 2003, Longo & Finch 2003). At the cellular level, it is clear that IGF-1 signalling inhibits apoptosis and stimulates proliferation (Jones & Clemmons 1995). Paradoxically, life expectancy of several model organisms increases with reduced IGF-related signalling (Tatar et al 2003, Arantes-Oliveira et al 2003, Longo & Finch 2003).

One potential application of this research is the development of novel antineoplastic therapies that target the IGF-1 receptor or downstream signalling molecules. Another is the characterization of potentially modifiable IGF-1 and insulin-related cancer risk factors that may underlie certain trends in the global patterns of cancer incidence.

Structural features of the IGF-1 receptor and details of downstream signalling pathways have been the subject of recent reviews (De Meyts & Whittaker 2002, Nakae et al 2001, Jones & Clemmons 1995, Pollak 2001) and will not be described here.

Inter-individual variation in circulating IGF-1 levels

There is evidence that both lifestyle and genetic factors contribute to the large variation in circulating IGF-1 and IGF binding protein (IGFBP) levels between normal individuals (Harrela et al 1996). Dozens of proteins are involved in the physiological systems that regulate IGF-1 levels, and polymorphic variation of the genes encoding each of these may contribute to the interindividual variability in circulating concentrations. Examples include IGF-1 itself, IGFBPs and their proteases, growth hormone (GH) and its receptor, and somatostatin and GH-releasing hormone (GHRH) and their receptors. To date, only a few of these have been studied in the context of their influence on variation of IGF-1 levels within the normal range (Le Marchand et al 2002, Johnston et al 2003, Deal et al 2001, Bonafe et al 2003), but some are mutated in growth disorders that are associated with abnormal IGF-1 levels (Laron 1995, Maheshwari et al 1998). Some (but not all; Schernhammer et al 2003) early reports (for example Ho et al 2003, Le Marchand et al 2002, Wang et al 2003) suggest that polymorphic variation of some of these genes influences cancer risk or prognosis.

The measurement of circulating levels of IGF-1 and/or IGFBP3 to aid in the diagnosis of GH deficiency and acromegaly is well established in clinical endocrinology. Recent results have challenged the traditional view that there is no biological or medical significance to the substantial interindividual variation in serum IGF-1 and IGFBP3 levels that fall within the broad normal range between pathological extremes. We review below evidence that the risk of common cancers is elevated in individuals with higher circulating levels of IGF-1 relative to those at the lower end of the normal range. There is also separate evidence linking risk of cardiac disease inversely to circulating IGF-1 levels (Juul et al 2002, Vasan et al 2003).

Nutritional factors are important lifestyle influences on circulating IGF-1 levels (Thissen et al 1994). Starvation is well known to be associated with substantially reduced IGF-1 levels in humans and animal models, and there is evidence that this explains at least in part the well known protective effect of caloric restriction against carcinogenesis in rodent models (Dunn et al 1997). More recent studies suggest that modest increases in IGF-1 levels are associated with high levels of energy or protein intake (Holmes et al 2002, Giovannucci et al 2003). In several studies, IGF-1 levels were seen to increase with increasing dairy product intake (Gunnell et al 2003, Giovannucci et al 2003, Holmes et al 2002). The underlying mechanism and significance of this relationship deserves further study, particularly in view of evidence that prostate cancer risk increases with both IGF-1 level (Pollak 2001) and dairy intake (Chan et al 2001). There is evidence that micronutrients including retinoids influence circulating IGFBP3 levels, and that this modified by a polymorphism (Deal et al 2001). It is likely that ongoing research will uncover additional genetic modifiers of nutritional influences on IGF physiology. This research may be relevant to the identification of certain individuals for whom specific dietary patterns have particularly important implications with respect to disease risk.

Racial factors also influence IGF-1 and IGFBP3 levels. It is important not to over-interpret what may be a coincidence, but black men, who have a higher risk for prostate cancer than other groups, were observed to have higher levels of IGFBP3 (Platz et al 1999), while black women have higher IGF-1 levels than racial groups with lower breast cancer risk (Jernstrom et al 2001a, DeLellis et al 2003).

Other hormones, including endogenous and exogenous steroids, have important influences on the GH–IGF-1 axis. Both tamoxifen and diethyl stilbestrol are effective breast cancer treatments, and while both have multiple mechanisms of action, it is of interest that both suppress IGF-1 levels (Pollak et al 1990a, Helle et al 2001).

It is often assumed that IGF-1 serum level can be used as a surrogate for IGF-1 receptor signalling or IGF-1 levels in interstitial fluid. Direct evidence to test this reasonable hypothesis is lacking, but may become available as methodology for measuring IGF-1 receptor activation in tissues improves. However, it is likely that the relationship between circulating level and tissue bioactivity will be found to be complex. For example, higher levels of IGF binding proteins may on the one hand increase the serum binding capacity for IGFs, and increase IGF-1 concentration by increasing its circulating half-life, but this may not reflect an increase at the tissue level. Oral oestrogen replacement therapy reduces IGF-1 circulating levels; this probably is a consequence of direct delivery to the liver of pharmacological oestrogen concentrations that suppress IGF-1 gene expression (Jernstrom et al 2001b). This lowers circulating IGF-1 levels, but may not reflect reduced IGF-1 signalling in tissues. Oestrogen delivery by the transdermal route does not lower circulating IGF-1 levels, and in several experimental systems physiological oestrogen concentrations enhance IGF signalling (Yee & Lee 2000). Polymorphisms that influence function of the IGF-1 receptor itself

(Abuzzahab et al 2003) or downstream signalling proteins would also be expected to add complexity to the relationship between circulating IGF-1 levels and IGF-1 receptor signalling.

IGF-1 physiology and cancer risk: indirect evidence

Circumstantial evidence

Studies concerning body size, birthweight and mammographic density are consistent with the possibility that IGF-1 physiology influences cancer risk. Small but significant increases in cancer risk with increasing height have been documented in many studies (Lawlor et al 2003, Mellemkjaer et al 2003, Engeland et al 2003, Gunnell et al 2001). Height *per se* is unlikely to be a risk factor, but it is possible that hormonal determinants of height also influence cancer risk. While circulating IGF-1 levels are related weakly or not at all to adult height (which may be influenced by factors such as osteoporosis), they are related to height early in life (Juul et al 1994). Thus, height may be weakly related to risk because it is weakly related to IGF-1 exposure over the first decades of life.

Birth weight and size have been associated with risk of breast cancer (Stavola et al 2000, McCormack et al 2003), colorectal (Sandhu et al 2002), prostate (Tibblin et al 1995) and childhood cancers (Von Behren & Reynolds 2003), and are positively correlated with cord blood IGF-1 level (Vatten et al 2002a). Conversely, pre-eclampsia is associated with reduced IGF-1 and reduced breast cancer risk (Altinkaynak et al 2003, Vatten et al 2002b).

Mammographic density is strongly related to breast cancer risk (reviewed in Boyd et al 2002), but the mechanisms involved are unclear. There is evidence (Byrne et al 2000, Maskarinec et al 2003) for a positive relation between circulating IGF-1 levels (or the ratio of IGF-1 to IGFBP3 levels) and mammographic density. This raises the possibility that the relation between mammographic density and breast cancer risk exists, at least in part, because variability in density functions as a surrogate for variability in IGF-1 physiology.

Experimental models

Several *in vivo* carcinogenesis models have provided data compatible with an effect of host IGF-1 physiology on cancer risk. These models are to be distinguished from those that study the influence of variations in IGF-1 levels or IGF-1 signalling on behaviour of established cancers. IGF-1 deficiency models related to expression of a GH antagonist or to liver-specific deletion of the IGF-1 gene both provide evidence that lower circulating levels of IGF-1 are associated with significant reduction in breast cancer following exposure to chemical carcinogens (Pollak et al 2001, Wu et al 2003). Prostate cancer incidence in the well-characterized TRAMP carcinogenesis model (Majeed et al 2003) is substantially reduced in IGF-1-deficient mice, while organ-specific overexpression of the IGF-1 receptor increased prostate neoplasia (DiGiovanni et al 2000). Another example concerns hepatocarcinogenesis: overexpression of IGFBP1, which can attenuate IGF-1 receptor activation by sequestering ligands, inhibited carcinogenesis following exposure to diethylnitrosamine (Lu & Archer 2003). It is also of interest to note that certain cancers are more frequent in large breeds of dogs, which have higher circulating IGF-1 levels (Eigenmann et al 1988, Withrow et al 1991). It is important to recognize that all these models involve perturbations of the IGF system that are large relative to the more subtle variations in IGF-1 physiology between normal human subjects. However, it is reasonable to employ models of large differences over relatively short times to simulate more subtle differences that may influence human carcinogenesis over decades.

IGF physiology and cancer risk: evidence from population studies

Methodological issues

In order to examine the possibility that levels of a circulating analyte predict risk of a future cancer diagnosis, a nested case–control study design is useful. This involves blood sampling of a large number of apparently healthy subjects prior to subsequent long-term clinical observation. After years of follow-up, subjects who have developed a particular cancer can be identified and assays performed on their stored blood samples together with samples from an appropriate control group from the same cohort. The distribution of levels between the cases and controls is used to reach conclusions concerning the association of the analyte with risk. This method is useful because it minimizes the possibility that conclusions will be biased by effects of the disease itself on the analyte. This is an important consideration for studies of IGF-1 and cancer risk, as it is known that the malnourishment associated with cancer cachexia lowers IGF-1 levels. A non-prospective study design, where IGF-1 levels are compared in blood samples from cases sampled after diagnosis and from a cancer-free control group, presents potential difficulties in interpretation.

Assay technology for measuring IGF-1, IGFBPs and related analytes is evolving rapidly (Pollak 2001). Epidemiological research involving small differences between groups requires greater sensitivity than the traditional clinical applications of the assays — diagnosis of GH deficiency and acromegaly. It is necessary to ensure that a particular assay method is appropriate for a given set of samples, as varying amounts of proteolysis may occur between the time of veinopuncture and assay, and antibodies vary in their specificity for different molecular species. This issue is particularly important for IGFBP3, which is present in the circulation as a mixture of proteins of varying lengths (due to proteolytic cleavage) and varying glycosylation and phosphorylation modifications, all of which may have physiologic significance. Some of the discrepancies in the literature regarding relationships of IGFBP3 levels to subsequent cancer risk may relate to technical issues concerning assay methodology.

Epidemiological data

Earlier reviews (Pollak 2000, 2001, Pollak et al 1999, Khandwala et al 2000, Yu & Rohan 2000) summarized both prospective and non-prospective studies in this area. Overall, the trend towards increasing risk with increasing levels of IGF-1 is clear. In the occasional study, results are dramatic—for example, within the Physician's Health Study Cohort, the association between IGF-related analytes and prostate cancer risk was stronger than the association between cholesterol and cardiovascular disease; Stampfer et al (1991), Stampfer (2000), Chan et al (1998)—but overall the associations are modest. Of course, the impact of a risk factor that is common in a population and associated with modestly increased risk may exceed the disease burden attributable to strong risk factors that are encountered rarely.

It is important to point out that some studies did not detect an association of IGF-1 levels with risk, particularly in the case of lung cancer. This may be because IGF-related risk is insignificant for a cancer where risk in carcinogen exposure is very high, bearing in mind that the lung cancer cohort studies differed from those used for the other cancer studies, in that they were comprised of heavy smokers. Among heavy smokers, no association was seen between prostate cancer and IGF-related analytes. This remains unexplained, but a mechanism involving an effect of heavy smoking on IGF-1 levels cannot be ruled out.

The IGF-1 receptor as a target for cancer treatment

The paradigm of receptor targeting is now well established in Oncology therapeutics. Androgen and oestrogen receptors are 'classic' targets which have led to widely used therapies for prostate and breast cancer. More recently, trastuzumab (Herceptin™), imitrib (Gleevec™), and compounds that interfere with epidermal growth factor receptor function have demonstrated that the paradigm of receptor targeting can be extended beyond steroid hormone receptors.

Not long after the initial report of the presence of IGF-1 receptors (IGF-1Rs) on surgically resected tumour specimens and speculation that IGF-1R might represent a therapeutic target (Pollak et al 1987), it was shown that administration of a blocking antibody directed against this receptor slowed the *in vivo* proliferation of human breast cancer xenografts (Arteaga et al 1989). This experimental result did not lead to immediate translational research, as it was obtained years prior to the now-widespread therapeutic use of antibodies and also antedated current interest in tyrosine kinase receptors as molecular targets in oncology. Nearly 15 years later, interest in targeting IGF-1R has become widespread (Surmacz 2003,Wang & Sun 2002).

Preclinical models

Work with transgenic mice (e.g. Wu et al 2002) adds to prior evidence (Yang et al 1996, Pollak et al 1990b, Khandwala et al 2000) that IGF-1 provided by the host stimulates aggressive behaviour of established cancers. Further research has shown that targeting the IGF-1 receptor leads to impressive antineoplastic activity in many *in vitro* and *in vivo* models of common human cancers. Strategies employed include:

- Measures to prevent ligand binding, including IGFBPs, peptide or small molecule competitive binding antagonists, or blocking anti-receptor antibodies (Maloney et al 2003).
- Antisense or siRNA strategies to reduce receptor expression (Bohula et al 2003).
- Introduction of a dominant negative IGF-1R to interfere with receptor action (Sachdev et al 2003, Lee et al 2003, Min et al 2003, Hongo et al 2003).
- Use of small molecule IGF-1R-specific tyrosine kinase inhibitors (Garcia-Echeverria et al 2003).
- Targeting signalling downstream of the IGF-1R, with agents much as AKT inhibitors or rapamycin (Houghton & Huang 2004).

Evidence that functional IGF-1Rs are necessary for transformation induced by a variety of means including oncogene activation or chemical carcinogens has led to optimism that IGF-1R blockade may be of therapeutic value in a broad spectrum of malignancies (Surmacz 2003, LeRoith & Roberts 2003, Sell et al 1994). Apart from possible activity as a single agent, IGF-1R blockade may potentiate various existing therapies, including cytotoxic agents, radiotherapy, and therapies that target various steroid or peptide hormone receptors. There is, for example, *in vitro* evidence that reduction of IGF-1R signalling enhances the efficacy of therapies that target HER2/neu (Lu et al 2001, Camirand et al 2002).

Towards clinical trials

Recent results from preclinical studies of IGF-1R targeting strategies have provided evidence of efficacy comparable or superior to that obtained for other antineoplastic strategies subsequently found to be useful clinically. Some methods that successfully targeted IGF-1R experimentally, such as the dominant negative receptor approach, are not immediately ready for clinical evaluation due to general issues related to optimization of gene therapy methods. Others, such as the use of orally active small molecule IGF-1R kinase inhibitors, are expected to be evaluated in phase I/II clinical trials that may be initiated shortly.

The design of such trials will be challenging: there is a need to consider single agent activity, but on the other hand preclinical research suggests that some of the most promising applications may involve combinations with current cytotoxic or endocrine therapies. With respect to anticipated toxicity, the possibility that therapies directed against the IGF-1R will lack sufficient specificity to avoid co-targeting the insulin receptor must be considered, and careful assessment of glucose metabolism will be required. However, dose-limiting diabetogenic toxicity has not been seen in preclinical studies to date.

It will be important to discover molecular predictors of therapeutic response in order to allow the identification of those patients for whom IGF-1R targeting may be useful. Early research in this area suggests that IGF-1R overexpression in biopsy specimens may not be a useful predictor of responsivity to IGF-1R targeting drugs. This is in contrast to experience in prediction of efficacy of agents that block HER2/neu signalling, where receptor level has been found to be useful. Phosphorlyated IGF-1R levels and levels of IGF-2 expression (suggesting presence of an active IGF-2–IGF-1R autocrine loop) are examples of candidate predictors of response to IGF-1R targeting therapies that are now being evaluated.

It would not be surprising if effective IGF-1 receptor blockade were associated with a compensatory increase in circulating IGF-1 levels, as receptors involved in IGF-1 homeostatic control would likely be blocked in parallel with the target receptors present on neoplasms. However, early experimental results indicate that the increase in IGF-1 level is insufficient to overcome the pharmacological blockade. Furthermore, this phenomenon may be useful: experimental results raise the possibility that IGF-1 levels, as well as IGF-1R phosphorylation level in skin biopsies (analogous to similar studies used in evaluating EGFR blockade; Baselga et al 2002) may be useful as endpoints in early dose-finding studies.

Another challenge in the clinical evaluation of IGF-1R targeting strategies will be the choice of suitable patient populations. Preclinical evidence provides a rationale for clinical trials in multiple myeloma, breast cancer, prostate cancer, colon cancer, sarcoma and others. IGF-1R targeting may have important anti-metastatic and anti-angiogenic properties (Sachdev et al 2003). This implies the possibility of antineoplastic activity that might be easier to detect in adjuvant trials than in trials for advanced disease. However, it is clear that advanced disease trials represent necessary first steps to establish dose and toxicity.

Further research directions

GH therapy, IGF-1, cancer and ageing

GH replacement therapy for GH deficiency represents an important medical advance that offers major benefits to patients with low IGF-1 levels secondary to low GH levels. On the other hand, GH supplementation to achieve IGF-1 levels higher than age-specific population norms is controversial (Giovannucci & Pollak 2002). Short-term studies have suggested that GH therapy may have short-term anabolic or 'anti-ageing' effects (Rudman et al 1990), but these benefits have been questioned (Vance 2003). It is sobering to recognize that while pharmacological measures to raise IGF-1 levels have been proposed to retard ageing, results from model organisms suggest that over the long-term such measures may have the opposite effect (Longo & Finch 2003, Tatar et al 2003).

The evidence concerning a relationship between cancer risk and IGF-1 levels would suggest that a cautious approach to growth hormone therapy is wise, and that efforts should be made to titrate the growth hormone dose to achieve levels near the age-specific mean in an appropriate reference population (Wetterau & Cohen 2000, Swerdlow et al 2002).

In animal models ranging from *Caenorhabditis elegans* to mice, life expectancy has been found to be inversely related to IGF signalling (Longo & Finch 2003, Tatar et al 2003). Homozygosity for the *lit* mutation, which inactivates the GHRH receptor, results in small mice with subnormal levels of circulating IGF-1 (Yang et al 1996). Interestingly, these animals provide an environment less permissive for neoplastic proliferation than controls (Majeed et al 2003, Yang et al 1996), and also have a longer expectancy than controls (Flurkey et al 2001). Consistent with these results, mice heterozygous for the IGF-1 receptor were recently shown to have extended life expectancy (Holzenberger et al 2002). These examples provide an interesting contrast to mice with enhanced p53 activity (Tyner et al 2002), which are resistant to carcinogenesis but show premature ageing.

What mechanisms might underlie the experimental results indicating increased life expectancy and reduced cancer risk in animals with low IGF-1, and be compatible with the anti-apoptotic and proliferation-stimulating effects of IGF-1 at the cellular level? One concept which deserves re-examination is the notion of 'rate of living'. It is plausible that somatic cell DNA damage, which contributes to both carcinogenesis and ageing, accumulates as a function of the number of cell divisions following ovum fertilization. In individuals with higher IGF-1 levels, the rate of cell division in renewing somatic tissues may be somewhat greater than in individuals with lower levels. In a Darwinian sense, this would be expected to be associated with certain advantages, such as more rapid wound healing and earlier achievement of adult body size. At the cellular level, a consequence of the hypothesized higher rate of cell division associated with higher IGF-1 level would be that at any arbitrary organism age, those with higher IGF-1 levels would have undergone a higher number of somatic cell divisions in renewing epithelial cell populations. By the 'clock' of number of cell divisions, those with higher IGF-1 levels would be ageing faster. Those with lower IGF-1 levels, by spacing cell divisions more widely, would be ageing more slowly with reference to an external clock. Evidence that mice strains that grow to larger sizes have shorter life expectancies (Miller et al 2002) is consistent with this model. The fact that cancer risk increases with age while IGF-1 levels decline with age does not represent evidence against this concept, because in stepwise carcinogenesis DNA damage accumulates over decades: important determinants of cancer risk late in life operate in early and midlife.

Also consistent with the model is early evidence from murine, primate and human studies that epithelial cell turnover rates vary with IGF-1 levels (Cats et al 1996, Pollak et al 1999, Ng et al 1997). Quantitative studies of this important issue are limited by precision of current methods. For example, between person variability in mean half life of colon epithelial cells by as little as a few hours would result in a huge difference in number of cell divisions over decades of life.

Conclusion

More than a decade has passed since the hypothesis that IGF-1 signalling may be relevant to human neoplasia was formulated. While laboratory research provides evidence that many molecular signals are relevant to neoplasia, the IGF system provides a rare example where evidence is accumulating from both population and laboratory research. In the coming years it is likely that conclusions with potential relevance to cancer prevention and treatment will emerge from large-scale population studies concerning risk, clinical trials of IGF-1R targeting therapies, and ongoing laboratory research.

References

Abuzzahab MJ, Schneider A, Goddard A et al 2003 IGF-1 receptor mutations resulting in intrauterine and postnatal growth retardation. N Engl J Med 349:2211–2222

Altinkaynak K, Aksoy HH, Bakan E, Kumtepe Y 2003 Serum IGF-I and IGFBP-3 in healthy pregnancies and patients with preeclampsia. Clin Biochem 36:221–223

Arantes-Oliveira N, Berman JR, Kenyon C 2003 Healthy animals with extreme longevity. Science 302:611

Arteaga CL, Kitten LJ, Coronado EB et al 1989 Blockade of the type 1 somatomedin receptor inhibits growth of human breast cancer cells in athymic mice. J Clin Invest 84: 1418–1423

Baselga J, Rischin D, Ranson M et al 2002 Phase I safety, pharmacokinetic, and pharmacodynamic trial of ZD1839, a selective oral epidermal growth factor receptor tyrosine kinase inhibitor, in patients with five selected solid tumor types. J Clin Oncol 20: 4292–4302

Baserga R, Peruzzi F, Reiss K 2003 The IGF-1 receptor in cancer biology. Int J Cancer 107: 873–877

Bohula EA, Salisbury AJ, Sohail M et al 2003 The efficacy of small interfering RNAs targeted to the type 1 insulin-like growth factor receptor (IGF1R) is influenced by secondary structure in the IGF1R transcript. J Biol Chem 278:15991–15997

Bonafe M, Barbieri M, Marchegiani F et al 2003 Polymorphic variants of insulin-like growth factor I (IGF-I) receptor and phosphoinositide 3-kinase genes affect IGF-I plasma levels and human longevity: cues for an evolutionarily conserved mechanism of life span control. J Clin Endocrinol Metab 88:3299–3304

Boyd NF, Stone J, Martin LJ et al 2002 The association of breast mitogens with mammographic densities. Br J Cancer 87:876–882

Burroughs KD, Dunn SE, Barrett JC, Taylor JE 1999 Insulin-like growth factor-I: a key regulator of human cancer risk? J Natl Cancer Inst 91:579–581

Byrne C, Colditz GA, Willett WC, Speizer FE, Pollak M, Hankinson SE 2000 Plasma insulin-like growth factor-I, insulin-like growth factor-binding protein-3 and mammographic density. Cancer Res 60:3744–3748

Camirand A, Lu Y, Pollak M 2002 Co-targeting HER2/ErbB2 and insulin-like growth factor-1 receptors causes synergistic inhibition of growth in HER2-overexpressing breast cancer cells. Med Sci Monit 8:BR521–BR526

Cats A, Dullaart RP, Kleinbeuker JH et al 1996 Increased epithelial cell proliferation in the colon of patients with acromegaly. Cancer Res 56:523–526

Chan JM, Stampfer MJ, Giovannucci E et al 1998 Plasma insulin-like growth factor-I and prostate cancer risk: a prospective study. Science 279:563–566

Chan JM, Stampfer MJ, Ma J, Gann PH, Gaziano JM, Giovannucci EL 2001 Dairy products, calcium, and prostate cancer risk in the Physicians' Health Study. Am J Clin Nutr 74:549–554

De Meyts P, Whittaker J 2002 Structural biology of insulin and IGF-1 receptors: implications for drug design. Nat Rev Drug Discov 1:769–783

Deal C, Ma J, Wilkin F et al 2001 Novel promoter polymorphism in insulin-like growth factor-binding protein-3: correlation with serum levels and interaction with known regulators. J Clin Endocrinol Metab 86:1274–1280

DeLellis K, Ingles S, Kolonel L et al 2003 IGF1 genotype, mean plasma level and breast cancer risk in the Hawaii/Los Angeles multiethnic cohort. Br J Cancer 88:277–282

DiGiovanni J, Kiguchi K, Frijhoff A et al 2000 Deregulated expression of insulin-like growth factor 1 in prostate epithelium leads to neoplasia in transgenic mice. Proc Natl Acad Sci USA 97:3455–3460

Dunn SE, Kari FW, French J et al 1997 Dietary restriction reduces IGF-I levels, which modulates apoptosis, cell proliferation, and tumor progression in p53 deficient mice. Cancer Res 57:4667–4672

Eigenmann JE, Amador A, Patterson DF 1988 Insulin-like growth factor I levels in proportionate dogs, chondrodystrophic dogs and in giant dogs. Acta Endocrinol (Copenh) 118:105–108

Engeland A, Tretli S, Bjorge T 2003 Height, body mass index, and prostate cancer: a follow-up of 950000 Norwegian men. Br J Cancer 89:1237–1242

Flurkey K, Papaconstantinou J, Miller RA, Harrison DE 2001 Lifespan extension and delayed immune and collagen aging in mutant mice with defects in growth hormone production. Proc Natl Acad Sci USA 98:6736–6741

Garcia-Echeverria C, Brueggen J, Capraro H-G et al 2003 Characterization of potent and selective kinase inhibitors of IGF-1R. Proc Am Assoc Cancer Res 44:1008

Giovannucci E, Pollak M 2002 Risk of cancer after growth-hormone treatment. Lancet 360:268–269

Giovannucci E, Pollak M, Liu Y et al 2003 Nutritional predictors of insulin-like growth factor-I and their relationships to cancer in men. Cancer Epidemiol Biomarkers Prev 12:84–89

Giudice LC 2002 Maternal–fetal conflict — lessons from a transgene. J Clin Investig 110:307–309

Gunnell D, Okasha M, Smith GD, Oliver SE, Sandhu J, Holly JM 2001 Height, leg length, and cancer risk: a systematic review. Epidemiol Rev 23:313–342

Gunnell D, Oliver SE, Peters TJ et al 2003 Are diet–prostate cancer associations mediated by the IGF axis? A cross-sectional analysis of diet, IGF-I and IGFBP-3 in healthy middle-aged men. Br J Cancer 88:1682–1686

Harrela M, Koinstinen H, Kaprio J et al 1996 Genetic and environmental components of interindividual variation in circulating levels of IGF-I, IGF-II, IGFBP-1, and IGFBP-3. J Clin Invest 98:2612–2615

Helle SI, Geisler J, Anker GB, Leirvaag B, Holly JM, Lønning PE 2001 Alterations in the insulin-like growth factor system during treatment with diethylstillboestrol in patients with metastatic breast cancer. Br J Cancer 85:147–151

Ho GY, Melman A, Liu SM et al 2003 Polymorphism of the insulin gene is associated with increased prostate cancer risk. Br J Cancer 88:263–269

Holly JM 1998 Insulin-like growth factor-I and new opportunities for cancer prevention. Lancet 351:1373–1375

Holmes MD, Pollak MN, Willett WC, Hankinson SE 2002 Dietary correlates of plasma insulin-like growth factor-I and insulin-like growth factor binding protein-3 concentrations. Cancer Epidemiol Biomarkers Prev 11:852–861

Holzenberger M, Dupont J, Ducos B et al 2002 IGF-I receptor regulates lifespan and resistance to oxidative stress in mice. Nature 421:125–126

Hongo A, Kuramoto H, Nakamura Y et al 2003 Antitumor effects of a soluble insulin-like growth factor-I receptor in human ovarian cancer cells: advantage of recombinant protein administration *in vivo*. Cancer Res 63:7834–7839

Houghton PJ, Huang S 2004 mTOR as a target for cancer therapy. Curr Top Microbiol Immunol 279:339–359

Jernstrom H, Chu W, Vesprini D et al 2001a Genetic factors related to racial variation in plasma levels of insulin-like growth factor-I: implications for pre-menopausal breast cancer risk. Mol Genet Metab 72:144–154

Jernstrom H, Wilkin F, Deal C et al 2001b Genetic and non-genetic factors associated with variation of plasma levels of insulin-like growth factor-I and insulin-like growth factor binding protein-3 in healthy premenopausal women. Cancer Epidemiol Biomarkers Prev 10:377–384

Johnston LB, Dahlgren J, Leger J et al 2003 Association between insulin-like growth factor 1 (IGF-1) polymorphisms, circulating IGF-1, and pre- and postnatal growth in two European small for gestational age populations. J Clin Endocrinol Metab 88:4805–4810

Jones JI, Clemmons DR 1995 Insulin-like growth factors and their binding proteins: biological actions. Endocr Rev 16:3–34

Juul A, Main K, Blum WF, Lindholm J, Ranke MB, Skakkebaek NE 1994 The ratio between serum levels of insulin-like growth factor (IGF)-1 and the IGF binding proteins (IGFBP)-1, 2 and 3 decreases with age in healthy adults and is increased in acromegalic patients. Clin Endocrinol 41:85–93

Juul A, Scheike T, Davidsen M, Gyllenborg J, Jorgensen T 2002 Low serum insulin-like growth factor-1 is associated with increased risk of ischemic heart disease: a population-based case-control study. Circulation 106:939–944

Khandwala HM, McCutcheon IE, Flyvbjerg A, Friend KE 2000 The effects of insulin-like growth factors on tumorigenesis and neoplastic growth. Endocr Rev 21:215–244

Laron Z 1995 Prismatic cases: Laron syndrome (primary growth hormone resistance) from patient to laboratory to patient. J Clin Endocrinol Metab 80:1526–1531

Lawlor DA, Okasha M, Gunnell D, Smith GD, Ebrahim S 2003 Associations of adult measures of childhood growth with breast cancer: findings from the British Women's Heart and Health Study. Br J Cancer 89:81–87

Le Marchand L, Donlon T, Seifried A, Kaaks R, Rinaldi S, Wilkens LR 2002 Association of a common polymorphism in the human GH1 gene with colorectal neoplasia. J Natl Cancer Inst 94:454–460

Lee CT, Park KH, Adachi Y et al 2003 Recombinant adenoviruses expressing dominant negative insulin-like growth factor-I receptor demonstrate antitumor effects on lung cancer. Cancer Gene Ther 10:57–63

LeRoith D, Roberts CT Jr 2003 The insulin-like growth factor system and cancer. Cancer Lett 195:127–137

Longo VD, Finch CE 2003 Evolutionary medicine: from dwarf model systems to healthy centenarians? Science 299:1342–1346

Lu S, Archer MC 2003 Insulin-like growth factor binding protein-1 over-expression in transgenic mice inhibits hepatic preneoplasia. Mol Carcinog 36:142–146

Lu Y, Zi X, Zhao Y, Mascarenhas D, Pollak M 2001 Insulin-like growth factor-I receptor signaling and resistance to trastuzumab (Herceptin). J Natl Cancer Inst 93:1852–1857

Maheshwari HG, Silverman BL, Dupuis J, Baumann G 1998 Phenotype and genetic analysis of a syndrome caused by an inactivating mutation in the growth hormone-releasing hormone receptor: Dwarfism of Sindh. J Clin Endocrinol Metab 83:4065–4074

Majeed N, Kaplan P, Blouin M-J, Greenberg N, Pollak M 2003 Lit is the first germ-line mutation to reduce prostate cancer risk and prolong survival in the TRAMP transgenic model. Proc Am Assoc Cancer Res 44:877

Maloney EK, McLaughlin JL, Dagdigian NE et al 2003 An anti-insulin-like growth factor-I receptor antibody that is a potent inhibitor of cancer cell proliferation. Cancer Res 63:5073–5083

Maskarinec G, William AE, Kaaks R 2003 A cross-sectional investigation of breast density and insulin-like growth factor 1. Int J Cancer 107:996

McCormack VA, dos Santos Silva I, De Stavola BL, Mohsen R, Leon DA, Lithell HO 2003 Fetal growth and subsequent risk of breast cancer: results from long term follow up of Swedish cohort. Br Med J 326:248

Mellemkjaer L, Olsen ML, Sorensen HT, Thulstrup AM, Olsen J, Olsen JH 2003 Birth weight and risk of early-onset breast cancer (Denmark). Cancer Causes Control 14:61–64

Miller RA, Harper JM, Galecki A, Burke DT 2002 Big mice die young: early life body weight predicts longevity in genetically heterogenous mice. Aging Cell 1:22–29

Min Y, Adachi Y, Yamamoto H et al 2003 Genetic blockade of the insulin-like growth factor-I receptor: a promising strategy for human pancreatic cancer. Cancer Res 63:6432–6441

Nakae J, Kido Y, Accili D 2001 Distinct and overlapping functions of insulin and IGF-I receptors. Endocr Rev 22: 818–835

Ng ST, Zhou J, Adesanya OO, Wang J, LeRoith D, Bondy CA 1997 Growth hormone treatment induces mammary gland hyperplasia in aging primates. Nat Med 3:1141–1144

Platz EA, Pollak M, Majeed N, Tao Y, Willett WC, Giovannucci E 1999 Racial variation in insulin-like growth factor-I and binding protein-3 concentrations in middle-age men. Cancer Epidemiol Biomarkers Prev 8:1107–1110

Pollak M 2000 Insulin-like growth factor physiology and cancer risk. Eur J Cancer 36:1224–1228

Pollak M 2001 Insulin-like growth factors (IGFs) and prostate cancer. Epidemiol Rev 23:59–66

Pollak M, Perdue JF, Margolese RG, Baer K, Richard M 1987 Presence of somatomedin receptors on primary human breast and colon carcinomas. Cancer Lett 38:223–230

Pollak M, Costantino J, Polychronakos C et al 1990a Effect of tamoxifen on serum insulin-like growth factor I levels in stage I breast cancer patients. J Natl Cancer Inst 82:1693–1697

Pollak M, Polychronakos C, Richard M 1990b Insulin like growth factor 1: a potent mitogen for human osteogenic sarcoma. J Natl Cancer Inst 82:301–305

Pollak M, Beamer W, Zhang JC 1999 Insulin-like growth factors and prostate cancer. Cancer Metastasis Rev 17:383–390

Pollak M, Blouin MJ, Zhang JC, Kopchick JJ 2001 Reduced mammary gland carcinogenesis in transgenic mice expressing a growth hormone anatgonist. Br J Cancer 85:428–430

Rudman D, Feller AG, Nagraj HS et al 1990 Effects of human growth hormone in men over 60 years old. New Engl J Med 323:1–6

Sachdev D, Hartell JS, Lee AV, Zhang X, Yee D 2003 A dominant negative type I insulin-like growth factor receptor inhibits metastasis of human cancer cells. J Biol Chem 279:5017–5024

Sandhu MS, Luben R, Day NE, Khaw KT 2002 Self-reported birth weight and subsequent risk of colorectal cancer. Cancer Epidemiol Biomarkers Prev 11:935–938

Schernhammer ES, Hankinson SE, Hunter DJ, Blouin M-J, Pollak MN 2003 Polymorphic variation at the -202 locus in IGFBP3: influence on serum levels of insulin-like growth factors, interaction with plasma retinol and vitamin D and breast cancer risk. Int J Cancer 107:60–64

Sell C, Dumenil G, Deveaud C et al 1994 Effect of a null mutation of the insulin-like growth factor I receptor gene on growth and transformation of mouse embryo fibroblasts. Mol Cell Biol 14:3604–3612

Stampfer MJ 2000 The study of cancer risks in populations. Growth Horm IGF Res 10:S4–S5

Stampfer MJ, Sacks FM, Salvini S, Willett WC, Hennekens CH 1991 A prospective study of cholesterol, apolipoproteins, and the risk of myocardial infarction. New Engl J Med 325:373–381

Stavola BL, Hardy R, Kuh D, Silva IS, Wadsworth M, Swerdlow AJ 2000 Birthweight, childhood growth and risk of breast cancer in British cohort. Br J Cancer 83:964–968

Surmacz E 2003 Growth factor receptors as therapeutic targets: strategies to inhibit the insulin-like growth factor-I receptor. Oncogene 22:6589–6597

Swerdlow AJ, Higgins CD, Adlard P, Preece MA 2002 Risk of cancer in patients treated with human pituitary growth hormone in the UK, 1959–85: a cohort study. Lancet 360:273–277

Tatar M, Bartke A, Antebi A 2003 The endocrine regulation of aging by insulin-like signals. Science 299:1346–1351

Thissen JP, Ketelslegers JM, Underwood LE 1994 Nutritional regulation of the insulin-like growth factors. Endocr Rev 15:80–101

Tibblin G, Eriksson M, Cnattingius S, Ekbom A 1995 High birthweight as a predictor of prostate cancer risk. Epidemiology 6:423–424

Tyner SD, Venkatachalam S, Choi J et al 2002 p53 mutant mice that display early ageing-associated phenotypes. Nature 415:45–53

Vance ML 2003 Can human growth hormone prevent aging? N Engl J Med 348:779–780

Vasan RS, Sullivan LM, D'Agostino RB et al 2003 Serum insulin-like growth factor I and risk for heart failure in elderly individuals without a previous myocardial infarction: the Framingham Heart Study. Ann Intern Med 139:642–648

Vatten LJ, Nilsen ST, Odegard RA, Romundstad PR, Austgulen R 2002a Insulin-like growth factor-I and leptin in umbilical cord plasma and infant birth size at term. Pediatrics 109:1131–1135

Vatten LJ, Romundstad PR, Trichopoulos D, Skjaerven R 2002b Pre-eclampsia in pregnancy and subsequent risk for breast cancer. Br J Cancer 87:971–973

Von Behren J, Reynolds P 2003 Birth characteristics and brain cancers in young children. Int J Epidemiol 32:248–256

Wang Y, Sun Y 2002 Insulin-like growth factor receptor-1 as an anti-cancer target: blocking transformation and inducing apoptosis. Curr Cancer Drug Targets 2:191–207

Wang L, Habuchi T, Tsuchiya N et al 2003 Insulin-like growth factor-binding protein-3 gene -202 A/C polymorphism is correlated with advanced disease status in prostate cancer. Cancer Res 63:4407–4411

Wetterau L, Cohen P 2000 Role of insulin-like growth factor monitoring in optimizing growth hormone therapy. J Pediatr Endocrinol Metab 13:1371–1376

Withrow SJ, Powers BE, Straw RC, Wilkins RM 1991 Comparative aspects of osteosarcoma. Dog versus man. Clin Orthop 270:159–168

Wu Y, Yakar S, Zhao L, Hennighausen L, LeRoith D 2002 Circulating insulin-like growth factor-1 levels regulate colon cancer growth and metastasis. Cancer Res 62:1030–1035

Wu Y, Cui K, Miyoshi K et al 2003 Reduced circulating insulin-like growth factor I levels delay the onset of chemically and genetically induced mammary tumors. Cancer Res 63:4384–4388

Yang XF, Beamer W, Huynh HT, Pollak M 1996 Reduced growth of human breast cancer xenografts in hosts homozygous for the 'lit' mutation. Cancer Res 56:1509–1511

Yee D, Lee AV 2000 Crosstalk between the insulin-like growth factors and estrogens in breast cancer. J Mammary Gland Biol Neoplasia 5:107–115

Yu H, Rohan T 2000 Role of the insulin-like growth factor family in cancer development and progression. J Natl Cancer Inst 92:1472–1489

DISCUSSION

Laron: We have evidence that patients with no IGF-1 can still live a long time. On the Krk island some patients lived up to the age of 90 even though they lacked GH and also gonadotrophins. In fact, we found them to have a mutation in the *PROP1* transcription factor gene (Krzisnik et al 1999). Of our Laron syndrome patients, the oldest one is 78. As far as I know from the cohort in Ecuador, they also have patients who lived up to the age of 90.

LeRoith: Do you have a sufficient number of patients to make this observation?

Laron: We follow a large cohort. When you go back to your data on energy, nowadays many people follow the Atkins diet, in which they have a high energy intake mainly in the form of protein. Years ago, in the US you couldn't eat a lunch without a glass of milk. Is there really evidence that this is promoting cancer?

Pollak: No, there is only speculation. But certainly in terms of the relationship to the IGF axis, I believe that one of the few things we have learned without any contradiction is that a higher intake of milk increases IGF-1 levels. Even a few years ago, the only thing we knew for certain was looking in the other direction at the effects of starvation, which decreases IGF levels.

Laron: Did they become shorter with less cancer?

Pollak: That's a possibility, but I would favour the examination of the following hypothesis: why do IGF-1 levels fall with starvation? I don't think it is an accident:

rather, it is an adaptive response. In those situations IGF-1 levels may fall with starvation rather profoundly as a way of saving energy and protein specifically by reducing cellular turnover. If this is true, then it is possible that these control systems, which evolved over millennia when you were either barely surviving or starving, are now dealing with a situation where people are eating too much. So we could not a priori predict how such control systems will behave under situations so different from the circumstances under which they evolved. Now it seems that when we eat too much we may be turning up the cellular turnover rate, which may be deleterious. But we only have clues now, and not conclusions.

Lønning: I'd like to raise the issue of cancer risk and IGF levels. You mentioned that cervical cancer was related to IGF. This was quite surprising to me, because cervical cancer is largely caused by papilloma virus. Along with lung cancer, this is one of the cancers I would not expect to be related to IGF because it is so clearly related to an external carcinogenic effect. I know this is not your work, but would you like to comment on this?

Pollak: One model that could account for this is the survival of the partially damaged cell model. Yes, the dominant factor for cervical cancer is viral. The question is, are there a large number of women with viral infections but low IGF environments such that the partially transformed cells die? As you say, it is not my study and I have an open mind on it.

LeRoith: Surely this would fit the model we discussed earlier, that IGF-1 is not the major cause of this cancer but it is bringing out the cancer in these patients. The primary oncogenic hit could still be the virus.

Holly: There is no problem at all here: most cancer is caused by gene mutations, but gene mutation is not the system going wrong. It is a natural frequent event. The thing that goes wrong is the safeguard, which is apoptosis. It is the same safeguard whether you have a mutation or an infected cell: damaged cells should commit suicide. This going wrong is what gives you cancer. If a cell survives inappropriately because of excess signalling of a survival factor, this will shift your risk of getting cancer. The argument is no different whether a viral infection or a gene mutation is the insult.

Lønning: When you look at the family germline syndromes, this illustrates how strong particular genetic events are. What you are talking about with these viral infections in the inactivation of p53 is an event, as strong as a germline mutation happening somewhat later, to the cervix.

Holly: If you look at the prevalence of HPV infection in sexually active women it is quite high, but most of these don't go on to get cervical cancer. The problem with most cancers is their progression, not the original hit.

Lønning: I have a second question, relating to what you mentioned about breast cancer. You said that high IGF levels at the early stage also predict for postmenopausal breast cancer at a later stage. As we are all aware of, there have been a number of studies showing that the oestrogen levels after the menopause are a severe risk factor for breast cancer. Interestingly, in the latest update on these studies published in *JNCI* in August, they looked at body mass index (BMI) in relation to oestrogen levels in post-menopausal women. The claim was that the increased risk in post-menopausals related to increased BMI could be mostly explained by the influence on oestrogen levels. Do you have any plans to look at the IGF in relation to the oestrogen levels and see how early life IGF levels and subsequent body mass and oestrogen levels could fit into a sort of model?

Pollak: That is an interesting project. I think that the person sitting to your right, Dr Kaaks, probably has the largest population set in which to analyse multiple hormones and anthropomorphic measurements together.

Werner: We were talking about locally-produced versus endocrine factors. I understand that IGF-1 is a risk factor in breast and prostate cancer whereas IGF-2 is not a risk factor. However, most of the really important players in cancer biology, including tumour suppressors and oncogenes, are not necessarily risk factors. We know that IGF-2 is expressed very early in the transformation process. A number of years ago Doug Hanahan showed that focal expression of IGF-2 is a very early event in cancer. This is consistent with the fact that, in ontogenetic terms, IGF-2 is more primitive than IGF-1. There are a number of molecular mechanisms that explain the increased expression of IGF-2 in tumours and overgrowth syndromes. I don't know whether there is a good IGF and a bad IGF but, in my opinion, if there is a bad IGF that is most probably IGF-2.

Pollak: In our first study we measured IGF-2, because a priori we would have thought that IGF-2 might be important. We had no reason to speculate that IGF-1 would be related to cancer and IGF-2 would not be. We were surprised, but this finding has been consistent. I agree that loss of imprinting of IGF-2 is crucially important in early cancer progression. A recent paper in *Science* by the Feinberg group showed that loss of imprinting of IGF-2 is an independent risk factor for colon cancer (Cui et al 2003): forget about circulating IGF-1 levels. This is very interesting and suggests that if there is a loss of imprinting of IGF-2 there is a risk that is independent of the circulating IGF-1 level. If we put those subjects to the side, the relationship of IGF-1 level to risk would actually be strengthened. IGF-2 loss of imprinting is an important issue, but somehow this is not manifest in circulating IGF-2 levels. I can only wonder whether there is any meaning to the fact that IGF-1 turns out to be more of a risk factor for cancer and IGF-2 circulating levels seem less important, and in the clinical growth deficiency situation IGF-2 doesn't seem to substitute for IGF-1 in stimulating somatic growth. These are two parallel mysteries which may be linked.

Roberts: Jeff Holly, don't you have some data on IGF-2 that suggest that it is also a positive risk factor?

Holly: Yes, in our study in prostate cancer it is a risk factor, although not as strong as IGF-1.

Kaaks: We also saw this in a prospective study of colorectal cancer. I am not quite sure what this means, because the levels found in the circulation may be high or low as a secondary effect of the amount of IGFBP3 circulating.

Yee: It seems that there are at least a couple of interrelated factors that explain the observations. One is caloric restriction, in terms of both ageing and cancer. This was one of the older models. The other is IGF's action on its receptor. The third is just body size. In the Nurse's Health Study, don't they have some dietary history, anthropomorphic measurements and IGF levels? At least in terms of trying to correlate which of these come up, have you looked at this?

Pollak: The Nurse's Health Study predominantly involves older women. That is why I mentioned that our confidence in the negative results for postmenopausal women was statistically far more certain than for our positive results in the younger women. To look at the interactions in a multivariate model between the factors you have mentioned is very important, but in the Nurse's Health Study we are limited by the number of premenopausal cancers. The EPIC study that Rudolf Kaaks runs is larger. If we are doing the subset analysis or the interaction analysis we need more people, but what you suggest is a great idea. With the small numbers we have power is limited, but IGF-1 was the stronger predictor of premenopausal risk than any of the conventional breast cancer risk factors.

LeRoith: People have suggested that the dietary component was removed as a player in this study, but what you are saying is that it hasn't really been excluded.

Pollak: We are not claiming that IGF-1 is *necessarily* causatively related to premenopausal breast cancer. The data are consistent with the possibility that there is a dietary risk factor that influences breast cancer and also influences IGF-1.

LeRoith: That wasn't suggested in the early presentations of the study. People said that they had excluded diet as being an issue so IGF-1 is important. But I think the dietary component wasn't excluded totally.

Pollak: Absolutely, but the diet could be acting through IGF-1, or there could be a dietary variable that is correlated with IGF-1.

Holly: Sandy Dunn did an elegant experiment in p53 deficient mice, showing that calorie restriction does reduce the incidence of progression of tumours induced by a bladder carcinogen (Dunn et al 1997). Then she showed that the calorie restriction reduced the circulating IGF-1 and if you replaced the IGF-1 you completely negated any benefits of the reduced calorie restriction, suggesting that in that model all the benefit of calorie restriction was mediated by IGF-1.

Kaaks: Just a word about methodological difficulties in epidemiology, trying to link lifestyle factors such as diet to intermediate metabolism and cancer risk. First of all, there is usually an enormous amount of measurement error in these questionnaire assessments of what people eat. You can't really calculate balances between energy intake and energy expenditure, because it is usually very small differences that lead to obesity. This is out of the question. Only anthropometrical or other indices of adiposity can give you an idea of the long term energy imbalance in the past. With regard to foods or nutrients that may have an effect on circulating levels of IGF, we see the same thing as Michael Pollak has reported: dairy products increase the circulating levels of IGF-1. Their effect is significant and has been observed in a number of studies, but the percentage variation among subjects that can be explained by this association is very small. It is just a few percent of the overall variance. If one postulated that IGF-1 was an intermediate between milk consumption and cancer risk, then you would need a much larger proportion of variance in IGF explained by this factor, just in view of the observed association of risk with IGF itself. Otherwise it is not possible to have such a pathway explain the relationship. It may be that IGF is just a bystander—a marker for high or low intakes of specific foods. The truth is that from dietary epidemiology very few dietary risk factors come out as strong risk factors. Although it cannot be ruled out, in my view it is very unlikely that we are looking at a phenomenon here that is confounded by some dietary behaviour which is the true risk factor that explains the risk of cancer and as a secondary phenomenon also leads to high or low IGF levels. I think it is much more likely that IGF itself plays a role, also in view of all the biology that we have heard about today.

Pollak: Derek LeRoith was saying that in the original papers we perhaps did not give equal space to the dietary intermediate possibility and the direct effect of IGF possibility. We didn't give equal space because we favoured the direct hypothesis, just as you do. But in a formal sense all that we know is that there is a relationship.

Kaaks: In a formal sense nothing is ever proven. It is just a matter of plausibility and likelihood. In terms of plausibility the IGF hypothesis is strong, in my opinion.

Holly: You played down the association with IGF-1, but I would agree with Michael Pollak: a few years ago we all knew that big changes in dietary input had an impact. But none of us would have thought that we could identify a single component. Think of the variation in dietary intake among all of us in this room: in this variation in diet milk is a fairly small component, and to identify one small component of your dietary variation having a robust and significant association is surprising. I am surprised that one component came up with such a strong association.

Kaaks: The association is significant but it is not strong. The *P* value is low but the association is weak.

Clark: I think the most impressive data today were those showing the effects of different nutrition in various countries on the incidence of cancer. Clearly this isn't all via IGF-1. Japanese don't have zero IGF and Americans don't have 1000 ng/ml. These diseases are driven by diet.

Laron: You made a very wise statement saying that one should individualize any manipulation of the GH–IGF-1 axis. Could you go one step further and say how you would do this?

Pollak: I stated this because sometimes as a result of the data that we have generated I am presented as an individual who thinks that GH or IGF therapies are poison and should never be given to anyone. I wanted to make it clear that in clinical deficiency states these are valuable drugs. But I also wanted to make it clear that I believe you can have too much of a good thing. The off-label use of GH far exceeds its use in correcting GH deficiency. There are many people who are playing in a pseudoscientific way with their health by maintaining adolescent levels of GH as adults. This is dangerous and is not to be condoned by proper scientists. As a way of expressing this notion, I thought that a positive way to say this is that to ask what should we do for each patient. Perhaps one could envisage the possibility that in a decade or so we can take an IGF-1 serum measurement or do a chip for gene polymorphisms so we could recognize that a titration upwards or downwards might be useful in some cases. For example, someone aged 60 at risk of heart disease might want a different level than someone with a strong risk for cancer. This is a research direction and not something that is ready for prime time.

Laron: I agree, but we have so many experts here that I wonder whether, because use of GH is increasing tremendously at all ages, we should try to get a sort of consensus on this. Perhaps size at birth is important, or IGF-1 levels at puberty. You showed that if you have a higher intake of proteins that you have higher IGF-1 levels.

LeRoith: I think it's too early to try to get a consensus. As long as 'maybe' and 'perhaps' are prefacing each statement, we can't reach consensus.

Pollak: We could ask the question, who in the audience feels that chronic supplementation of GH to adolescent levels is a good thing?

LeRoith: If you take oral preparations of GH like those advertised on the internet, then I think it has no side effects! That is the only one I'd prescribe!

Laron: If you take it by mouth you may suppress ghrelin.

LeRoith: I don't think it is functional when it gets into the stomach.

Clark: On the GH story, GH physiologists know that the best way to increase GH levels is via exercise. Are you are going to inject GH, or should you just exercise?

LeRoith: There are data suggesting that the exercise effect is limited and short-lived. Exercise has very good cardiovascular effects which long-term GH treatment does not offer.

Kaaks: We have reviewed the literature on this recently. There are a huge number of studies looking at the short-term effects of a bout of exercise. Although these studies do systematically show increases in GH levels, there is generally only a very modest increase in circulating levels of IGF-1. The increase in IGF-1 is difficult to interpret because exercise-induced dehydration changes concentrations, and many analytes go up.

Clark: I am talking about the effects of exercise on releasing GH (Godfrey et al 2003). Traditional exercise to maintain cardiac function is sufficient to increase GH levels.

Kaaks: The long-term effects haven't been established. There are very few good studies on exercise and GH levels over more than just a day or two.

Pollak: The *NEJM* editorial (Vance 2003) more than a decade after the Rudman study (Rudman et al 1990) pointed out that the benefits that Rudman observed by GH treatment were better achieved by a simple exercise programme.

Rosenfeld: In fact the field is moving in the direction of trying to maintain serum IGF levels within some reasonable range, whatever that means. It is important to point out that this is a very conservative step to take. In a way, it is like Pascal's wager. He was asked whether he believed in God, and he reasoned that although he didn't know whether God existed it was safer to say he does! No one knows whether there is a long-term risk to humans of elevated IGF-1 in terms of cancer. There are epidemiological correlations but no definitive causality studies. The conservative approach is that if you can get a therapeutic benefit by maintaining IGF-1 levels within the physiological range for age, this is the appropriate thing to do. It would be dangerous for us to make recommendations beyond that.

Holly: Coming back to the issue of ageing and extending lifespan with GH, I am still unsure about the validity of extrapolating from animal models. Evolution has been driven by Darwinian selection pressure. For most animals, lifespan is linked to reproductive competence, because as soon as they have reproduced they are in competition with offspring for resources. Somewhere up in higher mammals it became a selective advantage for the parents to stay around, and then the limitations on lifespan extended beyond reproductive age. The reasons for the length of the lifespan are not always ageing; there are other considerations that come into it. There is a lot of mixing up of the concepts of ageing and limitations of lifespan. I am not at all clear that we can extrapolate anything from animal models such as *Drosophila* and *Caenorhabditis elegans*, because we are talking about humans for who the rules are completely different, and which age long after their reproductive competence has finished.

LeRoith: Are you arguing that the age-related decline in GH and IGF-1 is a good thing?

Holly: I think it was designed for a purpose.

LeRoith: So we should leave it well alone.

Holly: Unless we understand it better, then yes, we shouldn't mess with it. We certainly shouldn't extrapolate from worms and flies which die for very different reasons.

Yee: If we think about this in the context of post-menopausal HRT, we didn't really know the answer for HRT and cancer or cardiovascular risk until we did the controlled clinical trial. Everything prior to this was anecdotal, suggesting benefit for HRT. This argument about GH–IGF supplementation will go on for ever unless one of the endocrinologists supports a proposed randomised clinical trial with enough power to look at cancer events.

Pollak: We should remember that in the case of post-menopausal oestrogen replacement therapy there was optimisim and speculation, and we certainly have precedent for hormone supplementation having negative effects.

LeRoith: Take the optimism with Rudman's trial, and then there was a study by Mark Blackman (Blackman et al 2002) in the aged population where he gave GH and saw some benefit in terms of fat distribution and muscle mass. But he showed quite significant side effects, including increased arthritis, diabetes and insulin resistance. His conclusion after many years of trying GH in the Baltimore aged population was that the side effects outweigh the benefits. This has put a dampener on GH. Are you suggesting we try IGF-1? There have been some studies on this from the VA in Stanford by Andy Hoffman (Friedlander et al 2001). There again the results have been mixed.

Rosenfeld: I don't think that is what Doug Yee is saying. He is saying until we really have data that really address causality rather than correlation, we will be in the ether.

LeRoith: But who is going to take on these trials when some of the studies have suggested that the side effects outweigh the benefits.

Pollak: The possibility of long term toxicity may not arise if there is no evidence of health benefits; if there are benefits then they have to be evaluated in relationship to risks.

Rosenfeld: The data will come from long-term trials of GH and IGF-1 therapy. They are just not going to be available to us a year from now.

LeRoith: But the trials are going to be in adults with low GH.

Yee: As we see now, there are many adults who are choosing to self-administer GH.

LeRoith: They aren't in trials. We won't get results from them.

Yee: As long as people continue to report single-arm trials of people who select one therapy over no treatment, we will never know.

Pollak: Even Ron Rosenfeld's populations won't give us the answers. I think you are referring to people who have a clinical indication because of deficiency, which is very different. This is actually a minor use of GH.

Rosenfeld: But if 10 years from now these studies indicate an increased risk of cancer in patients with certain IGF-1 levels, these are the studies that will be most comparable to the HRT replacement studies.

Yee: When the Women's Health Initiative trial was planned, it was understood that breast cancer risk was going to be increased by HRT, but they thought this risk would be outweighed by the bone and cardiovascular benefits. The fact that there are some negative data for GH–IGF-1 and cancer doesn't mean that you couldn't do a randomised trial.

Kaaks: I have been surprised by this whole argument. We have heard that there may be a risk of cancer associated with high GH and IGF-1 levels. If one was to do an intervention from this perspective one should rather think of lowering IGF-1 or GH. It may be that for cardiovascular disease it is different, although I have some questions about this. To me it is not clear what benefit one should hope for with GH replacement therapy, except for some concept of reducing age-related degeneration phenomena.

Yee: Don't get me wrong: I am not suggesting it is a good idea. I am just presenting the argument that we don't know for sure. The benefits of improvement in quality of life, bone density and cardiovascular risk might outweigh an increased risk of some cancers.

Pollak: That's why I thought the most diplomatic way of summarizing the situation was the notion of individualization. There might be individuals who could benefit, despite the risks. Whether we will ever be able to conduct the studies that will allow us to select a subpopulation of people with IGF-1 levels in the normal range who deserve a little extra GH is not clear. I would see ethical problems in offering GH supplementation to people with IGF levels in the normal range, though, because we have some short term documented risks and some theoretical long-term risks. These have to be weighed against benefits that are largely theoretical. Or, if you go by the Rudman paper, benefits that are easily achievable by non-pharmacological means, namely exercise. Given the current picture, large-scale HRT-type trials for GH would be difficult to execute.

References

Blackman MR, Sorkin JD, Munzer T et al 2002 Growth hormone and sex steroid administration in healthy aged women and men: a randomized controlled trial. JAMA 288:2282–2292

Cui H, Cruz-Correa M, Giardiello FM et al 2003 Loss of IGF2 imprinting: a potential marker of colorectal cancer risk. Science 299:1753–1755

Dunn SE, Kari FW, French J et al 1997 Dietary restriction reduces insulin-like growth factor I levels, which modulates apoptosis, cell proliferation, and tumor progression in p53-deficient mice. Cancer Res 57:4667–4672

Friedlander AL, Butterfield GE, Moynihan S et al 2001 One year of insulin-like growth factor I treatment does not affect bone density, body composition, or psychological measures in postmenopausal women. J Clin Endocrinol Metab 86:1496–1503

Godfrey RJ, Madgwick Z, Whyte GP 2003 The exercise-induced growth hormone response in athletes. Sports Med 33:599–613
Krzisnik C, Kolacio Z, Battelino T, Brown M, Parks JS, Laron Z 1999 The 'Little People' of the island of Krk — revisited. Etiology of hypopituitarism revealed. J Endocr Genet 1:9–19
Rudman D, Feller AG, Nagraj HS et al 1990 Effects of human growth hormone in men over 60 years old. N Engl J Med 323:1–6
Vance ML 2003 Can growth hormone prevent aging? N Engl J Med 348:779–780

Loss of *IGF2* imprinting: mechanisms and consequences

Rolf Ohlsson

Department of Development & Genetics, Evolution Biology Centre, Uppsala University, Norbyvägen 18A, S-752 36 Uppsala, Sweden

Abstract. Although the leading dogma for the origin of the diversity in cancer cell subpopulations is based on a stepwise selection and accumulation of genetic changes that allow uncontrollable malignant growth, there is an emerging understanding that the variability of heritable phenotypes in cancer and cancer-prone cells may also involve epigenetic mechanisms. This is exemplified by the unscheduled activation of the normally repressed maternal *IGF2* allele in a wide range of human cancers. The notion that this so-called loss of imprinting (LOI) provides a proliferative advantage by increasing the levels of the IGF-2 ligand available to its receptors is supported by the overgrowth symptoms of neonatal mice, which has been genetically manipulated to express *Igf2* biallelically. Although the mechanisms underlying *IGF2* LOI in human cancer remains unknown, it is likely to directly or indirectly involve the *H19* imprinting control region (ICR). This stretch of 2 kb sequence just upstream of the *H19* promoter functions to block enhancer-*Igf2* promoter communications by means of a DNA methylation-sensitive chromatin insulator. We discuss here the possibility that pathological mechanisms leading to *IGF2* LOI use different strategies with the neutralization of the *H19* ICR insulator function as a common denominator.

2004 Biology of IGF-1: its interaction with insulin in health and malignant states. Wiley, Chichester (Novartis Foundation Symposium 262) p 108–124

Epigenetic marks establish active or inactive states of genes in a heritable manner (Ohlsson 1999). The epigenetic state can be laid down and faithfully propagated within a lineage, in a developing fetus or in the regenerating tissues of the adult. In the normal context, epigenetic mechanisms are likely to manifest developmental decisions by laying down cellular memories. For example, genome-wide remethylation of the genome during early postimplantation development accompanies the allocation of the three germ layers and the loss of totipotency of embryonic stem cell derivatives. There is a general consensus, therefore, that *de novo* CpG methylation stabilizes chromatin structures that result from developmental decisions (Kafri et al 1992).

Genomic imprinting is a form of epigenetic inheritance that distinguishes maternal and paternal alleles (Horsthemke et al 1999). Imprinting, and epigenetic alterations in general, are commonly studied in the context of gene silencing, but the intrinsic definition refers to the heritable modification itself. This modification may have consequences beyond gene expression changes, such as pairing of homologous chromosomes, or organization of chromatin (Pardo-Manuel de Villena et al 2000). The paradigm of genomic imprinting is represented by the *IGF2* (insulin-like growth factor 2) and the *H19* genes, which are expressed monoallelically from opposite parental alleles and are both members of the same cluster of imprinted loci at the distal part of chromosome 7 (Horsthemke et al 1999). The imprinted states of these two genes are coordinated at a 2 kb imprinting control region (ICR) in the 5′-flank of *H19* (Pant et al 2003), which is maintained paternally methylated and maternally unmethylated during development (Horsthemke et al 1999).

The unravelling of the molecular function of the *H19* ICR depended on several key observations. First, the insertion of a second endodermal-specific *H19* enhancer (Leighton et al 1995a) in the intergenic region between *Igf2* and *H19* overrides the maternal-specific repression of *Igf2* (Webber et al 1998). Second, the *H19* 5′-flanking sequence containing the ICR has chromatin insulator functions, i.e. it blocks enhancer-promoter communications in a position-dependent manner (Bell et al 2001, Ohlsson et al 2001). Third, the chromatin conformation of the *H19* ICR displays several unusual features, including multiple nuclease hypersensitive sites that map specifically at linker regions flanked by positioned nucleosomes in the maternally inherited allele (Kanduri et al 2000a). The most prominent hypersensitive sites map to a 21 bp element which is repeated several times in both mouse *H19* ICR and in the human counterpart (Kanduri et al 2000a). When comparing the 21 bp repeat elements with the functional *cis* elements of the β-globin chromatin insulator which interacts with a factor, CTCF (Bell et al 1999), we and others observed strong sequence similarity (Bell & Felsenfeld 2000, Hark et al 2000, Kanduri et al 2000b).

The CTCF — imprinting connection

The *in vivo* link between chromatin insulators and imprinting was first determined by chromatin immunopurification analyses revealing that CTCF interacts with only the maternal allele of the *H19* ICR (Kanduri et al 2000b). DNase I footprinting analyses revealed that CTCF interacts with the entire linker regions (Kanduri et al 2000b), which have the 21 bp repeat element strategically positioned in the middle between positioned nucleosomes (Kanduri et al 2000a). This arrangement is vital to make CTCF target sites constitutively available, since insertional mutagenesis to shift nucleosome positioning resulted in loss of CTCF binding and chromatin insulator function (Kanduri et al 2002). The functional link between CTCF and the *H19* chromatin insulator was further determined in several independent approaches. Initially, we inserted mutated versions—by point-mutating the G residues within each of the 21 bp repeats that were demonstrated to represent contact points for CTCF (Kanduri et al 2000b)—into the episomal insulator vector, pREP*H19*. Our results show that these GTGG→ATAT mutations completely abolished not only CTCF binding, but also the insulator function (Kanduri et al 2000b). Moreover, the observation that the interaction between CTCF and the *H19* ICR is methylation-sensitive (Kanduri et al 2000b) is paralleled by the demonstration that the chromatin insulator function is methylation-sensitive (Holmgren et al 2001). Finally, the targeted mutations of three of the four CTCF target sites at the endogenous *H19* ICR locus led not only to complete loss of CTCF binding *in vivo*, but also to loss of imprinting and methylation protection when maternally inherited (Pant et al 2003). These data prove that CTCF has a dual role in both interpreting and maintaining the epigenetic status of the *H19* chromatin insulator domain.

H19 function

While the function of IGF-2 as a growth factor has been firmly established in numerous reports (see elsewhere in this volume), the function of the *H19* gene remains enigmatic. For example, the *H19* transcript does not display an open reading frame common between mouse and human prompting suggestions that the cytoplasmic *H19* transcript does not display any function. It is surprising, therefore, that the *H19* transcript co-sediments with polysomes in a variety of cell types in both mouse and man (Li et al 1998). A possible *trans* function of the *H19* gene is suggested by a reciprocal correlation in *trans* between cytoplasmic *H19* and *IGF2* mRNA levels (Li et al 1998). Specifically, in a patient suffering from the Beckwith–Wiedemann syndrome (BWS) and who displayed mosaic deletions of the maternal *H19* allele, the *H19* expression inversely correlated with cytoplasmic *IGF2* mRNA levels (Fig. 1). Moreover, there exists an inverse relationship between cytoplasmic levels of *H19* transcripts and apparent polysome association of *IGF2* mRNAs in a Wilms' tumour (Li et al 1998).

This conclusion was rendered possible by the strategy outlined in Fig. 2, where the parental alleles (A and B) are distinguishable by a sequence polymorphism. The generally silent *IGF2* allele B (discriminated by an *Apa* I polymorphism in exon 9) was only expressed in *H19*-negative cells marked by a green dot as determined by allele-specific *in situ* hybridization (see below), whereas the majority of the tumour cells expressed only the normally active allele A in *H19*-positive cells (Fig 2A,B). If *H19* expression modifies the translatability of *IGF2* mRNAs, we would predict that the overall sedimentation properties of transcripts derived from alleles A and

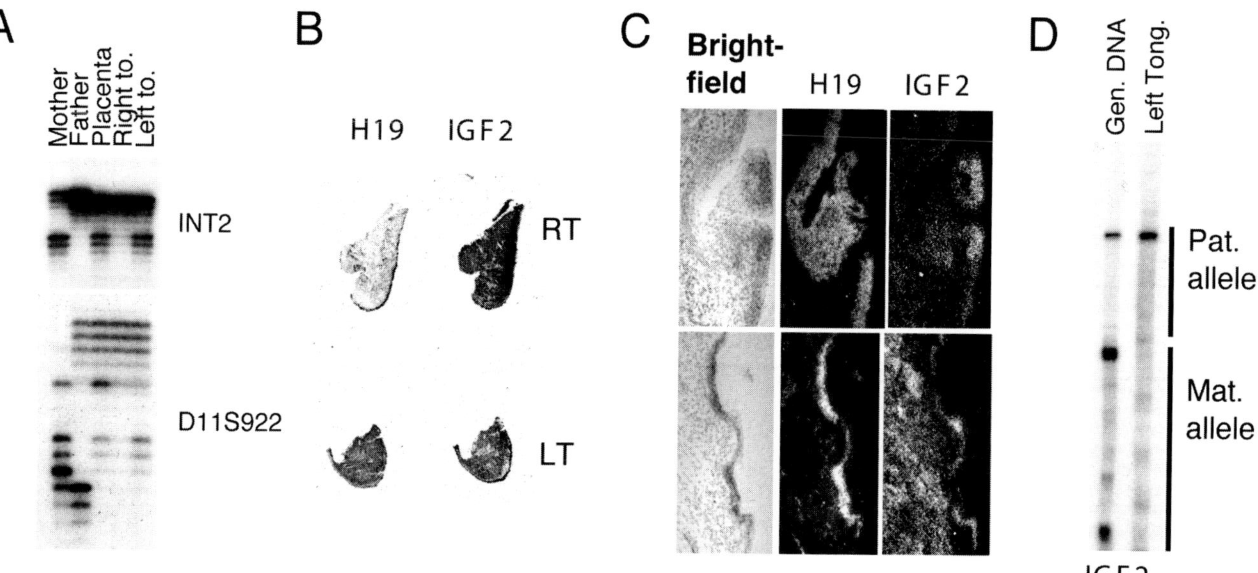

FIG. 1. Inverse correlation between *IGF2* and *H19* gene expression in a BWS patient displaying hemohypertrophy. (A) PCR analysis shows that the maternal alleles for D11S922 and INT2 markers for chromosome 11 are deleted specifically in the right-hand tongue specimen of a BWS patient. (B) *In situ* hybridization shows that *H19* expression is much reduced in the right-hand tongue compared to the left-hand tongue. (C) shows the spatial patterns of *IGF2* and *H19* expression in adjacent sections of right-hand tongue of the BWS patient. (D) RNase protection analysis (Ohlsson et al 1993) to show that *IGF2* is expressed from only the paternally derived allele of *IGF2* in the left-hand tongue (left). Reproduced with permission from Feinberg et al 2002.

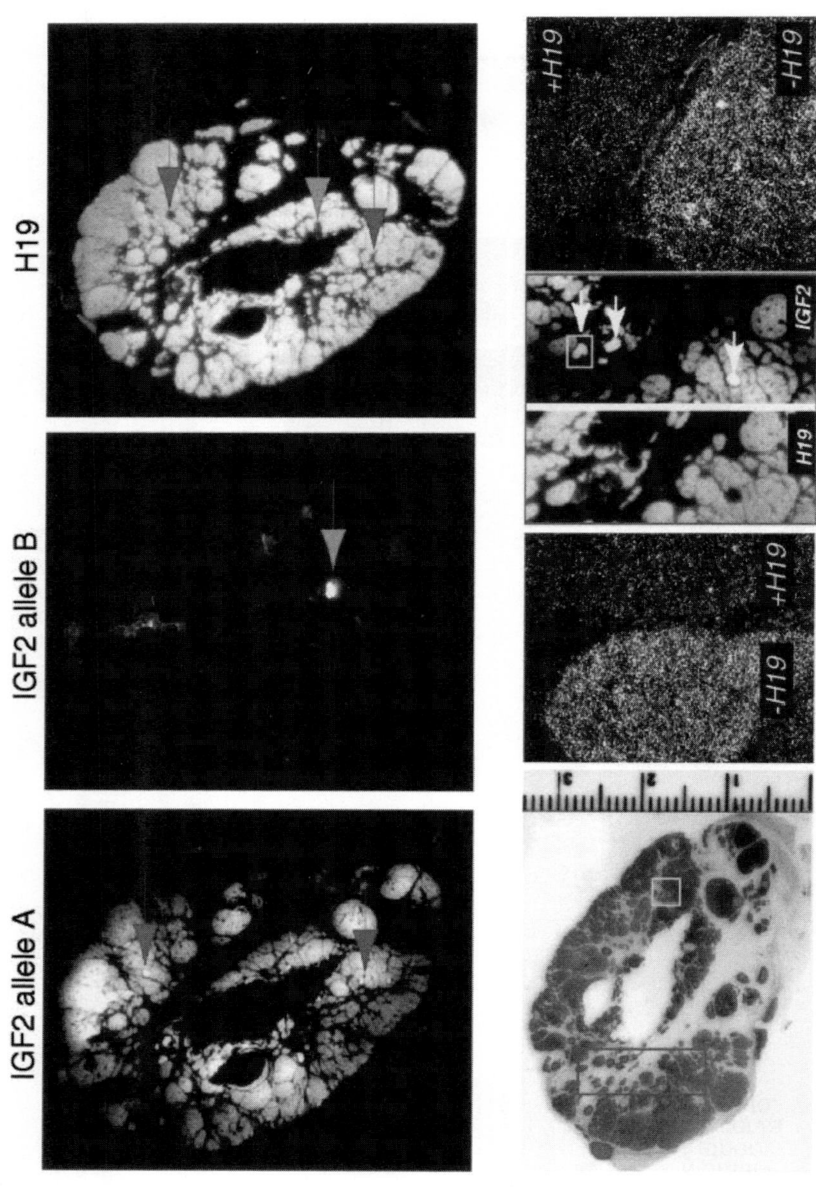
A
IGF2 allele A
IGF2 allele B
H19
-H19
+H19
H19
IGF2
+H19
-H19

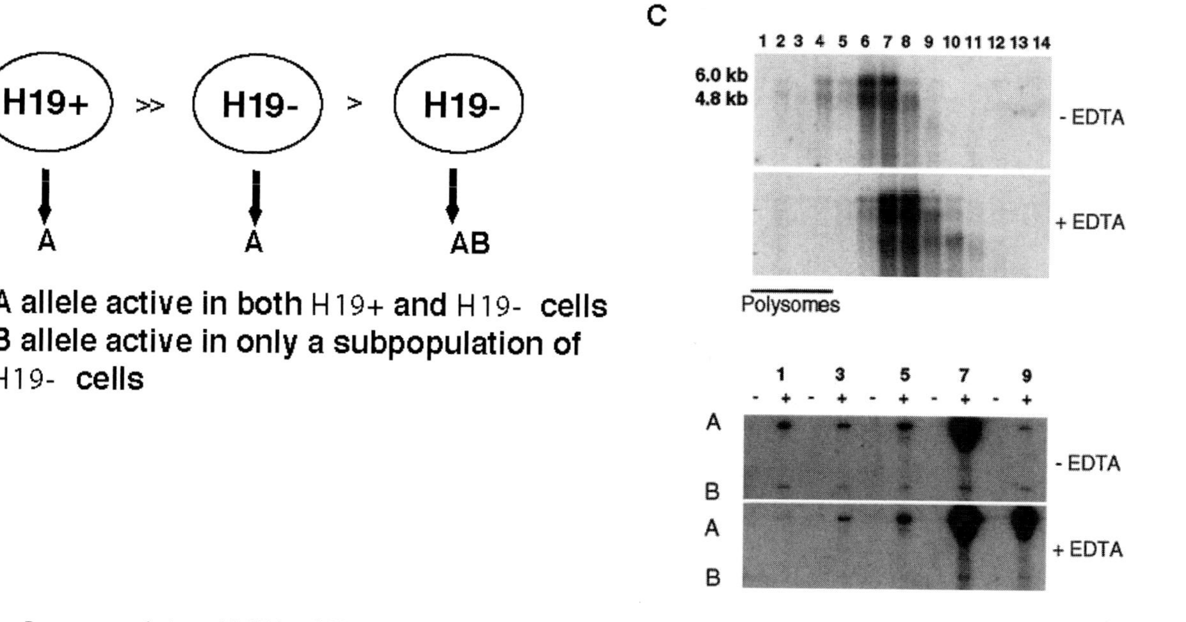

FIG. 2. Inverse correlation of *IGF2* and *H19* transcripts in a Wilms' tumour as analysed by *in situ* hybridization. (A) The upper three panels provide an overview of cells which lack *H19* expression but express *IGF2* monoallelically and cells which lack *H19* expression and express *IGF2* biallelically, as determined by allele-specific *in situ* hybridization. The lower five panels show an overview and close-up of the boxed area to demonstrate that a *H19*-negative focus expresses higher levels of *IGF2* transcripts than a neighbouring, *H19*-positive focus and to demonstrate that *H19* expression inversely correlates with *IGF2* expression. (B) The rationale for examining the effect of *H19* expression on the association of *IGF2* RNA with polysomes in the Wilms' tumour. (C) Parent of origin-dependent sedimentation properties of Wilms' tumour-derived *IGF2* mRNAs in sucrose gradients. The upper panel shows Northern blot analysis of *IGF2* mRNA species extracted from every second fraction, while the lower panel shows selected fractions of the sucrose gradient that were subjected to RT-PCR analysis to examine allelic origin of *IGF2* transcripts. A and B denote the *Apa* I non-cutting and cutting alleles, respectively. −RT and +RT denote minus and plus reverse transcriptase, respectively. Reproduced with permission from Li et al 1998.

B, respectively, would differ in a sucrose gradient analysis (Fig. 2C). Figure 2D shows that the various *IGF2* mRNAs appeared to be poorly translated in this Wilms' tumor, as examined by Northern blot hybridization analysis of the sucrose gradient fractions. We next examined whether or not the presence or absence of *H19* transcripts correlated with the sedimentation properties of *IGF2* transcripts, as outlined above. Figure 2D shows that the *IGF2* transcripts derived from the allele A, which is predominantly expressed in *H19*-positive cells, is poorly translated, while *IGF2* transcripts derived from the allele B (exclusively expressed in *H19*-negative cells) sediment generally as larger complexes. Hence, the translatibility of *IGF2* mRNA is inversely correlated with *H19* expression.

H19 and regulation of *IGF2* expression in *trans* — a model

These observations provide yet another glimpse into the complex regulation of the function of *IGF2*. This involves multiple steps of controls from gene dosage, differential promoter usage, splicing patterns, translational control(s) to post-secretory attenuation of *IGF2* function by IGF-binding proteins (Ohlsson et al 2001). Whereas some of the cytoplasmic and extracellular levels of control appear to be uncoordinated with *IGF2* activity, the expression of *H19* and hence the antagonistic function of *H19* in *trans*, is expected to be coordinated (Ohlsson et al 1994). This allows us to formulate a model in which *H19* serves to prevent overshoot of *IGF2* expression in *trans*. In this model, an increase in *H19* expression would accompany an increase in *IGF2* expression since their expression patterns are coordinated (Ohlsson et al 1994, Leighton et al 1995b) (Fig. 3). This coordination would be of particular importance in cases where the high levels of *IGF2* expression could be expected to saturate the uncoordinated types of negative cytoplasmic and/or extracellular controls, such as IGF-binding proteins. In practice, this would mean that the higher levels of *IGF2* expression, the more important the *H19* regulatory pathway would become. According to this model, a loss of the *H19* function in *trans* would be expected to be a key event in cells expressing high levels of *IGF2* mRNAs to subsequently and significantly increase production of free IGF-2 ligands. Our model would highlight the consequences of losing the *H19* function in *trans* when *IGF2* is overexpressed either from one or both parental alleles. In this regard, loss of *H19* expression is an early event to potentially predispose for Wilms' tumours (Cui et al 1997a).

Cancer and loss of imprinting

Loss of imprinting (LOI) is defined as a parental origin-specific epigenetic modification that is disrupted, and can include gain or loss of methylation or

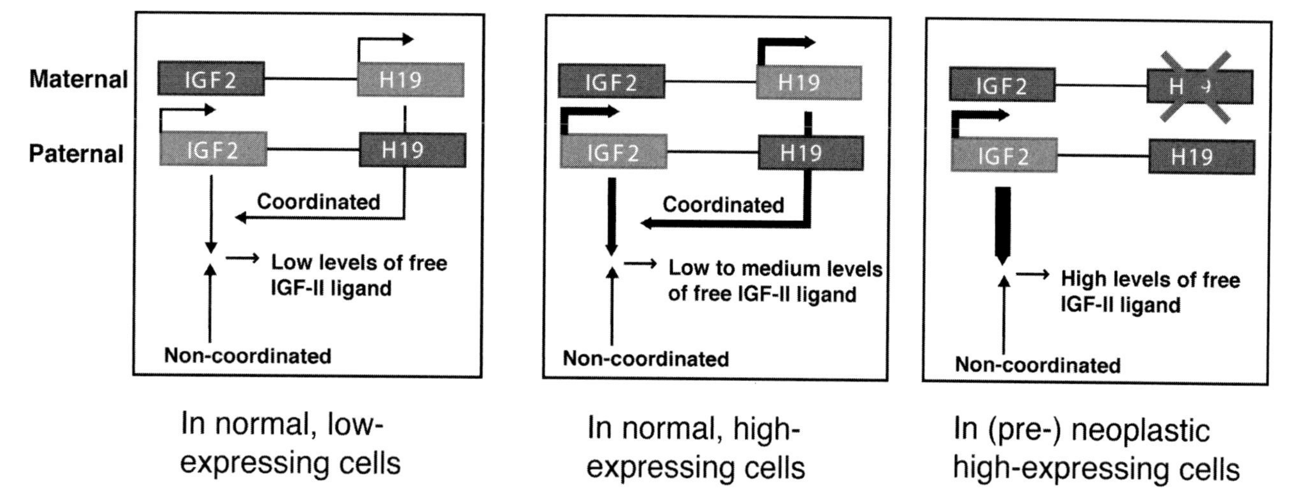

FIG. 3. A model of the postulated *H19*-specific control loop. Whereas the *H19*-specific control would be coordinated with *IGF2* activity, other levels of controls, represented by IGF-binding proteins, for example, may be uncoordinated. In the event of abnormal activity of *IGF2*, and therefore of *H19*, the uncoordinated controls would become saturated. In this scenario, the coordinated *H19* control would gain importance in direct proportion to the inability of the uncoordinated controls to deal with abnormal levels of *IGF2* activity (see also Fig.1). Reproduced with permission from Li et al 1998.

other chromosomal marks, or loss of the normal pattern of parental origin-specific gene expression (Feinberg et al 2002). *IGF2* LOI was first discovered in Wilms' tumour (Rainier et al 1993, Ogawa et al 1993), an embryonal kidney cancer, and it is the most common molecular alteration in these tumours, occurring in 50–70% of tumours, compared to mutations in the *WT1* gene, which occur in only 5% of tumours. These observations were first extended to other embryonal tumours of childhood, including hepatoblastoma and rhabdomyosarcoma (Rainier et al 1995, Li et al 1995, Zhan et al 1995). LOI was then also found commonly in most adult solid tumours (Douc-Rasy et al 1996, Hibi et al 1996, Hashimoto et al 1995).

Interestingly, Cui et al (1998) found that about one-third of colorectal cancers undergo LOI, and that LOI is also found in the matched normal colon of the same patients. In order to prove that LOI was not simply a developmental alteration unrelated to cancer *per se*, these authors analysed the normal colon of patients without colorectal cancer, and found that the frequency of LOI was threefold greater in cancer patients (Cui et al 1998). Moreover, LOI was a constitutional abnormality also present in lymphocytes of many of these individuals (Cui et al 1998). The perception that this might lead to a simple blood test for cancer risk was recently borne out by the demonstration that diagnosis of *IGF2* LOI in leukocytes might provide a predictive marker for colorectal cancer (Cui et al 2003). Although these results suggest that epigenetic lesions in normal tissue set the stage for neoplasia, we cannot exclude the possibility that *IGF2* LOI is diagnostic of a more general epigenetic disruption in the 'normal' colon of the affected patients.

This issue is compounded by the fact that while methylation patterns are very stable in the normal context, it is becoming increasingly clear that methylation disturbance in neoplasia involves not only a range of novel target sequences, but also a loss of the fidelity of the epigenetic states. In the absence of a selective force, therefore, the methylation pattern may become mosaic to generate variegated expression patterns. On this note, allelic *IGF2* expression patterns are mosaic during Wilms' tumorigenesis, as determined by allele-specific (Fig. 4) (Ohlsson et al 1999a). Specifically, The *IGF2* LOI appeared stochastically in both premalignant and malignant cells suggesting that its appearance cannot be linked with a specific stage during Wilms' tumorigenesis (Ohlsson et al 1999a). This observation is not without precedence since the *IGF2* and *H19* genes are randomly (in)activated in complete hydatidiform moles, which are bipaternally derived, as documented by the ASISH approach (Ohlsson et al 1999b). In addition, there are hypervariable and uncoupled allelic expression patterns of the *IGF2* and *H19* genes in a human tumour cell line (Cui et al 1997b). It is conceivable, therefore, that the coordination of allelic expression status of clustered genes, such as *IGF2* and *H19*, is lost upon pathological neutralization of parental imprints.

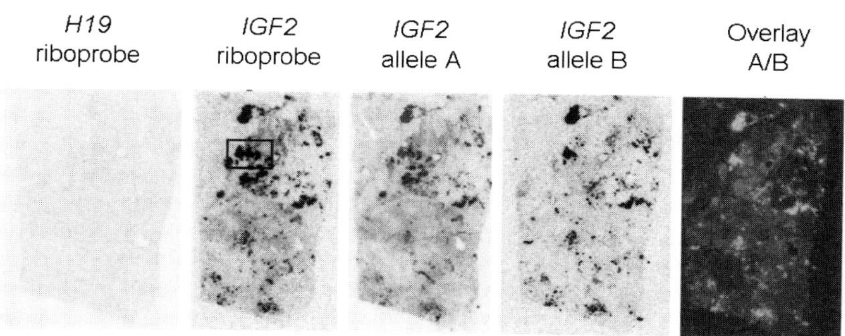

FIG. 4. *IGF2* allele usage in a Wilms' tumour relapse as resolved by autoradiographic images of allelic expression patterns of *IGF2*. *Right*, a computer-coloured overlay (not visible in this grey-scale reproduction) to illustrate the variable allelic expression patterns of *IGF2* in this Wilms' tumour. The various shades depict monoallelic A, B, and biallelic expression (magnification, 1.3-fold). Reproduced with permission from Ohlsson et al 1999a.

Such a heterogenous epigenetic state has been postulated to pave the way for selection mechanisms that lead to biallelically active growth-promoting genes and inactivate imprinted tumour suppressor genes, respectively (Ohlsson et al 1998). This model is outlined in some detail in Fig. 5. Random monoallelic expression in epigenetically unstable (pre)neoplastic cells sets the stage for selection in these tumours. If a tumour suppressor gene is relevant to that particular tumour type, then cell populations with both alleles inactive would be selected for. Conversely, if a randomly activated gene encodes a growth-promoting activity, cell populations with both alleles active will have a selective growth advantage.

In the case of *IGF2*, there is ample evidence that overexpression is a selectable marker in overgrowth and neoplasia. For example, point mutation of the maternal *H19* ICR allele to destroy the CTCF target sites leads to biallelic expression in a wide range of tissues from neonatal offspring that were 17% larger than control offspring (Pant et al 2003). BWS patients with either loss of *IGF2* imprinting or uniparental disomy display organomegaly (Hedborg et al 1994), in all likelihood due to IGF II overdosage (Sun et al 1997). Moreover, the range of organs displaying organomegaly in BWS patients is very similar to the range of organs expressing *IGF2* at high levels during prenatal development. Finally, BWS patients displaying hemihypertrophy which can lead to higher levels of *IGF2* expression on one of the body halves (see Fig. 1), is strongly linked with increased risk for cancer (Green et al 1993).

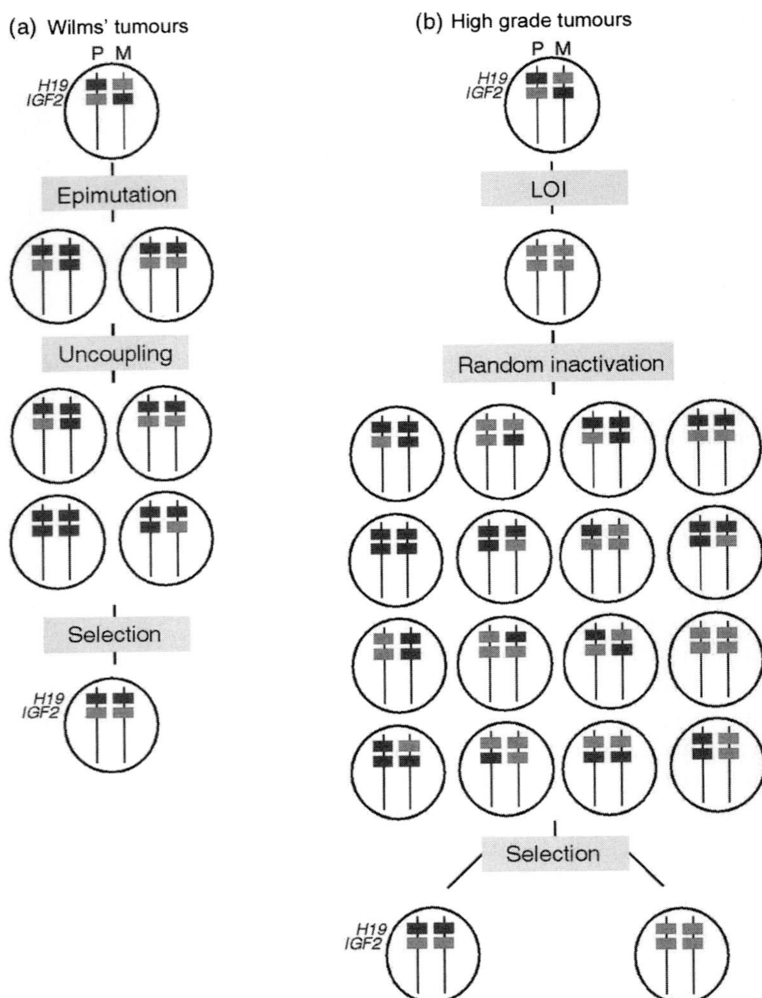

FIG. 5. Model to explain LOI and selection of biparental repression/activation of the *H19* and *IGF2* genes, respectively, during the initiation of Wilms' tumorigenesis (a) or the progression of high grade tumours (b). Epimutation is an early event in preneoplastic kidney development that results in biallelic methylation and silencing of *H19*. LOI refers to erasure of the imprint of the *IGF2*/*H19* region to generate biallelic hypomethylation in *H19*, which might occur in an epigenetically unstable tumour cell. The final outcome of the allelic gene expression patterns depends on biological selection factors specific to each tumour type. The active alleles are in light grey and the silent alleles are in dark grey. P and M depict paternal and maternal alleles, respectively. The data are consistent with an innate tendency of these two imprinted loci to engage in random monoallelic expression when released from the constraints of the parental imprint. Reproduced with permission from Ohlsson et al 1998.

Mechanisms of loss of imprinting — an outlook

Given the fundamental role of the methylation-sensitive insulator segment in maintaining the repressed status of the maternal *IGF2* allele, it is not surprising that biallelic *IGF2* expression is frequently associated with biallelic methylation of the *H19* ICR. While this explanation is straightforward, it does not address the underlying reason for the epigenetic lesion. Even though our ignorance of the involved mechanisms is substantial, we can discern several, not mutually exclusive possibilities. First, the possibility that the ICR-CTCF association is a postreplicative phenomenon suggests that inappropriate expression of the methylation machinery during a window of the S phase (Kanduri et al 2002) could facilitate *de novo* methylation. Second, although rare mutations of CTCF zinc fingers have been demonstrated to lead to selective loss of binding capacity to the *H19* ICR (Fillippova et al 2002), in the absence of the protective features of CTCF, *de novo* methylation of the maternal allele ensues. Third, CTCF might be removed by the product of a second *CTCF* gene, termed *BORIS* (Loukinov et al 2002). While this gene is normally expressed only in male germline cells undergoing epigenetic reprogramming (Loukinov et al 2002), inappropriate expression in somatic cells might lead to epigenetic lesions at a wide range of CTCF target sites, including the *H19* ICR. These and a number of additional events might collaborate in different combinations to break down the methylation privilege character of the *H19* ICR.

Acknowledgements

This overview is based in part on the work by numerous present and past members of my lab during several years. I would like to express my sincere gratitude to in particular Drs Gail Adam, Hengmi Cui, Gary Franklin, Chandra Kanduri, Yi-Ming Li and Vinod Pant. I would also like to acknowledge that parts of the ideas presented here stem from many discussions with Drs Ben Tycko, Carmen Sapienza, Andy Feinberg and Victor Lobanenkov. This work has been supported by Swedish Science Research Council, the Swedish Cancer Research Foundation, The Swedish Pediatric Cancer Research Foundation, the Lundberg Foundation and the Wallenberg Foundation.

References

Bell AC, Felsenfeld G 2000 Methylation of a CTCF-dependent boundary controls imprinted expression of the *Igf2* gene. Nature 405:482–485

Bell A, West A, Felsenfeld G 1999 The protein CTCF is required for the enhancer blocking activity of vertebrate insulators. Cell 98:387–396

Bell AC, West AG, Felsenfeld G 2001 Insulators and boundaries: versatile regulatory elements in the eukaryotic genome. Science 291:447–450

Cui H, Hedborg F, He L et al 1997a Inactivation of *H19*, an imprinted and putative tumor repressor gene, is a preneoplastic event during Wilms' tumorigenesis. Cancer Res 57:4469–4473

Cui H, He L, Walsh C, Anneren G, Pfeifer-Ohlsson S, Ohlsson R 1997b Hypervariable allelic expression patterns of *IGF2* in tumor cells. Oncogene 16:113–120

Cui H, Horon IL, Ohlsson R, Hamilton SR, Feinberg AP 1998 Loss of imprinting in normal tissue of colorectal cancer patients with microsatellite instability. Nat Med 4: 1276–1280

Cui H, Cruz-Correa M, Giardiello F et al 2003 Loss of *IGF2* imprinting: a potential marker of colorectal cancer risk. Science 299:1753–1755

Douc-Rasy S, Barrois M, Fogel S et al 1996 High incidence of loss of heterozygosity and abnormal imprinting of *H19* and *IGF2* genes in invasive cervical carcinomas. Uncoupling of *H19* and *IGF2* expression and biallelic hypomethylation of H19. Oncogene 12:423–430

Feinberg A, Cui H, Ohlsson R 2002 DNA methylation and genomic imprinting: Insights from cancer into epigenetic mechanisms. Sem Cancer Biol 12:389–398

Fillippova G, Qi C, Ulmer J et al 2002 Tumor-associated zing finger mutations in the CTCF transcription factor selectively alter its DNA-binding specificity. Cancer Res 62:48–52

Green D, Breslow N, Beckwith J, Norkool P 1993 Screening of children with hemihypertrophy. aniridia, and Beckwith-Wiedemann syndrome in patients with Wilms' tumor: a report from the National Wilms' Tumor Study. Med Pediat Oncol 21:188–192

Hark AT, Schoenherr CJ, Katz DJ et al 2000 CTCF mediates methylation-sensitive enhancer-blocking activity at the *H19/Igf2* locus. Nature 405:486–489

Hashimoto K, Azuma C, Koyama M et al 1995 Loss of imprinting in choriocarcinoma. Nat Genet 9:109–110

Hedborg F, Holmgren L, Sandstedt B, Ohlsson R 1994 The cell type-specific *IGF2* expression during early human development correlates to the pattern of overgrowth and neoplasia in the Beckwith-Wiedemann syndrome. Am J Path 145:802–817

Hibi K, Nakamura H, Hirai A et al 1996 Loss of *H19* imprinting in esophageal cancer. Cancer Res 56:480–482

Holmgren C, Kanduri K, Dell G et al 2001 CpG methylation regulates the *Igf2/H19* insulator. Curr Biol 11:1128–1130

Horsthemke B, Surani MA, James TC, Ohlsson R 1999 The mechanisms of genomic imprinting. In: Ohlsson R (ed) Genomic imprinting: an interdisciplinary approach. Springer-Verlag, Berlin, Heidelberg, NewYork, p 91–118

Kafri T, Ariel M, Brandeis M et al 1992 Developmental pattern of gene-specific DNA methylation in the mouse embryo and germ line. Genes Dev 6:705–714

Kanduri C, Holmgren C, Franklin G et al 2000a The 5′-flank of the murine *H19* gene in an unusual chromatin conformation unidirectionally blocks enhancer-promoter communication. Curr Biol 10:449–457

Kanduri C, Pant V, Loukinov D et al 2000b Functional interaction of CTCF with the insulator upstream of the *H19* gene is parent of origin-specific and methylation-sensitive. Curr Biol 10:853–856

Kanduri M, Kanduri C, Mariano P et al 2002 Multiple nucleosome positioning sites regulate the CTCF-mediated insulator function of the *H19* imprinting control region. Mol Cell Biol 22:3339–3344

Leighton PA, Saam JR, Ingram RS, Stewart CL, Tilghman SM 1995a An enhancer deletion affects both H19 and Igf2 expression. Genes Dev 9:2079–2089

Leighton PA, Ingram RS, Eggenschwiler J, Efstratiadis A, Tilghman SM 1995b Disruption of imprinting caused by deletion of the H19 gene region in mice. Nature 375:34–39

Li X, Adam G, Cui H, Sandstedt B, Ohlsson R, Ekstrom TJ 1995 Expression, promoter usage and parental imprinting status of insulin-like growth factor II (*IGF2*) in human hepatoblastoma: uncoupling of *IGF2* and *H19* imprinting. Oncogene 11:221–229

Li Y-M, Franklin G, Cui HM et al 1998 The *H19* transcript is associated with polysomes and may regulate *IGF2* expression in *trans*. J Biol Chem 273:28247–28252

Loukinov D, Pugacheva E, Vatolin S et al 2002 BORIS, a novel male germline-specific protein associated with epigenetic reprogramming events, shares the same 11 Zn-finger domain with CTCF, the insulator protein involved in reading imprinting marks in the soma. Proc Natl Acad Sci USA 99:6806–6811

Ohlsson R 1999 Gemonic imprinting, an interdisciplinary approach. Springer, Berlin, Heidelberg-New York, p 1–330

Ogawa O, Eccles M, Szeto J et al 1993 Relaxation of insulin-like growth factor II gene imprinting implicated in Wilms' tumour. Nature 362:749–751

Ohlsson R, Nyström A, Pfeifer-Ohlsson S et al 1993 *IGF2* is parentally imprinted during human embryogenesis and in the Beckwith-Weidemann syndrome. Nat Genet 4:94–97

Ohlsson R, Hedborg F, Holmgren L, Walsh C, Ekström TJ 1994 Overlapping patterns of *IGF2* and *H19* expression during human development: biallelic *IGF2* expression correlates with a lack of *H19* expression. Development 120:361–368

Ohlsson R, Tycko B, Sapienza C 1998 Monoallelic expression: 'there can only be one'. Trends Genet 14:435–438

Ohlsson R, Cui H, He L et al 1999a Mosaic allelic *IGF2* expression patterns reveal a link between Wilms' tumorigenesis and epigenetic heterogeneity. Cancer Res 59:3889–3892

Ohlsson R, Cui H, Flam F et al 1999b Absence of discriminative parental imprints is linked with epigenetic mosaicism of the *IGF2* and *H19* genes. Dev Genes Evol 209:113–119

Ohlsson R, Renkawitz R, Lobanenkov V 2001 CTCF is a uniquely versatile transcription regulator linked to epigenetics and disease. Trends Genet 17:520–577

Pant V, Mariano P, Kanduri C et al 2003 The nucleotides responsible for the direct physical contact between the chromatin insulator protein CTCF and the *H19* imprinting control region manifest parent of origin-specific long-distance insulation and methylation-free domains. Genes Dev 17:586–590

Pardo-Manuel de Villena F, de la Casa-Esperon E, Sapienza C 2000 Natural selection and the function of genome imprinting: beyond the silenced minority. Trends Genet 16:573–579

Rainier S, Johnson L, Dobry C et al 1993 Relaxation of imprinted genes in human cancer. Nature 362:747–749

Rainier S, Dobry C, Feinberg A 1995 Loss of imprinting in hepatoblastoma. Cancer Res 55:1836–1838

Sun F, Dean W, Kelsey G, Allen N, Reik W 1997 Transactivation of *Igf2* in a mouse model of Beckwith-Wiedemann syndrome. Nature 389:809–815

Webber A, Ingram R, Levorse J, Tilghman S 1998 Location of enhancers is essential for the imprinting of *H19* and *Igf2* genes. Nature 391:711–715

Zhan S, Shapiro D, Helman L 1995 Loss of imprinting of *IGF2* in Ewing's sarcoma. Oncogene 11:2503–2507

DISCUSSION

LeRoith: In the old days we thought there was this negative regulation of *H19* just at the gene expression level, and everyone was asking what *H19* did, because it doesn't get translated. Do you know how it interferes with the translation of IGF-2?

Ohlsson: We don't know, but we can guess. We know that *H19* mRNA is associated with polysomes in a translation-dependent manner, despite the absence of a suitable open reading frame. We think it is sitting on the polysomes and stalling IGF-2 translation (Li et al 1998).

LeRoith: It must be something more specific than that.

Ohlsson: David Haig once showed me that there is an inverted repeat present in both the *IGF2* and *H19* loci, suggesting the formation of a duplex that could antagonize translation. Since then, other reports have shown there are three other genes might be similarly regulated by H19.

Thomas: If you do RNAi experiments and knock out *H19*, does this up-regulate *IGF2*?

Ohlsson: I don't think this has been done, because some important players in the field thought it had no function. I think that this experiment should be done, since IGF-2 expression is increased even if you knock out only the *H19* transcriptional unit.

Werner: Do you believe that relaxation of imprinting of the *IGF2* gene is the real cause or an innocent bystander of the neoplastic process? You mentioned that LOI of the *IGF-2* gene has been implicated in both overgrowth and cancer cases. What else will affect the net outcome? Why does LOI of the IGF-2 gene result 'only' in overgrowth in certain cases and full blown cancer in other cases?

Ohlsson: I can only give you my own impression, which is to a degree supported by published data. The loss of *IGF2* imprinting is by and large a predisposition phenomenon. We have looked at different types of tumours, including Wilms' tumours, and found a considerable degree of epigenetic heterogeneity. From this perspective, we have reasoned that *IGF2* LOI may have a reduced role to play in the tumorigenic process as such, but it may very well set the stage for cancer formation.

De Meyts: In the case of hemi hypertrophy where only one side of the body is overgrowing, is there some kind of chimeric status? Or is it possible that in one individual with a uniform genetic background that genetic regulation can change in different parts of the body?

Ohlsson: I would think that you need to start off with a trisomy to get that. Of course, the maternal chromosome 11, for example, could still be around, although I would expect that you select for cells deleting the maternal copy, because this expresses growth inhibitory functions that are repressed on the paternal copy. This, on the other hand, expresses growth-promoting functions which can be repressed on the maternal copy. The end-point effect is uniparental (paternal) isodisomy although the intervening steps would be expected to be mosaic within a given tissue with respect to the presence of the maternal chromosome.

Werner: Three papers were published last year that showed that children conceived by means of IVF showed an increased risk of developing Beckwith–Wiedemann syndrome (Gicquel et al 2003, DeBaun et al 2003, Gosden et al 2003). Taken together, these reports suggested that the imprinting process may be affected during the IVF procedure.

Ohlsson: This is a warning to everyone using cell lines. One of the hallmarks of epigenetic states is their stability in the living organism. Out of context, such as in *in vitro* cultures, the epigenetic states have a tendency to become destabilized. Oocytes in culture are no exception to this rule, which might definitively account for developmental problems of children conceived by IVF. Moreover, many of you used cultured cells to transfectants by scoring for an effect. If you are unlucky, such effects can depend on epigenetic heterogeneity present either in the parent cells or induced during the selection procedure. A partial remedy to this problem is to isolate many transfectants showing the same effect.

Laron: What happens in syndromes where you have overgrowth?

Ohlsson: I don't think the story is complete yet. To some degree this is linked with *GRB10*, which is also imprinted and is maternally expressed.

Laron: Do you have an increase in cancer?

Ohlsson: No. But is interesting with respect to this audience because *GRB10*, which is implicated in Silver–Russel syndrome has been considered to modulate IGF-1 receptor function. There could be a different physiological status of IGF-2 and IGF-1 in those patients.

Pollak: A recent *Science* paper (Cui et al 2003) recently made the point that LOI of *IGF2* in leukocytes is a strong predictor of risk of colon cancer. The part that confuses me about this finding relates to the tissue specificity. In other words, is there a particular relationship to the imprinting status in leukocytes and colon mucosa? This would be unexpected. If the relationship between LOI in leukocytes and colon is true, wouldn't you expect that the LOI status in the blood would be a general marker for epithelial cancer risk? This was not found.

Ohlsson: There are two explanations for these data. One is that there is systemic LOI, in which case it would have to be manifested early in the patient's life with problems similar to those of the Beckwith–Wiedemann syndrome. Another, more interesting possibility is that the tumour is able to re-programme neighbouring cells, changing the imprinting state of neighbouring tissue and infiltrating blood cells to potentially be recruited into the carcinogenic process. We know that most cancers are polyclonal, but we don't know why.

Pollak: By extension from the colon specificity, which is an interesting model without precedent, in principal a breast cancer could do the same to alter the imprinting status of leukocytes. In the *Science* paper, where we see a particular relationship between LOI of *IGF2* in leukocytes being related to risk of future colon cancer, even with the mechanism you propose this could apply to breast cancer or prostate cancer.

Ohlsson: One of the hallmarks of colon cancer is the hypomethylated genome. This is an important lesion, since DNA methylation normally stabilizes the other epigenetic marks. In other words, developmental cues can be stabilized by DNA methylation removing the need to sustain those cues. By erasure of methylation marks and with the relevant cues no longer around there is a clear danger that a whole range of genes might become aberrantly activated to contribute to the neoplastic process. In the absence of DNA methylation, many factors normally present in only pluripotent stem cells and aberrantly expressed in the colon cancer progenitor cells, might reprogram the genome to facilitate the selection of cells with unrestrained proliferation potential. With respect to the LOI of *IGF2* in the leukocytes, this could be just an innocent bystander and have no direct effect on the cancer process.

Holly: I was fascinated by the anecdote about the famine in northern Sweden with the speculation that the nutritional status is affecting the sperm, and the *IGF2* gene is outside the imprinting machinery. I was expecting you to go on and say that the grandchildren were predisposed to cancer but you said they were predisposed to diabetes. Do you think this is the insulin?

Ohlsson: Yes, it could be.

Holly: Was there any change in their predisposition to cancer?

Ohlsson: Not to my knowledge.

Kaaks: Does LOI in leukocytes mark a systemic LOI? Has anyone been looking at correspondence in LOI measures for the *IGF2* gene in colon and a completely different tissue?

Ohlsson: I don't have full coverage of the literature, but I recall that there are differences. In many cases LOI may not play a role. It could simply be a marker of a general epigenetic lesion involving IGF-2 as an innocent bystander.

References

Cui H, Cruz-Correa M, Giardiello FM et al 2003 Loss of IGF2 imprinting: a potential marker of colorectal cancer risk. Science 299:1753–1755

DeBaun MR, Niemitz EL, Feinberg AP 2003 Association of in vitro fertilization with Beckwith–Wiedemann syndrome and epigenetic alterations of LIT1 and H19. Am J Hum Genet 72:156–160

Gicquel C, Gaston V, Mandelbaum J, Siffroi JP, Flahault A, Le Bouc Y 2003 In vitro fertilization may increase the risk of Beckwith-Wiedemann syndrome related to the abnormal imprinting of the KCN1OT gene. Am J Hum Genet 72:1338–1341

Gosden R, Trasler J, Lucifero D, Faddy M 2003 Rare congenital disorders, imprinted genes, and assisted reproductive technology. Lancet 361:1975–1977

Li Y-M, Franklin GC, Cui H et al 1998 The H19 transcript is associated to polysomes and may regulate IGF2 expression in trans. J Biol Chem 273:28247–28252

Insulin and IGF-1 receptor trafficking and signalling

Michelangelo Foti, Moulay Ahmed Moukil, Pierrick Dudognon and Jean-Louis Carpentier[1]

Department of Cell Physiology and Metabolism, Faculty of Medicine, University of Geneva, Geneva, Switzerland

Abstract. Receptor-mediated endocytosis governs the entry of receptors inside the cells. In the case of signalling receptors, e.g. tyrosine kinase receptors, the process is ligand-dependent and includes a series of surface events which determines the specificity of the internalization process and the activation of distinct signal transduction pathways. Tyrosine kinase receptors, e.g. the insulin/IGF-1 receptors, are initially located outside the internalization gates (the clathrin-coated pits) and concentrated on thin digitations of the cell surface: the microvilli. In the case of the insulin receptor, specific motifs of the β subunit are responsible for anchoring the receptor to microvilli. However, the molecular mechanisms by which this motif mediates this anchoring are poorly understood and necessitate further studies. In particular, the association of insulin receptors with cytoskeletal elements or specific lipidic domains concentrated on microvilli (e.g. lipid rafts) are under investigation as these interactions may provide the appropriate environment for the transduction of the insulin metabolic effects. Upon ligand binding, activated insulin receptors complexed to insulin are released from microvilli, segregate in clathrin-coated pits and enter the cells. In endosomes, insulin is uncoupled from its receptor and recycles back to the cell surface, whereas the hormone is degraded in lysosomes thus terminating the wave of signalling. These steps participate in the biological activity of the hormone via: (1) a regulation of cell sensitivity to the hormone through a fine tuning of the number of surface receptors; (2) termination of the signalling by intracellular degradation of the ligands; and (3) giving the receptors access to plasma membrane domains and intracellular compartments from which distinct signalling pathways originate. Current studies are designed to compare the behaviour of IGF-1 receptors to that of insulin receptors to establish whether different localization on the plasma membrane, trafficking pathways and/or kinetics of signalling might explain the different biological activities of these two receptors.

2004 Biology of IGF-1: its interaction with insulin in health and malignant states. Wiley, Chichester (Novartis Foundation Symposium 262) p 125–147

[1]This paper was presented at the symposium by Jean-Louis Carpentier, to whom correspondence should be addressed.

Insulin and insulin-like growth factor 1 (IGF-1) are closely related polypeptides. While the first one is secreted uniquely by the β-cells of islets of Langerhans, the second one is widely expressed, although the majority of circulating IGF-1 derives from the liver. The two hormones produce their biological effects by binding to the insulin receptor (IR) and the IGF-1 receptor (IGF-1R), two transmembrane receptors belonging to the large family of growth factor receptors with intrinsic tyrosine kinase activity.

Upon ligand binding, insulin/IGF-1 receptors undergo a conformational change, which enables them to bind ATP and be autophosphorylated (Hubbard 1997, Wei et al 1995). Autophosphorylation increases the kinase activity of the receptors, enabling them to phosphorylate a variety of intracellular substrates which initiate signalling cascades, leading to the activation of multiple downstream effectors and resulting ultimately in distinct biological actions. These actions are pleiotropic and commonly divided into two distinct categories: mitogenic and metabolic responses. The IR and IGF-1R share redundant functions in cell growth, differentiation and metabolism but they show also predominant physiological roles: IR activation leads primarily to metabolic effects whereas activation of IGF-1R results in stimulation of mitogenic pathways. Since, insulin and IGF-1 receptor structures share considerable homologies and are activating many common intracellular pathways, the question of the specificity of their terminal biological effect is the subject of intense investigation. Several hypotheses have been raised to explain these different specificities such as the ligand affinities which might modulate the strength and duration of the signals, differential tissue distribution of the two receptors, different ability to activate distinct intracellular pathways and distinct spatial/temporal compartmentalization of signalling. In this review, we will briefly summarize the major advances outlining the importance of insulin/IGF-1 and their cognate receptors trafficking from the plasma membrane to intracellular compartments as a means to control the specificity of signalling generated by the IR and IGF-1R.

Insulin/IGF-1 receptor trafficking

Insulin/IGF-1 receptors, like most signalling tyrosine kinase receptors, are internalized via receptor-mediated endocytosis through the classical clathrin-coated pit (CCP) endocytic gates (Goldstein et al 1985). In contrast to transport protein receptors, e.g. LDL and transferrin receptors, tyrosine kinase signalling receptors are not trapped in CCPs unless they have bound their ligand (Brown et al 1983, Carpentier 1994). They exhibit ligand occupancy-induced endocytosis which frequently requires the stimulation of the intrinsic tyrosine kinase (Carpentier 1993, 1994, Carpentier et al 1992, 1993, Welsh et al 1994, Wiley et al 1991). This activation triggers the translocation of the receptors from surface domains where they are maintained in an unoccupied state towards surface areas where CCPs are present (Carpentier & McClain 1995, Carpentier et al 1992, 1993, Hamer et al 1997).

Localization of unstimulated insulin/IGF-1 receptors

Unstimulated IR preferentially associates with thin digitations of the cell surface called microvilli. The cytoplasmic domain of the receptor is required for this anchoring and in particular the kinase domain is crucial for IR localization to microvilli (Carpentier & McClain 1995, Hamer et al 1997). Serial mutational studies of the IR led to the conclusions that sequences mediating anchoring of the IR to microvilli were contained within exon 17. In particular, a dileucine motif ($LL^{986/987}$) and a sequence of 12 amino acids (extending from position 1001 to position 1012) encompassing a diisoleucine motif ($II^{1006/1007}$) play a pivotal role in this anchoring function (Carpentier & McClain 1995, Hamer et al 1997, Shackleton et al 2002) (see Fig. 1). The integrity of other domains within the IR is also required for a correct microvillar localization as evidenced by mutations in the transmembrane domain of the IR which affect its localization on microvilli (probably indirectly via a conformational change of the molecule) (Hamer et al 2002). Similarly to the IRs, IGF-1Rs are also localized on microvilli in their free conformation, but determinants required to anchor these receptors to microvilli have not been investigated (Zapf et al 1994).

The receptor localization on microvilli might reflect and be dependent on their tight coupling to the cytoskeleton. Indeed, microvilli are actin-filled extensions enriched in a panel of actin-associated cytoskeletal proteins (Condeelis 1993, Louvard 1989). In this regard, cytoskeletal proteins such as talin and α-actinin have been proposed to participate in the microvillar localization of a series of adhesion molecules, but this function has recently been questioned (Abitorabi et al 1997, Moore et al 1995, Pavalko et al 1995, Picker et al 1991). Other candidates are the members of the ERM (ezrin–moesin–radixin) family (Tsukita & Yonemura 1997). Unfortunately, except for the EGF receptor which has been shown to bind actin (den Hartigh et al 1992, van Bergen en Henegouwen et al 1992), little information is available on the cytoskeletal potential partner involved in IR/IGF-1R localization on microvilli.

In cell types displaying almost no microvilli, such as mature adipocytes, localization of IRs and IGF-1Rs is still a controversial issue. In particular, it remains to be established whether these receptors are concentrated in caveolae. Caveolae are 50–100 nm flask-shaped invaginations of the plasma membrane enriched in cholesterol and sphingolipids which are distinct from CCPs since they possess a characteristic striated coat consisting of oligomerized caveolin proteins (Anderson 1998). These structures are found in the plasma membrane of many cell types, but are particularly abundant in adipocytes where they increase in number during the course of fibroblast differentiation to mature adipocytes (Fan et al 1983a, Kandror et al 1995, Scherer et al 1994). Recent studies have suggested through both qualitative morphological and/or biochemical analyses an association of insulin and IGF-1 receptors with caveolae in adipocytes (Gustavsson et al 1999, Huo et al 2003), but these results have been challenged by others who failed to find any preferential association, at least for the IR, with purified caveolae (Mastick et al 1995, Souto et al 2003). Independently of the initial localization of these receptors, it still remains that following ligand binding, internalization occurs through clathrin-coated pits (Fan et al 1983b), although the fact that caveolae may function both as signal transduction platforms and endocytic units (Anderson 1998, Gilbert et al 1999, Hooper 1999, Kurzchalia & Parton 1999). Interestingly, studies with another tyrosine kinase receptor, i.e. the EGF-R, have led to the hypothesis that tyrosine kinase signalling receptors may associate with caveolae for signalling, then exit these structures, and migrate in the bulk plasma membrane until they are finally captured by CCPs (Mineo et al 1999).

Insulin/IGF-1 receptor internalization

Receptor activation mediates the release of the brake maintaining unoccupied IRs on microvilli by a mechanism which remains poorly understood. Up to now, the only indications are that the intrinsic kinase activation is not sufficient since specific mutations in the IR prevent the insulin-induced receptor shift from microvilli in spite of a normal autophosphorylation of the receptor (Hamer et al 2002).

On reaching the non-villous domain of the cell surface, IRs segregate into clathrin-coated pits, via two types of motifs present in the juxtamembrane region of its cytoplasmic tail. The first motifs are the tyrosine-based motifs, $NPEY^{953}$ and $GPLY^{960}$, which are exposed following ligand-induced receptor activation (Backer et al 1990, 1992, Rajagopalan et al 1991) and bind to the $\mu 2$ subunit of the adaptor protein, AP2, present in CCPs (Ohno et al 1995). The second motif is a dileucine sequence ($LL^{986-987}$), which does not require activation of the receptor to enable association with CCPs and may also associate with AP2 molecules (Haft

FIG. 1. Structural domains and motifs in the insulin receptor. The insulin receptor is a tetramer formed by two α and two β subunits linked by disulfide bridges in their extracellular portions. Distinct functional domains within the α and β subunits of the insulin receptor are shown. Although the kinase domain and sites of phosphorylation play a role in the receptor internalization process, important determinants, allowing the receptor to localize to microvilli and to associate with clathrin-coated pits upon activation, are contained in the juxtamembrane domain. The IGF-1R displays a structure very close to that of the IR. Similarities, in term of percentage of identity within each domain of the two receptors, are indicated on the left side of the panel.

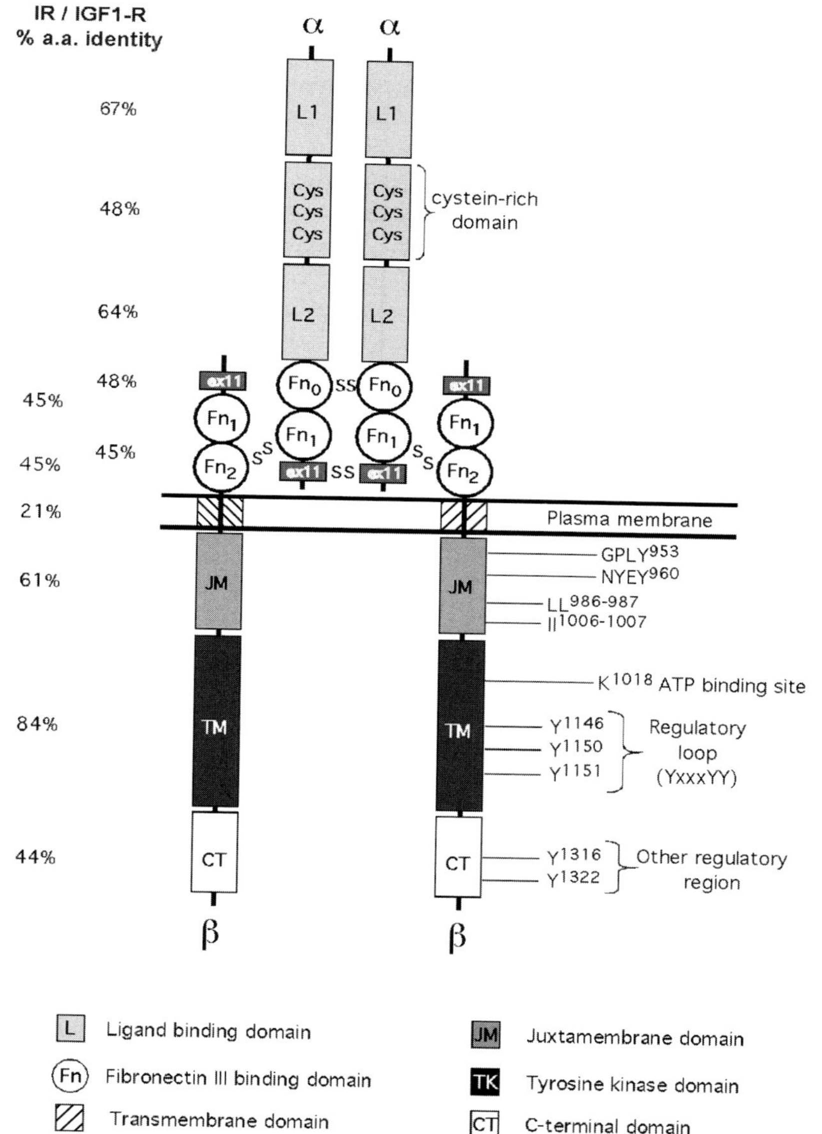
IR / IGF1-R
% a.a. identity
67%
48%
64%
48%
45%
45%
45%
21%
61%
84%
44%
α
α
L1
Cys
Cys
Cys
cystein-rich domain
L2
Fn0
Fn1
Fn2
ex11
SS
Plasma membrane
JM
TM
CT
β
GPLY953
NYEY960
LL986-987
II1006-1007
K1018 ATP binding site
Y1146
Y1150
Y1151
Regulatory loop (YxxxYY)
Y1316
Y1322
Other regulatory region
Ligand binding domain
Fibronectin III binding domain
Transmembrane domain
Juxtamembrane domain
Tyrosine kinase domain
C-terminal domain
S S Disulfide bridge

et al 1994, Hamer et al 1997, Heilker et al 1996) (see Fig. 1). Although the kinetics of IGF-1R internalization upon activation might not be similar to those of activated IR in specific cell types (Wiley & Cunningham 1982, Zapf et al 1994), the IGF-1R also presents a tyrosine-based motif, similar to the IR NPXY^{960} motif, which is crucial to the ligand-induced internalization of the receptor (Hsu et al 1994). However, in contrast to the IR, mutations of this motif and surrounding amino acids affect not only the ligand-induced internalization but also the kinase activity of the IGF-1R (Backer et al 1990, Berhanu et al 1991, Rajagopalan et al 1991, Thies et al 1990, Yamasaki et al 1992).

In addition to internalization motifs which have been shown to bind directly to adaptin complexes within CCPs, other potential connector molecules have been suggested recently to specifically promote internalization of the insulin or IGF-1 receptors. pp120, a membrane glycoprotein phosphorylated by the IR upon activation, has been shown to specifically stimulate the internalization of the IR, and not the IGF-1R, through mechanisms dependent on the NPXY^{960} motif in the β-subunit of the receptor (Formisano et al 1995, Najjar et al 1998). On the other hand, both β-arrestin, which acts as a clathrin adaptor (Ferguson et al 1996, Goodman et al 1996), and EHD1, a functional homologue of Eps15 (Mintz et al 1999), have been described as playing a role in IGF-1R internalization (Dalle et al 2002, Lin et al 1998, Rotem-Yehudar et al 2001). It is interesting to note that Shc, which binds both the insulin and IGF-1Rs upon activation by their respective ligands, has been shown to interact specifically with proteins closely involved in the formation of CCPs, such as dynamin and a/β subunits of adaptin complexes (Baron et al 1998, Okabayashi et al 1996). However, whether Shc can act as a connector molecule between activated insulin/IGF-1 receptors and CCP components or whether Shc may modulate the endocytic machinery remains to be determined.

Interaction of insulin/IGF-1 downstream effectors with components of the endocytic machinery raises the question as to whether signalling by tyrosine kinase receptors, such as the insulin or IGF-1 receptors, may in turn modulate the transport machinery. Previous studies have suggested that EGF and NGF could increase the density of CCPs at the plasma membrane (Connolly et al 1984). Further studies highlighted a potential role for c-Src, which phosphorylates the clathrin heavy chain following cell activation by growth factors and thus allows clathrin recruitment to the plasma membrane (Ahn et al 2002, Beattie et al 2000). Activation of the EGF receptor also induces the phosphorylation and recruitment of Eps15, a CCP component, and apparently leads to the formation of CCPs specifically incorporating EGF receptors (Confalonieri et al 2000). *De novo* formation of CCPs specifically incorporating one particular membrane protein has also been previously observed for transferrin receptors, IgM receptors, mannose 6-phosphate receptors and CD4 (Foti et al 1997, Iacopetta et al 1988, Le

Borgne & Hoflack 1997, Miller et al 1991, Salisbury et al 1980), but no evidence for such mechanisms has been described for the insulin or IGF-1 receptors.

Finally, besides the importance of the kinase activity, internalization motifs and connector molecules for IR/IGF-1R internalization, other intra-molecular determinants in these receptors may also influence the efficiency of these processes. In particular mutations in the transmembrane domain or in extracellular *N*-glycosylation sites of IR the β-subunit impaired significantly the internalization of the receptor without necessarily affecting the kinase activity upon stimulation (Leconte et al 1994, Yamada et al 1995). Also, in the case of the IGF-1R, a unique amino acid mutation in the extracellular portion of the β-subunit has been reported to significantly affect the internalization of this receptor (Condorelli et al 1994).

IR/IGF-1R recycling and degradation

Following segregation of insulin/IGF-1 receptors into CCPs, the neck of the CCP constricts in a dynamin-dependent process and fission of the neck membranes occurs thus forming a free cytoplasmic clathrin-coated vesicle. The coat constituents are then released to allow for heterotypic membrane fusion with endosomal compartments. The acidic pH of endosomes allows the dissociation of ligands from their receptors and their sorting in different directions: classically dissociated ligands are targeted to lysosomes, where they are degraded, while membrane receptors are recycled back to the cell surface where they can be reused (see Fig. 2).

Both IGF-1 and insulin share the same intracellular itinerary to lysosomal compartments (Smith et al 1991). However, following internalization of activated receptors, insulin dissociates much faster than IGF-1 from its receptor and is almost completely degraded. This is presumably due to a weak dissociation of IGF-1 from its receptor at low endosomal pH as compared to insulin (Zapf et al 1994). Whereas ligand-free IRs are recycled back to the surface, the fate of IGF-1R still coupled to its ligand in endosomes is unclear since both recycling at the surface and degradation in lysosomes have been described (see Fig. 2).

Interestingly, targeting of receptor–ligand complexes to late endosomal/lysosomal compartments may be signal mediated. Indeed, when insulin is covalently cross-linked to its receptors, the activated ligand–receptor complexes are targeted to late endosomes and lysosomes, but the recycling capacities of the covalently-linked complex is significantly slowed as compared to free IRs (Carpentier et al 1986). In addition, degradation of activated IGF-1R seems to be regulated by additional mechanisms. Indeed, IGF-1Rs have been described to undergo ligand-induced ubiquitination by the ubiquitin protein ligase Nedd4 through interaction with Grb10, an interacting partner of the IGF-1R

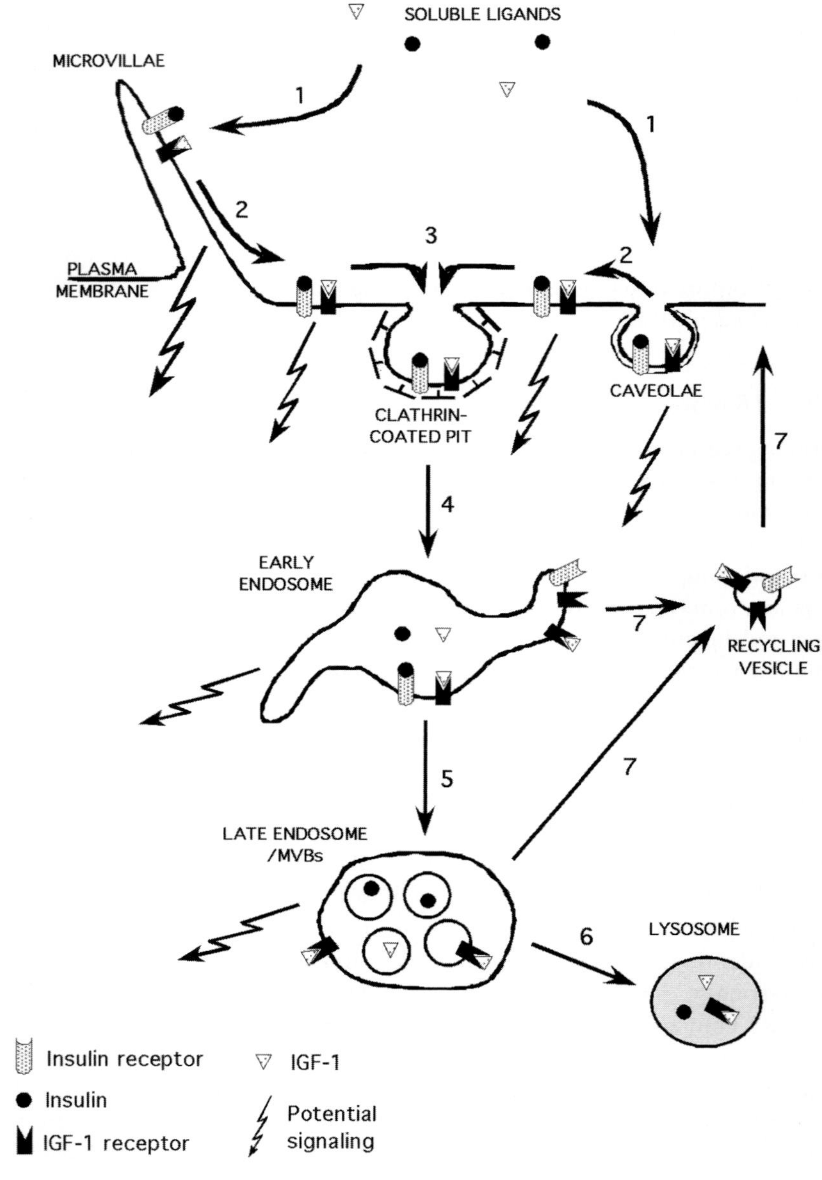
SOLUBLE LIGANDS
MICROVILLAE
1
1
2
3
2
PLASMA MEMBRANE
CLATHRIN-COATED PIT
CAVEOLAE
7
4
EARLY ENDOSOME
7
RECYCLING VESICLE
5
7
LATE ENDOSOME /MVBs
6
LYSOSOME
Insulin receptor
Insulin
IGF-1 receptor
IGF-1
Potential signaling

(Vecchione et al 2003). The ubiquitin–proteasome system is now well recognized as a regulator of endocytosis for selected membrane receptors in order to degrade signalling molecules and thus control the magnitude of signalling events (Strous & Govers 1999). It remains, however, to be established how much the ubiquitin–proteasome pathway contributes to the ligand-induced IGF-1R internalization and termination of IGF-1-induced signalling.

Spatial and temporal control of IR/IGF-1R signalling

It is commonly accepted that receptor-mediated endocytosis provides a mechanism for insulin/IGF-1 to be delivered to intracellular organelles involved in their degradation in order to terminate signaling transduction events (Carpentier 1993, 1994). It is also widely accepted that the modulation of both the internalization rate of the insulin/IGF-1 receptors and of the rate of recycling, determines the number of receptors present on the cell surface and hence available for ligand binding. This fine tuning of surface insulin/IGF-1 receptors number is crucial for the determination of the cell sensitivity to circulating hormones (Carpentier 1993, 1994). If these physiological functions of insulin/IGF-1 receptor internalization are well accepted, the question as to whether this process also permits a distinct spatial and temporal compartmentalization of signal transduction remains highly controversial. These issues are still the subject of intense investigations since differences in insulin- and IGF-1-induced signalling and terminal biological effects could be in part related to a distinct spatial and temporal activation of similar intracellular pathways by the two hormones (see above).

Concerning IR, several studies have suggested that it remains active for a while in endosomes and therefore some signalling might be mediated from these structures (Backer et al 1989, Burgess et al 1992). Similar conclusions were

FIG. 2. Internalization and sorting of ligand-bound insulin and IGF-1 receptors. Soluble circulating insulin and IGF-1 bind to their cognate receptors present on microvilli or caveolae depending on the cell type (step 1). Following their activation insulin/IGF-1 receptors translocate with their respective ligands to planar domains of the plasma membrane (step 2) in order to be incorporated into clathrin-coated pits (step 3) for their subsequent internalization (step 4). In early endosomes, insulin dissociates from its receptor, whereas IGF-1 stay bound more tightly to its receptor. Ligand-free receptors are efficiently recycled back to the plasma membrane from early endosomes (step 7) whereas free ligands and ligand-bound receptors are sorted to late endosomes/multivesicular bodies (step 5) in order to be routed for degradation in lysosomes (step 6). A significant portion of ligand-bound receptors can also recycle back to the plasma membrane from early and late endosomes. As long as the ligand is associated with its cognate receptor, intracellular signalling can be propagated if downstream effectors are locally available. Thus signalling may originate at each distinct subcellular location through which occupied insulin/IGF-1 receptors are travelling following their activation, such as microvilli or caveolae, planar plasma membrane domains, early endosomes and late endosomes/MVBs.

reached from comparative analysis of the kinetics and degree of IR kinase activation and of the subcellular localization of the active IR (by cellular fractionation) (Bevan et al 1997, Inoue et al 1998, Kublaoui et al 1995, Nave et al 1996, Wang et al 1996). On the other hand, IRS-1 phosphorylation is preserved at 4 °C (a temperature at which IR endocytosis is prevented) (Biener et al 1996, Heller-Harrison et al 1995, Maggi et al 1998) and is induced by insulin binding to cells expressing a dominant interfering dynamin which inhibits clathrin-coated pit mediated endocytosis (Ceresa et al 1998, Kao et al 1998). In the same study, Shc and ERK1/2 phosphorylation was impaired suggesting that IR internalization was necessary to propagate fully mitogenic signals. Further morphological and biochemical analyses of mutated IRs which are impaired for ligand-induced internalization and which remain hooked to microvilli (mutants of glycosylation side chain of the β subunit) suggest that IR interaction with IRS-1 and signal transduction can be initiated at the microvillus stage. In agreement with these observations, we reported the behaviour of a mutated IR (IR^{C860S}) which shows an inhibition of IR internalization but nevertheless is capable of some interaction with IRS-1 and can transduce limited insulin biological signals (Maggi et al 1998). More recently, we have analysed the behaviour of another mutated IR (IR^{R252C}) with a natural mutation accompanied with severe insulin resistance. This receptor showed a defect in insulin-induced internalization in spite of a normal autophosphorylation in response to insulin. This surface-located active receptor transduces normal signalling via IRS molecules but by contrast Shc phosphorylation was inhibited and thymidine incorporation was abolished (Hamer et al 2002). In another study, transfection of cells with antisense cDNA for pp120 prevented IR internalization and increased thymidine incorporation whereas overexpression of wild-type pp120 stimulated endocytosis of the IR and decreased thymidine overexpression (Formisano et al 1995). Along the same line, another report showed a comparable effect with a splice variant of the IGF-1R which displays an increased internalization rate associated with a decreased thymidine incorporation (Condorelli et al 1994). Thus, in terms of mitogenic signalling, results are contradictory (see below), while by contrast acute metabolic actions of insulin seem at least partly independent of IR endocytosis and to be mainly initiated by activation of IR at the plasma membrane.

As previously described, lipid rafts/caveolae might represent important plasma membrane compartments for insulin and IGF-1R signalling in adipocytes. In particular, disruption of caveolear structures using cholesterol-sequestering agents has been shown to affect insulin-mediated glucose transport (Gustavsson et al 1999, Khan & Pessin 2002, Parpal et al 2000), whereas IGF-1-induced adipocyte differentiation and mitotic clonal expansion are inhibited under similar conditions (Huo et al 2003). At the molecular level, caveolar disruption, prior to insulin/IGF-1 stimulation, does not affect autophosphorylation of the tyrosine kinase receptors, but IRS-1 and Akt activation by insulin are impaired whereas ERK1/2 phosphorylation proceeds normally. This is consistent with another study showing that inhibition of IR internalization by dominant-negative mutant dynamin prevents Shc and ERK1/2 activation upon insulin stimulation but not IRS-1 phosphorylation (Ceresa et al 1998). These results suggest that signalling through IRS proteins is potentially issued from caveolae at the plasma membrane whereas ERK1/2 and Shc activation necessitate internalization of the activated IR. Eventually, a combination of biochemical and morphological studies has clearly demonstrated the insulin-dependent association of elements of a new signalling pathway for IR in caveolae. This new signalling pathway involves the recruitment of a Cbl-CAP-TC10 complex into caveolae following insulin stimulation, which then triggers the translocation of GLUT4 vesicles at the plasma membrane. Although, this pathway of signalling initiates in caveolae and is dependent on the integrity of these plasma membrane invaginations, a direct association of IRs with caveolae has not been reported in these studies (Baumann et al 2000, Khan & Pessin 2002).

Within endosomal compartments, insulin dissociates from its receptor because their association is very sensitive to the low intraluminal pH of these organelles. Ligand-free IRs are then recycled back to the plasma membrane whereas insulin is degraded very rapidly, thus allowing termination of the insulin-induced signalling (Authier et al 1994). Importantly, the rapid insulin dissociation and degradation is consistent with hypophosphorylation of endosomal IRs as compared with plasma membrane IRs. In contrast, IGF-1 dissociation from its cognate receptor is much less sensitive to the low endosomal pH and a high proportion of ligand-bound IGF-1Rs are found in endosomes following their internalization from the plasma membrane (Zapf et al 1994). Within endosomes, ligand-bound tyrosine kinase receptors remain activated and keep their ability to phosphorylate downstream intracellular effectors (Bergeron et al 1995, Grimes et al 1996, Sorkin et al 1993). This may be of importance since Grb2, Shc and ERK/MAPK, the main downstream effectors for mitogenic terminal biological effects induced by insulin/IGF-1 signalling, co-localize on endosomal membranes (Di Guglielmo et al 1994, Oksvold et al 2001, Pol et al 1998, Rizzo et al 2000, Sorkin et al 2000). Therefore the pronounced effect of IGF-1, as compared to insulin, to induce mitogenic terminal cellular effects, may partially relate to signalling issued from endosomes. In this hypothesis, ligand-bound IGF-1Rs within endosomes may signal for a longer time than IRs, thus favouring propagation of mitogenic signals as opposed to acute metabolic signalling from the plasma membrane. Interestingly, a recent report evidences that IGF-1 could activate Shc and ERK kinases through transactivation of the EGF-receptor (Roudabush et al 2000). Thus, in addition to generating signalling from endosomal membranes directly,

IGF-1Rs may also generate endosomal signalling through transactivation of the EGF receptor (Sorkin & Von Zastrow 2002).

Conclusions

All together, the majority of data accumulated up to now support the general concept that insulin/IGF-1 receptors initiate metabolic signalling from the plasma membrane whereas mitogenic signalling originate from inside the cells following internalization of activated receptors. In addition, consistent with the acute action of the insulin this hormone appears to be rapidly internalized and degraded, whereas IGF-1, which mediates a stable chronic cellular action, is metabolized more slowly in order to achieve a constant level of the growth factor.

References

Abitorabi MA, Pachynski RK, Ferrando RE, Tidswell M, Erle DJ 1997 Presentation of integrins on leukocyte microvilli: a role for the extracellular domain in determining membrane localization. J Cell Biol 139:563–571

Ahn S, Kim J, Lucaveche CL, Reedy MC, Luttrell LM, Lefkowitz RJ, Daaka Y 2002 Src-dependent tyrosine phosphorylation regulates dynamin self-assembly and ligand-induced endocytosis of the epidermal growth factor receptor. J Biol Chem 277:26642–26651

Anderson RG 1998 The caveolae membrane system. Annu Rev Biochem 67:199–225

Authier F, Rachubinski RA, Posner BI, Bergeron JJ 1994 Endosomal proteolysis of insulin by an acidic thiol metalloprotease unrelated to insulin degrading enzyme. J Biol Chem 269: 3010–3016

Backer JM, Kahn CR, Cahill DA, Ullrich A, White MF 1990 Receptor-mediated internalization of insulin requires a 12-amino acid sequence in the juxtamembrane region of the insulin receptor beta- subunit. J Biol Chem 265:16450–16454

Backer JM, Kahn CR, White MF 1989 Tyrosine phosphorylation of the insulin receptor during insulin-stimulated internalization in rat hepatoma cells. J Biol Chem 264:1694–1701

Backer JM, Shoelson SE, Weiss MA et al 1992 The insulin receptor juxtamembrane region contains two independent tyrosine/beta-turn internalization signals. J Cell Biol 118:831–839

Baron V, Alengrin F, Van Obberghen E 1998 Dynamin associates with Src-Homology Collagen (Shc) and becomes tyrosine phosphorylated in response to insulin. Endocrinology 139:3034–3037

Baumann CA, Ribon V, Kanzaki M et al 2000 CAP defines a second signalling pathway required for insulin-stimulated glucose transport. Nature 407:202–207

Beattie EC, Howe CL, Wilde A, Brodsky FM, Mobley WC 2000 NGF signals through TrkA to increase clathrin at the plasma membrane and enhance clathrin-mediated membrane trafficking. J Neurosci 20:7325–7333

Bergeron JJ, Di Guglielmo GM, Baass PC, Authier F, Posner BI 1995 Endosomes, receptor tyrosine kinase internalization and signal transduction. Biosci Rep 15:411–418

Berhanu P, Ibrahim-Schneck RH, Anderson C, Wood WM 1991 The NPEY sequence is not necessary for endocytosis and processing of insulin-receptor complexes. Mol Endocrinol 5:1827–1835

Bevan AP, Krook A, Tikerpae J, Seabright PJ, Siddle K, Smith GD 1997 Chloroquine extends the lifetime of the activated insulin receptor complex in endosomes. J Biol Chem 272:26833–26840

Biener Y, Feinstein R, Mayak M, Kaburagi Y, Kadowaki T, Zick Y 1996 Annexin II is a novel player in insulin signal transduction. Possible association between annexin II phosphorylation and insulin receptor internalization. J Biol Chem 271:29489–29496

Brown MS, Anderson RG, Goldstein JL 1983 Recycling receptors: the round-trip itinerary of migrant membrane proteins. Cell 32:663–667

Burgess JW, Wada I, Ling N, Khan MN, Bergeron JJ, Posner BI 1992 Decrease in beta-subunit phosphotyrosine correlates with internalization and activation of the endosomal insulin receptor kinase. J Biol Chem 267:10077–10086

Carpentier JL 1993 Robert Feulgen Prize Lecture 1993 The journey of the insulin receptor into the cell: from cellular biology to pathophysiology. Histochemistry 100:169–184

Carpentier JL 1994 Insulin receptor internalization: molecular mechanisms and physiopathological implications. Diabetologia 37(suppl 2):S117–124

Carpentier JL, McClain D 1995 Insulin receptor kinase activation releases a constraint maintaining the receptor on microvilli. J Biol Chem 270:5001–5006

Carpentier JL, Paccaud JP, Backer J et al 1993 Two steps of insulin receptor internalization depend on different domains of the beta-subunit. J Cell Biol 122:1243–1252

Carpentier JL, Paccaud JP, Gorden P, Rutter WJ, Orci L 1992 Insulin-induced surface redistribution regulates internalization of the insulin receptor and requires its autophosphorylation. Proc Natl Acad Sci USA 89:162–166

Carpentier JL, Robert A, Grunberger G et al 1986 Receptor-mediated endocytosis of polypeptide hormones is a regulated process: inhibition of [^{125}I]iodoinsulin internalization in hypoinsulinemic diabetes of rat and man. J Clin Endocrinol Metab 63: 151–155

Ceresa BP, Kao AW, Santeler SR, Pessin JE 1998 Inhibition of clathrin-mediated endocytosis selectively attenuates specific insulin receptor signal transduction pathways. Mol Cell Biol 18:3862–3870

Condeelis J 1993 Life at the leading edge: the formation of cell protrusions. Annu Rev Cell Biol 9:411–444

Condorelli G, Bueno R, Smith RJ 1994 Two alternatively spliced forms of the human insulin-like growth factor I receptor have distinct biological activities and internalization kinetics. J Biol Chem 269:8510–8516

Confalonieri S, Salcini AE, Puri C, Tacchetti C, Di Fiore PP 2000 Tyrosine phosphorylation of Eps15 is required for ligand-regulated, but not constitutive, endocytosis. J Cell Biol 150:905–912

Connolly JL, Green SA, Greene LA 1984 Comparison of rapid changes in surface morphology and coated pit formation of PC12 cells in response to nerve growth factor, epidermal growth factor, and dibutyryl cyclic AMP. J Cell Biol 98:457–465

Dalle S, Imamura T, Rose DW et al 2002 Insulin induces heterologous desensitization of G-protein-coupled receptor and insulin-like growth factor I signaling by downregulating beta-arrestin-1. Mol Cell Biol 22:6272–6285

den Hartigh JC, van Bergen en Henegouwen PM, Verkleij AJ, Boonstra J 1992 The EGF receptor is an actin-binding protein. J Cell Biol 119:349–355

Di Guglielmo GM, Baass PC, Ou WJ, Posner BI, Bergeron JJ 1994 Compartmentalization of SHC, GRB2 and mSOS, and hyperphosphorylation of Raf-1 by EGF but not insulin in liver parenchyma. EMBO J 13:4269–4277

Fan JY, Carpentier JL, van Obberghen E, Grunfeld C, Gorden P, Orci L 1983a Morphological changes of the 3T3-L1 fibroblast plasma membrane upon differentiation to the adipocyte form. J Cell Sci 61:219–230

Fan JY, Carpentier JL, Van Obberghen E et al 1983b The interaction of 125I-insulin with cultured 3T3-L1 adipocytes: quantitative analysis by the hypothetical grain method. J Histochem Cytochem 31:859–870

Ferguson SS, Downey WE, Colapietro AM, Barak LS, Menard L, Caron MG 1996 Role of beta-arrestin in mediating agonist-promoted G protein-coupled receptor internalization. Science 271:363–366

Formisano P, Najjar SM, Gross CN, Philippe N et al 1995 Receptor-mediated internalization of insulin. Potential role of pp120/HA4, a substrate of the insulin receptor kinase. J Biol Chem 270:24073–24077

Foti M, Mangasarian A, Piguet V, Lew DP, Krause KH, Trono D, Carpentier JL 1997 Nef-mediated clathrin-coated pit formation. J Cell Biol 139:37–47

Gilbert A, Paccaud JP, Foti M, Porcheron G, Balz J, Carpentier JL 1999 Direct demonstration of the endocytic function of caveolae by a cell-free assay. J Cell Sci 112:1101–1110

Goldstein JL, Brown MS, Anderson RG, Russell DW, Schneider WJ 1985 Receptor-mediated endocytosis: concepts emerging from the LDL receptor system. Annu Rev Cell Biol 1:1–39

Goodman OB, Krupnick JG, Santini F et al 1996 Beta-arrestin acts as a clathrin adaptor in endocytosis of the β2-adrenergic receptor. Nature 383:447–450

Grimes ML, Zhou J, Beattie EC et al 1996 Endocytosis of activated TrkA: evidence that nerve growth factor induces formation of signaling endosomes. J Neurosci 16:7950–7964

Gustavsson J, Parpal S, Karlsson M et al 1999 Localization of the insulin receptor in caveolae of adipocyte plasma membrane. FASEB J 13:1961–1971

Haft CR, Klausner RD, Taylor SI 1994 Involvement of dileucine motifs in the internalization and degradation of the insulin receptor. J Biol Chem 269:26286–26294

Hamer I, Haft CR, Paccaud JP, Maeder C, Taylor S, Carpentier JL 1997 Dual role of a dileucine motif in insulin receptor endocytosis. J Biol Chem 272:21685–21691

Hamer I, Foti M, Emkey R, Cordier-Bussat M et al 2002 An arginine to cysteine (252) mutation in insulin receptors from a patient with severe insulin resistance inhibits receptor internalisation but preserves signalling events. Diabetologia 45:657–667

Heilker R, Manning-Krieg U, Zuber JF, Spiess M 1996 In vitro binding of clathrin adaptors to sorting signals correlates with endocytosis and basolateral sorting. EMBO J 15:2893–2899

Heller-Harrison RA, Morin M, Czech MP 1995 Insulin regulation of membrane-associated insulin receptor substrate 1. J Biol Chem 270:24442–24450

Hooper NM 1990 Detergent-insoluble glycosphingolipid/cholesterol-rich membrane domains, lipid rafts and caveolae (review). Mol Membr Biol 16:145–156

Hsu D, Knudson PE, Zapf A, Rolband GC, Olefsky JM 1994 NPXY motif in the insulin-like growth factor-I receptor is required for efficient ligand-mediated receptor internalization and biological signaling. Endocrinology 134:744–750

Hubbard SR 1997 Crystal structure of the activated insulin receptor tyrosine kinase in complex with peptide substrate and ATP analog. EMBO J 16:5572–5581

Huo H, Guo X, Hong S, Jiang M, Liu X, Liao K 2003 Lipid rafts/caveolae are essential for insulin-like growth factor-1 receptor signaling during 3T3-L1 preadipocyte differentiation induction. J Biol Chem 278:11561–11569

Iacopetta BJ, Rothenberger S, Kuhn LC 1988 A role for the cytoplasmic domain in transferrin receptor sorting and coated pit formation during endocytosis. Cell 54: 485–489

Inoue G, Cheatham B, Emkey R, Kahn CR 1998 Dynamics of insulin signaling in 3T3-L1 adipocytes. Differential compartmentalization and trafficking of insulin receptor substrate (IRS)-1 and IRS-2. J Biol Chem 273:11548–11555

Kandror KV, Stephens JM, Pilch PF 1995 Expression and compartmentalization of caveolin in adipose cells: coordinate regulation with and structural segregation from GLUT4. J Cell Biol 129:999–1006

Kao AW, Ceresa BP, Santeler SR, Pessin JE 1998 Expression of a dominant interfering dynamin mutant in 3T3L1 adipocytes inhibits GLUT4 endocytosis without affecting insulin signaling. J Biol Chem 273:25450–25457

Khan AH, Pessin JE 2002 Insulin regulation of glucose uptake: a complex interplay of intracellular signalling pathways. Diabetologia 45:1475–1483

Kublaoui B, Lee J, Pilch PF 1995 Dynamics of signaling during insulin-stimulated endocytosis of its receptor in adipocytes. J Biol Chem 270:59–65

Kurzchalia TV, Parton RG 1999 Membrane microdomains and caveolae. Curr Opin Cell Biol 11:424–431

Le Borgne R, Hoflack B 1997 Mannose 6-phosphate receptors regulate the formation of clathrin-coated vesicles in the TGN. J Cell Biol 137:335–345

Leconte I, Carpentier JL, Clauser E 1994 The functions of the human insulin receptor are affected in different ways by mutation of each of the four N-glycosylation sites in the beta subunit. J Biol Chem 269:18062–18071

Lin FT, Daaka Y, Lefkowitz RJ 1998 beta-arrestins regulate mitogenic signaling and clathrin-mediated endocytosis of the insulin-like growth factor I receptor. J Biol Chem 273: 31640–31643

Louvard D 1989 The function of the major cytoskeletal components of the brush border. Curr Opin Cell Biol 1:51–57

Maggi D, Andraghetti G, Carpentier JL, Cordera R 1998 Cys860 in the extracellular domain of insulin receptor beta-subunit is critical for internalization and signal transduction. Endocrinology 139:496–504

Mastick CC, Brady MJ, Saltiel AR 1995 Insulin stimulates the tyrosine phosphorylation of caveolin. J Cell Biol 129:1523–1531

Miller K, Shipman M, Trowbridge IS, Hopkins CR 1991 Transferrin receptors promote the formation of clathrin lattices. Cell 65:621–632

Mineo C, Gill GN, Anderson RG 1999 Regulated migration of epidermal growth factor receptor from caveolae. J Biol Chem 274:30636–30643

Mintz L, Galperin E, Pasmanik-Chor M et al 1999 EHD1 — an EH-domain-containing protein with a specific expression pattern. Genomics 59:66–76

Moore KL, Patel KD, Bruehl RE et al 1995 P-selectin glycoprotein ligand-1 mediates rolling of human neutrophils on P-selectin. J Cell Biol 128:661–671

Najjar SM, Choice CV, Soni P, Whitman CM, Poy MN 1998 Effect of pp120 on receptor-mediated insulin endocytosis is regulated by the juxtamembrane domain of the insulin receptor. J Biol Chem 273:12923–12928

Nave BT, Haigh RJ, Hayward AC, Siddle K, Shepherd PR 1996 Compartment-specific regulation of phosphoinositide 3-kinase by platelet-derived growth factor and insulin in 3T3-L1 adipocytes. Biochem J 318:55–60

Ohno H, Stewart J, Fournier MC et al 1995 Interaction of tyrosine-based sorting signals with clathrin-associated proteins. Science 269:1872–1875

Okabayashi Y, Sugimoto Y, Totty NF et al 1996 Interaction of Shc with adaptor protein adaptins. J Biol Chem 271:5265–5269

Oksvold MP, Skarpen E, Wierod L, Paulsen RE, Huitfeldt HS 2001 Re-localization of activated EGF receptor and its signal transducers to multivesicular compartments downstream of early endosomes in response to EGF. Eur J Cell Biol 80:285–294

Parpal S, Karlsson M, Thorn H, Stralfors P 2000 Cholesterol depletion disrupts caveolae and insulin receptor signaling for metabolic control via IRS-1, but not for MAP-kinase control. J Biol Chem 276:9670–9678

Pavalko FM, Walker DM, Graham L, Goheen M, Doerschuk CM, Kansas GS 1995 The cytoplasmic domain of L-selectin interacts with cytoskeletal proteins via alpha-actinin: receptor positioning in microvilli does not require interaction with alpha-actinin. J Cell Biol 129:1155–1164

Picker LJ, Warnock RA, Burns AR, Doerschuk CM, Berg EL, Butcher EC 1991 The neutrophil selectin LECAM-1 presents carbohydrate ligands to the vascular selectins ELAM-1 and GMP-140. Cell 66:921–933

Pol A, Calvo M, Enrich C 1998 Isolated endosomes from quiescent rat liver contain the signal transduction machinery. Differential distribution of activated Raf-1 and Mek in the endocytic compartment. FEBS Lett 441:34–38

Rajagopalan M, Neidigh JL, McClain DA 1991 Amino acid sequences Gly-Pro-Leu-Tyr and Asn-Pro-Glu-Tyr in the submembranous domain of the insulin receptor are required for normal endocytosis. J Biol Chem 266:23068–23073

Rizzo MA, Shome K, Watkins SC, Romero G 2000 The recruitment of Raf-1 to membranes is mediated by direct interaction with phosphatidic acid and is independent of association with Ras. J Biol Chem 275:23911–23918

Rotem-Yehudar R, Galperin E, Horowitz M 2001 Association of insulin-like growth factor 1 receptor with EHD1 and SNAP29. J Biol Chem 276:33054–33060

Roudabush FL, Pierce KL, Maudsley S, Khan KD, Luttrell LM 2000 Transactivation of the EGF receptor mediates IGF-1-stimulated shc phosphorylation and ERK1/2 activation in COS-7 cells. J Biol Chem 275:22583–22589

Salisbury JL, Condeelis JS, Satir P 1980 Role of coated vesicles, microfilaments, and calmodulin in receptor- mediated endocytosis by cultured B lymphoblastoid cells. J Cell Biol 87: 132–141

Scherer PE, Lisanti MP, Baldini G, Sargiacomo M, Mastick CC, Lodish HF 1994 Induction of caveolin during adipogenesis and association of GLUT4 with caveolin-rich vesicles. J Cell Biol 127:1233–1243

Shackleton S, Hamer I, Foti M, Zumwald N, Maeder C, Carpentier JL 2002 Role of two dileucine-like motifs in insulin receptor anchoring to microvilli. J Biol Chem 277:43631–43637

Smith RM, Seely BL, Shah N, Olefsky JM, Jarett L 1991 Tyrosine kinase-defective insulin receptors undergo insulin-induced microaggregation but do not concentrate in coated pits. J Biol Chem 266:17522–17530

Sorkin A, Von Zastrow M 2002 Signal transduction and endocytosis: close encounters of many kinds. Nat Rev Mol Cell Biol 3:600–614

Sorkin A, Eriksson A, Heldin CH, Westermark B, Claesson-Welsh L 1993 Pool of ligand-bound platelet-derived growth factor beta-receptors remain activated and tyrosine phosphorylated after internalization. J Cell Physiol 156:373–382

Sorkin A, McClure M, Huang F, Carter R 2000 Interaction of EGF receptor and grb2 in living cells visualized by fluorescence resonance energy transfer (FRET) microscopy. Curr Biol 10:1395–1398

Souto RP, Vallega G, Wharton J, Vinten J, Tranum-Jensen J, Pilch PF 2003 Immunopurification and characterization of rat adipocyte caveolae suggest their dissociation from insulin signaling. J Biol Chem 278:18321–18329

Strous GJ, Govers R 1999 The ubiquitin-proteasome system and endocytosis. J Cell Sci 112:1417–1423

Thies RS, Webster NJ, McClain DA 1990 A domain of the insulin receptor required for endocytosis in rat fibroblasts. J Biol Chem 265:10132–10137

Tsukita S, Yonemura S 1997 ERM proteins: head-to-tail regulation of actin-plasma membrane interaction. Trends Biochem Sci 22:53–58

van Bergen en Henegouwen PM, den Hartigh JC, Romeyn P, Verkleij AJ, Boonstra J 1992 The epidermal growth factor receptor is associated with actin filaments. Exp Cell Res 199:90–97

Vecchione A, Marchese A, Henry P, Rotin D, Morrione A 2003 The Grb10/Nedd4 complex regulates ligand-induced ubiquitination and stability of the insulin-like growth factor I receptor. Mol Cell Biol 23:3363–3372

Wang B, Balba Y, Knutson VP 1996 Insulin-induced in situ phosphorylation of the insulin receptor located in the plasma membrane versus endosomes. Biochem Biophys Res Commun 227:27–34

Wei L, Hubbard SR, Hendrickson WA, Ellis L 1995 Expression, characterization, and crystallization of the catalytic core of the human insulin receptor protein-tyrosine kinase domain. J Biol Chem 270:8122–8130

Welsh JB, Worthylake R, Wiley HS, Gill GN 1994 Specific factors are required for kinase-dependent endocytosis of insulin receptors. Mol Biol Cell 5:539–547

Wiley HS, Cunningham DD 1982 The endocytotic rate constant. A cellular parameter for quantitating receptor-mediated endocytosis. J Biol Chem 257:4222–4229

Wiley HS, Herbst JJ, Walsh BJ, Lauffenburger DA, Rosenfeld MG, Gill GN 1991 The role of tyrosine kinase activity in endocytosis, compartmentation, and down-regulation of the epidermal growth factor receptor. J Biol Chem 266:11083–11094

Yamada K, Carpentier JL, Cheatham B, Goncalves E, Shoelson SE, Kahn CR 1995 Role of the transmembrane domain and flanking amino acids in internalization and down-regulation of the insulin receptor. J Biol Chem 270:3115–3122

Yamasaki H, Prager D, Gebremedhin S, Melmed S 1992 Human insulin-like growth factor I receptor 950tyrosine is required for somatotroph growth factor signal transduction. J Biol Chem 267:20953–20958

Zapf A, Hsu D, Olefsky JM 1994 Comparison of the intracellular itineraries of insulin-like growth factor-I and insulin and their receptors in Rat-1 fibroblasts. Endocrinology 134:2445–2452

DISCUSSION

LeRoith: The IR 252 mutant binds insulin because insulin stimulates downstream pathways. It binds the insulin, stimulates the IRS and doesn't internalize so you don't get the mitogenic pathway. Do you understand the mechanism whereby 252 prevents the internalization?

Carpentier: No, I have no idea how it does. It is on the external domain of the receptor. Fortuitously we discovered these three mutants which have nothing to do with each other.

LeRoith: It is interesting that the external domain can affect the internalization.

Roberts: We have heard a bit in this meeting about the new appreciation of the alternative splicing of the insulin receptor making it either an IR or an IGF-2R. I think people have forgotten that about 10 years ago Robert Smith's group described alternative splicing of the IGF-1 receptor. This has been ignored since then. As I recall, this affected the region which, in the IR, you said determines association with clathrin-coated pits. Has anyone gone back to look to see whether there are different classes of the IGF-1 receptor that can or cannot associate with clathrin-coated pits?

Carpentier: No, but I think that any receptor will finally end up in clathrin-coated pits. The problem is knowing where they were before: in caveolae, on microvilli or somewhere else on the cell surface. In order to be internalized, finally they have to reach the clathrin-coated pits. I think it is a question of timing and knowing where they are to start with.

Holly: You raised the possibility of different classes of caveolae, and that there was only 25% co-localization of IGF-1 and the insulin receptor. Is that 25% the hybrid receptors? Are there insulin receptors in some caveolae and IGF-1 receptors in others and hybrids in a third class?

Carpentier: Perhaps. That is a good suggestion. I cannot distinguish the two. I can only localize the receptor with an antibody recognizing the external domain of the receptor.

Holly: It looked as if the receptors were enriched, but were not totally in those caveolae. You said that the MAP kinase signalling is dependent upon internalization. Do you get differential signalling whether they are in the caveolae or not in the caveolae, other than this raft signalling?

Carpentier: Again, I can't analyse this because the only way to analyse it is to find a condition where caveolae are absent. We could do this with cholesterol-destroying reagents, and then in this case we would maintain the activation of the receptor. In these conditions, we can't collect the activated receptor with the signalling machinery, especially in the case of IGF-1. This is an artificial way of getting rid of the caveolae.

Zick: I wanted to broaden the issue of internalization. You are talking about the very proximal event of getting into the coated pits. We know that in the case of the EGF receptor the signal is participating in driving EGF receptors to degradation in the proteasome. There are no data suggesting that the IR is degraded in the proteasome. What causes the differences between these two receptors?

Carpentier: I don't know. I can't even speculate about this.

De Meyts: I remember in the old days when Goldfine and colleagues proposed that insulin receptors got internalized into the nucleus (Goldfine et al 1982). Many of us were sceptical at the time. But today there are more and more reports of receptor typrosine kinases (RTKs), cytokine receptors and IGF-binding proteins going into the nucleus. What do you think of this?

Carpentier: I am very sceptical still. They'd have to cross a membrane at some stage. First you have to tell me how they would cross that membrane.

De Meyts: The number of reports is overwhelming, and from very good investigators.

LeRoith: There are reports, there's scepticism and controversy. It will probably go on for a long time.

Carpentier: It is outside the membrane and then it is inside a vesicle — it has to go through.

Pollak: To link some of the related questions, if we consider the overexpression of IGF-2 in a tumour cell, which is often suspected to drive an autocrine loop with

IGF-2 as a ligand for the IGF-1R, in that setting sometimes we speak vaguely of down-regulation of the IGF-1R numbers because of this chronic stimulation. But if we try to examine the kinetics of this more quantitatively, what do you think is going on in such a case? Does the receptor number fall because of the limitations of the receptor recycling speed, that the receptors cannot get back to the cell surface fast enough to maintain a steady state?

Carpentier: Yes, we have described this in many conditions. In fact, we can modulate the whole system. I am speaking about the IR. If we accelerate the internalization or if we block the recycling we can modulate the number of receptors at the cell surface. It is just a question of turnover and equilibrium between internalization rate, recycling rate, degradation and synthesis. This is what is happening in a hyperinsulinaemic state in patients with type II diabetes, with an increase of insulin in the blood. If you take monocytes they have a lower number of receptors. How do you get a lower number of receptors? In fact, the cell increases the internalization rate, and maintains the same recycling rate. As a result, more receptors are lost from the cell surface until the equilibrium is reached. The same thing happens in type I diabetes. If you take monocytes from type I diabetes, they have a higher number of receptors on the cell surface to compensate for the loss of circulating insulin. The internalization rate is lower in these cells.

LeRoith: There are some studies showing the level of IGF-1 in the circulation — high or low — will affect the gene expression of the IGF-1R (Eshet et al 1993) in addition to the internalization. The mechanism is not known but the mRNA was decreased with high IGF-1 and vice versa.

Laron: There is scant proof of an IGF-1 receptor defect in humans (Abuzzahab et al 2003). Would you imagine that if you could find more mutations, the same mechanism would act as you demonstrated with the mutations in the insulin receptor?

Carpentier: I think so. For the mutations that we described with the insulin receptor, only a few of them were natural mutations. Most of them were mutations that we introduced.

Laron: But we have natural mutations.

Carpentier: Yes. It should be the same for the IGF-1R.

Laron: Is there any activation of IGF-1Rs in patients with hyperinsulinaemia due to an insulin receptor defect?

LeRoith: You mean that in patients who have levels of insulin, is that sufficient to cross react with IGF-1R?

De Meyts: You would need to have levels about 500 times higher. I don't think this kind of level is ever reached. In the patients with receptor mutations perhaps it would be a possibility. But with regular hyperinsulinaemia like in type II diabetes I would say no.

LeRoith: It is interesting, though, that leprechauns are born small, funny looking children who fail to thrive. You would expect at that stage they were hyperinsulinaemic cross-reacting. Some people have suggested hyperinsulinaemia with pseudo-acromegalic patients.

Holly: Is the raised insulin crossing over on the growth factor receptor to cause the pseudo-acromegalic features?

LeRoith: That would explain the leprechaunism, but in the pseudo-acromegalics with hyperinsulinaemia there may be somatic enlargement. There may be occasional cases of this syndrome, but most diabetic patients don't get their levels high enough.

Zick: Earlier we discussed the hybrid receptors. Is the mechanism of internalization of the IGF-1 receptor similar or different to that of the insulin receptor? What is the mechanism of internalization of the hybrid receptors? Which pathway would they take, if the two are different?

LeRoith: Olefsky looked at the time course of the internalization, comparing insulin to IGF receptors (Sasaoka et al 1996). He found that insulin receptors internalize much faster.

Carpentier: Using transfected cells it can differ from one clone to the other. In CHO cells we got an internalization rate very similar for both receptor types, but I don't know whether this can be generalized. Also, the machinery may be slightly different. People have described that arrestin can be involved in the internalization as an adaptor for the association with clathrin-coated pits in the case of the IGF-1R, while for the insulin receptor it is an adaptor. This may be a difference, and there may be other differences along the pathway.

LeRoith: Can I extend the question to the IGF-2 receptor? The clathrin pits have the LDL and transferrin receptors, which are really just internalizing cholesterol, whereas the microvilli associate with tyrosine kinase receptors. In my understanding the IGF-2 receptor is just an internalizer of IGF-2 molecules. Is this associated with clathrin and not associated with the microvilli?

Carpentier: Yes, it is more a type 1 receptor.

LeRoith: Do they have the dileucine motifs?

Carpentier: I don't know that. In the case of the IGF-1 receptor one of the two dileucines is present but the second is not.

LeRoith: But it has the NPY. That commonality could help within the microvilli.

Thomas: There are data showing that the EGF receptor is not targeted to the proteasome but the lysosome. What happens to the insulin receptor?

Carpentier: It goes to the lysosomes.

Thomas: Is the inability of the receptor to signal to Shc due to localization of Shc, or phosphorylation of specific sites?

Carpentier: We couldn't find Shc associated with the caveolae. We are trying to localize Shc using EM techniques. There was a paper showing that Shc was associated with the endosome membrane. Thus a nice location for activating Shc is in the course of the internalization leaving the endosome.

Roberts: We have recently looked at Shc in prostate epithelial cells by confocal microscopy. In unstimulated cells there is no Shc at the plasma membrane: it is distributed in a punctate fashion throughout the cytoplasm. After 30 min of IGF treatment we see phospho Shc in a nuclear-adjacent location. It is not perinuclear, but in a glob next to the nucleus. 2 h later it goes away. There is never any at the surface, which would fit with your concept that Shc activation is significantly behind the initial plasma membrane events.

Zick: With regard to the question of Shc phosphorylation at the membrane, a couple of years back we published data suggesting that Shc phosphorylation depends on the temperature. At 4 °C presumably very little movement takes place. The IR does phosphorylate two of the isoforms, the 55 and 44 kDa. The phosphorylation of the 66 kDa Shc isoform by the insulin receptor is temperature dependent, suggesting that this isoform is distanced from the receptor. The other two isoforms might be in close proximity to the receptor even under conditions when it doesn't move a great deal. Namely, two of the isoforms might be part of what is called the initial signalling complex. So when we are talking about Shc localization and Rho, we should keep in mind that the various isoforms might differ in function.

LeRoith: Part of the question would be what antibody did you use?

Roberts: It actually sees all three isoforms of ShcA. There is also ShcB and C. ShcB is widely expressed and makes a p66 ShcA homologue. There was a poster presentation at the Endocrine Society meeting (De Tullio et al 2003) looking at a thyroid cancer line that either had all three Shc isoforms or only Shc46 and 52. The p66 version was necessary for IGF signalling through PI3K. Even though the other two were there, they were not sufficient.

Holly: In the first part of your talk I was fascinated by these spatial temporal differences in the receptor distributions. They are out on the microvilli and have to get down and into the clathrin-coated pits. MAP kinase signalling is dependent on the internalization but PKB can presumably occur prior to this. What is the mechanism of this trans-localization? Is it Rho GTPase dependent?

Carpentier: For the receptor to leave microvilli it has to be activated. The tyrosine kinase has to be activated. We showed several years ago that the 3 tyrosines within the kinase have to be phosphorylated. Whether other elements such as Rho GTPases are needed is unknown. If there is no internalization there is no Shc activation, MAP kinase activation or thymidine incorporation. We believe that internalization is necessary, but it is not clear whether there is something else at another stage. There may be something happening between the microvilli and the clathrin pits.

Holly: Is the movement within the membrane dependent on cytoskeletal reorganization?

Carpentier: You mean is it an active or passive movement? I would rather believe that it is a passive movement depending on the release of the constraint. Then the molecule is free on the cell surface and through the motif it recognizes clathrin-coated pits, where it gets segregated and is trapped.

Holly: What is the time frame?

Carpentier: I can't answer this.

Yee: There are a couple of monoclonal antibodies directed against the IGF-1R that we have been working with. They appear to cause internalization of the receptor but don't initiate any signalling events. We have been unable to show any tyrosine kinase activation of the receptor or phosphorylation of any downstream substrates. I wonder how this fits into your model. How can you get internalization with a non-natural ligand in the absence of any biochemical activation of the receptor? The same applies to the EGF receptor.

Carpentier: You have to distinguish between constitutive internalization and ligand-induced internalization. But there is always constitutive internalization of the receptor. In the case of the insulin receptor we have tracked it also with an antibody which was not activating the receptor. Let's say that after 30 minutes you have 20% of the receptor which internalizes. There are two different levels. First, there is a constitutive part, which is the one you are talking about, which can be modulated and inhibited. For example, if you apply PMA to cells, then you increase the whole internalization of the cell surface by large pieces of membrane, and then you will induce down-regulation of receptors and increase the constitutive internalization. Second, besides this there is also ligand-induced internalization, which is a specific pathway.

Holly: The antibodies enhance aggregation of the receptors by being divalent. Would this alter the constitutive internalization?

Carpentier: Yes, this is also a factor. It can have an effect at the level of the endosome, too. If you do not dissociate the ligands from the receptor at the level of the endosome, then the receptor is in trouble: it is targeted to the lysosome to be degraded. You need to detach your ligand from the receptor. This is what we observed when we were using a ligand that was covalently bound to the insulin receptor, and in this case you had a high degree of degradation. This has also been shown with other types of receptor: if you apply an antibody that doesn't detach from the receptor, then you degrade the receptor.

LeRoith: Some antibodies have been shown to activate the receptor. Aggregation can cause internalization, but sometimes it can actually activate. In your case it is not activating.

Yee: We had been working with a single chain antibody that is a full agonist but appears to internalize. We used the Novartis tyrosine kinase inhibitor and it still internalizes. At least for this phenotype the kinase activation wasn't required.

References

Abuzzahab MJ, Schneider A, Goddard A et al 2003 IGF-I receptor mutations resulting in intrauterine and postnatal growth retardation. N Engl J Med 349:2211–2222

De Tullio C, Montrone C, Natalicchio A, Martemucci S, Giorgino F 2003 The p66^{Shc} isoform modulates IGF-I stimulation of Akt phosphorylation in human thyroid carcinoma cells. Abstract P1-374, 85th annual meeting of the Endocrine Society, Philadelphia, PA

Eshet R, Werner H, Klinger B et al 1993 Upregulation of insulin-like growth factor-I (IGF-I) receptor gene expression in patients with reduced serum IGF-I levels. J Mol Endocrinol 10:115–120

Goldfine ID, Clawson GA, Smuckler EA, Purrello F, Vigneri F 1982 Action of insulin at the nuclear envelope. Mol Cell Biochem 48:3–14

Sasaoka T, Ishiki M, Sawa T et al 1996 Comparison of the insulin and insulin-like growth factor 1 mitogenic intracellular signaling pathways. Endocrinology 137:4427–4434

The mTOR/S6K signalling pathway: the role of the TSC1/2 tumour suppressor complex and the proto-oncogene Rheb

Takahiro Nobukini and George Thomas

Friedrich Miescher Institute, PO Box 2543, Maulbeerstrasse 66, CH-4002, Basel, Switzerland

Abstract. Gene deletion studies in mice and in *Drosophila* have shown that the 40S ribosomal protein S6 Kinases, dS6K in *Drosophila* and S6K1 and S6K2 in mice are important regulators of cell growth in response to insulin stimulation and nutrition availability. Here we chiefly focus on dS6k and S6K1, whose activities are regulated by an upstream kinase termed the mammalian target of rapamycin (mTOR, or dTOR in *Drosophila*). Our understanding of the mechanisms regulating the mTOR/S6K1-signalling pathway will be fundamental in determining the mechanisms which control cell growth in response to insulin signalling. Recent findings from this laboratory and others suggests that the tumour suppressor complex made of two proteins TSC1/hamartin and TSC2/tuberin, acts as a negative regulator of mTOR/S6K1 signalling. Mutations in either TSC1 or TSC2 are genetically linked to tuberous sclerosis complex (TSC) syndrome, which can lead to severe pathological consequences, including mental retardation, epilepsy and autism, as well as cardiac, pulmonary and renal failure. Despite a large number of initial reports on the TSC1/TSC2 complex, and the finding that its activity is regulated by protein kinase B (PKB), the direct target of the TSC1/TSC2 inhibitory complex was unknown until recently. Since TSC2 has a GTPase-activating domain, or GAP-like sequence, others and we searched for a small GTP binding protein, which may serve as the target of TSC1/TSC2 inhibitory complex. In our case we took advantage of a genome wide screen in *Drosophila* for effectors of cell growth and in parallel searched for a small GTPase whose activity is up-regulated in TSC2-deficient cells. The identified gene was a member of the Ras family of GTPases termed Ras homologue enriched in brain or Rheb. Here we review recent findings demonstrating that the TSC1/TSC2 inhibitory complex normally acts on Rheb to mediate mTOR/S6K1-signalling.

2004 Biology of IGF-1: its interaction with insulin in health and malignant states. Wiley, Chichester (Novartis Foundation Symposium 262) p 148–159

In brief, S6K1 is a Ser/Thr kinase, which was initially identified based on its ability to mediate the multiple phosphorylation of 40S ribosomal protein S6. Further studies provided evidence that the up-regulation of S6K1 was implicated in the translation and up-regulation of 5′ tandem oligo pyrimidine (TOP) mRNAs, which encode for components of the translational apparatus, most notably ribosomal proteins. This conclusion was based on the finding that a dominant interfering allele of S6K1 inhibited the mitogen-induced translational up-regulation of 5′TOP mRNAs to the same extent as rapamycin, a direct inhibitor of mTOR, whereas an activated allele of S6K1, which exhibits a substantial degree of rapamycin resistance, largely protected these transcripts from the inhibitory effects of rapamycin (Jefferies et al 1997, Schwab et al 1999). However recent studies in our group with mouse embryo fibroblasts derived from *S6k1*$^{-/-}$; *S6k2*$^{-/-}$ mice, suggest that the role of S6K1 in this response is more complicated (Pende et al 2004). Thus S6K1 is an important regulator of cell growth in response to both growth factor signalling and nutrition availability, but the mechanisms by which these effects are mediated are not yet established.

Activation of S6K1 is mediated by three critical residues; including Thr229 in the activation loop by phosphoinositide 3-dependent protein kinase 1 (PDK1) (Alessi et al 1998, Pullen et al 1998) and Ser371 (Saitoh et al 2002) and Thr389 (Burnett et al 1998, Isotani et al 1999, Dennis et al 2001) in the linker domain by mTOR. The phosphorylation of Thr229 is directly linked to kinase activation and requires phosphorylation at Thr389, which provides a docking site for PDK1 (Biondi et al 2001). Indeed, PDK1 appears to be constitutively active only requiring an acidic group at Thr229 to access the activation loop (Dennis et al 1998). Likewise, mTOR also appeared to be constitutively active (Dennis et al 2001), but was prevented from accessing Thr389 by one or more negative effectors.

Studies in *Drosophila* provided the initial evidence for such a negative effector. Genetic epistasis studies revealed that the dTsc1/2 tumour suppressor complex acted either on the dTOR/dS6K signalling pathway or on a common downstream target to control cell growth (Gao & Pan 2001, Potter et al 2001, Tapon et al 2001). Subsequent genetic and biochemical analyses showed that in the absence of either TSC1 or TSC2, S6K1 activity was constitutive and resistant to growth factor deprivation. These studies also suggested that the TSC1/2 complex either acted upstream of mTOR to inhibit kinase activity or prevented mTOR from signalling to its downstream substrates (Inoki et al 2002, Potter et al 2002, Jaeschke et al 2002, Gao et al 2002, Radimerski et al 2002a). Strikingly, earlier studies in *Drosophila* had demonstrated that dS6K acts negatively on dPKB signalling, such that dPKB activity is elevated in dS6K-deficient flies (Radimerski et al 2002b). Consistent with this finding, in dTsc1/2-deficient flies dPKB activity is suppressed and restored by removal of dS6K (Radimerski et al 2002a). As dPKB- and dTsc1/2-deficient flies die at second larval instar, it raised the possibility that dTsc1/2-deficient flies die because they have reduced dPKB activity. Indeed pharmacological or genetic reduction of mTOR/S6K1 signalling rescued dTsc1/2 deficient flies to viability (Radimerski et al 2002a) In parallel it was demonstrated that TSC2 is a direct target of PKB and that when phosphorylated, is reduced in its ability to suppress S6K1 activity, either due to its enhanced degradation (Inoki et al 2002) or reduced affinity for TSC1 (Manning et al 2002). Interestingly, Gao et al (2002) argue this is also true for amino acid signalling in both *Drosophila* and rodent cells deficient for either TSC1 or TSC2, arguing that both growth factors and amino acids converge on the TSC1/TSC2 inhibitory complex to mediate mTOR/S6K1 signalling.

We reported that TSC2-mediated suppression of S6 phosphorylation is potentiated by TSC1 and that this effect does not appear to be through inhibition of mTOR kinase activity in mammalian cells (Jaeschke et al 2002). Potentiation of the TSC2 inhibitory activity by TSC1 was also observed in *Drosophila* (Potter et al 2001, Gao & Pan 2001). Since the TSC1/TSC2 inhibitory complex may not regulate mTOR kinase activity by interacting directly to reduce its kinase activity, this raised the possibility that it exerted its inhibitory effects through a distinct signalling component. The severest forms of the TSC are associated with mutations in the C-terminus of TSC2 (Maheshwar et al 1997), which contains a domain highly homologous to Rap1 GAP (GTPase-activating protein). Although *in vitro* studies demonstrated that TSC2 has GAP activity towards Rap1, it is clear that Rap1 does not act on the mTOR/S6K1 signalling pathway. Thus we set out to search for the physiological target of TSC2.

To identify potential downstream effectors of TSC2 we took advantage of a genome wide screen in *Drosophila* in search of novel genes which effect cell proliferation or growth (Stocker et al 2003). In parallel, we searched for a small GTPase which binds elevated levels of GTP in extracts from *Tsc2*$^{-/-}$ MEFs as compared to *Tsc2*$^{+/+}$ MEFs. In the fly we took advantage of somatic recombination in the eye to screen for either positive or negative effectors of growth following treatment of flies with EMS (ethylmethane sulfonate). If the target gene is a positive regulator of growth loss-of-function would result in a pin-head phenotype (Oldham et al 2000). In a complementary gain-of-function screen, mutants were identified by random insertion of an EP element leading to specific overexpression of the target gene in the eye. In this case the enlarged eyes arise as a result of overexpression of a positive regulator of cell growth. In both screens a gene encoding a small GTPase was identified whose primary structure was most closely related to that of Rheb (Yamagata et al 1994). Although flies *trans*-heterozygous for Rheb EMS mutants were lethal, a *trans*-heterozygous line containing a Rheb EMS mutation and an imprecise EP excision produced a few flies that were dramatically reduced in body size. In contrast, targeted overexpression of Rheb in larvae endoreplicative tissues under conditions of amino acid deprivation resulted in an increase in size as compared to non-overexpressing cells.

Biochemical and genetic approaches were employed to determine whether dRheb acted on the dTOR/dS6K-signalling pathway and whether it was epistatic to dTsc1/2. Initially, dS6K activity was measured in larval extracts of dRheb mutants. In all of the *trans*-heterozygous combinations of EMS mutants examined, dS6K activity was dramatically reduced. Moreover, dRheb overexpression, driven by a heatshock promoter, resulted in activation of dS6K. Furthermore, dPKB activity was elevated in dRheb mutant larvae, whereas it was suppressed in larvae overexpressing dRheb (Stocker et al 2003), in agreement with dTsc1/2-deficient larvae having reduced dPKB activity (Radimerski et al 2002a). These findings were also compatible with the involvement of dRheb acting in the negative feedback loop to down-regulate dPKB activity through dS6K. In parallel, analysis in the eye of different genetic combinations of dRheb with specific components of dPI3K and dTOR signalling pathways revealed that enlarged ommatidia size, caused by Rheb overexpression, was reversed by overexpression of dTsc1/2 but not by dPten. Likewise, in a dS6K$^{-/-}$ or dTOR$^{-/+}$ background, but not in a dPKB$^{-/-}$ background, the Rheb overexpression phenotype was reversed, suggesting that dRheb function depends on dTOR and dS6K activity. Consistent with these findings dRheb was found to be epistatic over dTsc1/2, as the small eye phenotype of dRheb$^{-/-}$ mutants was not reversed by dTsc1/2 deficiency. These results argue that dRheb is a target of dTsc1/2, acting to control dTOR activity, but independent of dPI3K signalling in agreement with an earlier report that dPI3K and dTOR pathways are acting independently in *Drosophila* to control cell growth (Montagne et al 2001, Radimerski et al 2002a,b).

As mentioned above, in a second parallel approach to identify a small GTPase, we determined whether the GTP-bound form of any small GTPases, including Rheb, was elevated in *Tsc2*$^{-/-}$ MEFs (Garami et al 2003). GTP-bound GTPases were pulled-down employing activation-specific probes, GST fusion proteins containing the downstream GTPase target proteins (van Triest et al 2001). The results of such an analysis showed that there was no difference in the level of Ras, Ral or Rap2 bound GTP in *Tsc2*$^{-/-}$ MEFs as compared to *Tsc2*$^{+/+}$ MEFs. In parallel, we also attempted to pull down Rheb employing these same probes, including a GST fusion protein that contains the Ras binding domain of Raf1 (GST-RBD). These findings were inconclusive, apparently due to low affinity of Rheb for the RBD of Raf1 resulting from its markedly divergent effector region. However, consistent with the analysis in *Drosophila*, immunoprecipitated Rheb, but not Ras, had much higher activity in *Tsc2*$^{-/-}$ MEFs. This was confirmed in ectopic co-expression experiments of TSC1/2 together with Rheb in COS-7 cells. Although TSC1 alone did not have any impact on Rheb activity judged by GTP loading, TSC2 increased the amount of Rheb in the GDP bound state, an effect that was further potentiated by TSC1. Moreover the effect was specific, as co-expression of TSC1/2 had no effect on Rap2. These observations are consistent with the model that TSC2 is a GAP for Rheb. This was also in good agreement with our previous observation, that maximal suppression of S6K1 by TSC2 requires TSC1.

To determine whether Rheb also participates in regulation of S6Ks in mammalian systems as it does in *Drosophila*, we co-expressed Rheb ectopically with S6K1 and S6K2. The results showed that Rheb induced both S6K1 and S6K2 Thr389 phosphorylation to the same extent as insulin, although it had no effect on MAP kinase activation as previously reported (Im et al 2002). Also consistent with the observations in *Drosophila* (Radimerski et al 2002a), both basal and insulin stimulated PKB activity were down-regulated in cells in which Rheb was ectopically expressed (Garami et al 2003). If insulin stimulation leads to PI3K activation that relieves repression of S6K1 by repressing the GAP activity of TSC2, this should result in an increase in the GTP-bound form of Rheb. In agreement with this model, endogenous Rheb activity increased 1.8-fold after stimulation with insulin in A14 NIH 3T3. This stimulation was reversed by the treatment with a PI3K inhibitor, wortmannin, but not by an mTOR inhibitor, rapamycin. These observations argue that Rheb acts either upstream of mTOR or interferes with the ability of mTOR to signal, but downstream of PI3K in mammalian tissue.

If Rheb is upstream of mTOR or interferes with the ability of mTOR to signal, a second target of mTOR, such as 4E-BP1, might be expected to be effected in a similar manner to the S6Ks. The results of such an experiment showed that 4E-BP1 Thr70 phosphorylation, a target of mTOR (Gingras et al 1999), was also increased when 4E-BP1 was co-expressed with Rheb (Garami et al 2003). Consistent with these findings, rapamycin but not wortmannin counteracted activation of S6K1 by Rheb overexpression. Moreover, specific siRNAs to Rheb knocked down Rheb protein levels and in parallel lowered insulin-induced S6K1 Thr389 phosphorylation, arguing that insulin mediates S6K1 activation through Rheb. Amino acid withdrawal also eliminated insulin stimulation of S6K1, but did not have an impact on Rheb-induced S6K1 activation. In contrast to amino acids, 2-deoxyglucose (2-DG), which decreases intracellular ATP content, still had a negative impact on S6K1 activity in the presence of ectopically expressed Rheb. These results suggest that amino acids act on S6K1 through Rheb, but that ATP regulation of mTOR is not through Rheb. In fact, the latter finding is compatible with our earlier report, indicating that mTOR directly senses intracellular ATP concentrations (Dennis et al 2001).

Since the severest forms of TSC are associated with mutations at the C-terminus of TSC2, this raised the possibility that such mutations may alter GAP activity of TSC2. Indeed, when such a TSC2 mutant, associated with the human disease, was co-expressed with TSC1 it failed to increase the amount of the GDP-bound form of

Rheb, in contrast to wild-type TSC2. Consistent with this finding it also failed to block the ability of Rheb to activate S6K1. Taken together these studies demonstrate that Rheb is a physiological target of TSC2 both in *Drosophila* and in mammals, and that Rheb mediates the insulin signal to control the mTOR/S6K1 signalling pathway. Moreover, if the mutations in TSC patients are activating Rheb to cause the disease, rapamycin and its analogues may be powerful clinical tools.

References

Abraham RT 2002 Identification of TOR signaling complexes: more TORC for the cell growth engine. Cell 111:9–12

Alessi DR, Kozlowski MT, Weng QP, Morrice N, Avruch J 1998 3-Phosphoinositide-dependent protein kinase 1 (PDK1) phosphorylates and activates the p70 S6 kinase in vivo and in vitro. Curr Biol 8:69–81

Biondi RM, Kieloch A, Currie RA, Deak M, Alessi DR 2001 The PIF-binding pocket in PDK1 is essential for activation of S6K and SGK, but not PKB. EMBO J 20:4380–4390

Burnett PE, Barrow RK, Cohen N, Snyder SH, Sabatini DM 1998 RAFT1 Phosphorylation of the Translational Regulators p70 S6 Kinase and 4E-BP1. Proc Natl Acad Sci USA 95: 1432–1437

Dennis PB, Pullen N, Pearson RB, Kozma SC, Thomas G 1998 Phosphorylation sites in the autoinhibitory domain participate in p70s6k activation loop phosphorylation. J Biol Chem 273:14845–14852

Dennis PB, Jaeschke A, Saitoh M et al 2001 Mammalian TOR: a homeostatic ATP sensor. Science 294:1102–1105

Gao X, Pan D 2001 TSC1 and TSC2 tumor suppressors antagonize insulin signaling in cell growth. Genes Dev 15:1383–1392

Gao X, Zhang Y, Arrazola P et al 2002 Tsc tumour suppressor proteins antagonize amino-acid-TOR signalling. Nat Cell Biol 4:699–704

Garami A, Zwartkruis FJ, Nobukuni T et al 2003 Insulin activation of Rheb, a mediator of mTOR/S6K/4E-BP signaling, is inhibited by TSC1 and 2. Mol Cell 11:1457–1466

Gingras AC, Gygi SP, Raught B et al 1999 Regulation of 4E-BP1 phosphorylation: a novel two-step mechanism. Genes Dev 13:1422–1437

Im E, von Lintig FC, Chen J et al 2002 Rheb is in a high activation state and inhibits B-Raf kinase in mammalian cells. Oncogene 21:6356–6365

Inoki K, Li Y, Zhu T, Wu J, Guan KL 2002 TSC2 is phosphorylated and inhibited by Akt and suppresses mTOR signalling. Nat Cell Biol 4:648–657

Isotani S, Hara K, Tokunaga C et al 1999 Immunopurified mammalian target of rapamycin phosphorylates and activates p70 S6 kinase alpha in vitro. J Biol Chem 274:34493–34498

Jaeschke A, Hartkamp J, Saitoh M et al 2002 Tuberous sclerosis complex tumor suppressor-mediated S6 kinase inhibition by phosphatidylinositide-3-OH kinase is mTOR independent. J Cell Biol 159:217–224

Jefferies HBJ, Fumagalli S, Dennis PB et al 1997 Rapamycin suppresses 5′TOP mRNA translation through inhibition of p70s6k. EMBO J 12:3693–3704

Maheshwar MM, Cheadle JP, Jones AC et al 1997 The GAP-related domain of tuberin, the product of the TSC2 gene, is a target for missense mutations in tuberous sclerosis. Hum Mol Genet 6:1991–1996

Manning BD, Tee AR, Logsdon MN, Blenis J, Cantley LC 2002 Identification of the tuberous sclerosis complex-2 tumor suppressor gene product tuberin as a target of the phosphoinositide 3-kinase/akt pathway. Mol Cell 10:151–162

Montagne J, Radimerski T, Thomas G 2001 Insulin signaling: lessons from the Drosophila tuberous sclerosis complex, a tumor suppressor. Sci STKE 105:PE36

Oldham S, Montagne J, Radimerski T, Thomas G, Hafen E 2000 Genetic and biochemical characterization of dTOR, the Drosophila homolog of the target of rapamycin. Genes Dev 14:2689–2694

Pende M, Um S-H, Mieulet V et al 2004 $S6K1^{-/-}/S6K2^{-/-}$ mice exhibit perinatal lethality, rapamycin sensitive 5′TOP mRNA translation, and uncover a MAP kinase-dependent S6 kinase pathway. Mol Cell Biol 24:3112–3124

Potter CJ, Huang H, Xu T 2001 Drosophila tsc1 functions with tsc2 to antagonize insulin signaling in regulating cell growth, cell proliferation, and organ size. Cell 105:357–368

Potter CJ, Pedraza LG, Xu T 2002 Akt regulates growth by directly phosphorylating Tsc2. Nat Cell Biol 4:658–665

Pullen N, Dennis PB, Andjelkovic M et al 1998 Phosphorylation and activation of p70s6k by PDK1. Science 279:707–710

Radimerski T, Montagne J, Hemmings-Mieszczak M, Thomas G 2002a Lethality of Drosophila lacking TSC tumor suppressor function rescued by reducing dS6K signaling. Genes Dev 16:2627–2632

Radimerski T, Montagne J, Rintelen F et al 2002b dS6K-regulated cell growth is dPKB/dPI(3)K-independent, but requires dPDK1. Nat Cell Biol 4:251–255

Saitoh M, Pullen N, Brennan P, Cantrell B, Dennis PB, Thomas G 2002 Regulation of an activated S6K1 variant reveals a novel mTOR phosphorylation site. J Biol Chem 277:20104–20112

Schwab MS, Kim SH, Terada N et al 1999 p70(S6K) controls selective mRNA translation during oocyte maturation and early embryogenesis in xenopus laevis. Mol Cell Biol 19:2485–2494

Stocker H, Radimerski T, Schindelholz B et al 2003 Rheb is an essential regulator of S6 kinase in the control of cell growth in Drosophila. Nat Cell Biol 5:559–565

Tapon N, Ito N, Dickson BJ, Treisman JE, Hariharan IK 2001 The Drosophila tuberous sclerosis complex gene homologs restrict cell growth and cell proliferation. Cell 105:345–355

van Triest M, de Rooij J, Bos JL 2001 Measurement of GTP-bound Ras-like GTPases by activation-specific probes. Methods Enzymol 333:343–348

DISCUSSION

Roberts: I have a technical question. Early on you suggested that S6K action is going to regulate the activity of a very specific set of proteins. So why is rapamycin often used as a general global inhibitor of Cap-dependent translation?

Thomas: Because rapamycin also knocks out mTOR activity and blocks phosphorylation of 4E-BP1. 4E-BP1 is a repressor of initiation factor 4E. 4E is involved in regulating the expression of mRNAs with long 5′ UTRs. It is required more for these than ones that have short UTRs. The reason is that you have to unwind the secondary structure of these messages. But in the case of 4E-BP1 it doesn't look as if the phosphorylation is sufficient. It looks like it is also regulating levels of 4E-BP1, which might also be important in terms of titrating out 4E activity. In fact, some tumours are arising that are rapamycin resistant and have elevated levels of 4E-BP1. This suggests they could circumvent the effects of rapamycin. If you look at a lot of cell types and global translation, rapamycin has very selective effects.

Pollak: What do you know about the tissue specificity of a conventional immunosuppressive dose of rapamycin, where action on lymphocytes is important? What is being perturbed in other cell lineages?

Thomas: mTOR is ubiquitously expressed. I have never done an organ Northern blot so I can't say this for sure, but it seems to be everywhere. This is an ancient system: a recent paper (Matsuo et al 2003) showed that in *Schizosaccharomyces pombe* this ancient triad of TOR/PDK1 and a protein called Gad8, an S6K orthologue are present. They also showed that Tor will phosporylate all the same conserved sites in Gad8 as it does in S6K1. This is a nutrient-sensing pathway that has been out there forever. So what happens when we give rapamycin as an immunosuppressant reagent? We see very strong effects on translation of certain transcripts, but they are not dominant. If I take 3T3 cells and add rapamycin I suppress the translation of 5′TOP messages, but I don't abolish it. There is a decrease in G1 but then the cells progress through the cell cycle. It appears that there are other mechanisms that can operate. Maybe it is just global translation which is sufficient. In T cells, rapamycin blocks interleukin (IL)2 signalling. There, we have to up-regulate ribosome biogenesis tremendously. There we totally abolish the up-regulation of 5′TOP messages. They are completely dependent on this pathway in T cells. If you can't make ribosomes you are not going to grow and proliferate. It also works in smooth muscle cells, which is why it has been used to coat stents, blocking the chronic invasion of muscle cells into the stent. For tumours it turns out that you don't need these kinds of doses, because rapamycin stays around for a long time. My naïve interpretation has always been that T cells are turning over very rapidly but the tumour isn't, so you don't need weekly doses for efficacious treatment of solid tumours. It appears that the mTOR pathway might also be driving angiogenesis. TOR will regulate HIF-1α which will regulate vascular endothelial growth factor (VEGF) expression (Semenza 2000). Down-regulating TSC up-regulates VEGF expression and drives angiogenesis. There are no gross side effects at the doses given to patients.

Pollak: In terms of looking without a microscope, if you give the immunosuppressive doses the dominant effect is on the IL2-driven pathway.

Thomas: That is why it works well with cyclosporine, which acts on a different pathway.

Pollak: To my knowledge, people haven't excluded more subtle effects. There is no gross toxicity, but we don't know for sure that there are no subtle effects on cell turnover or other parameters which might be measured.

Thomas: Now that we have an efficacious drug, we will start to see these things emerging.

Zick: Are you implying that the TSCs act as the GAPs of RheB?

Thomas: Yes.

Zick: So what is the exchange factor that stimulates it?

Thomas: We have some candidates. Several years ago we began to take advantage of *Drosophila* for doing genetic screens. As an aside, when I was a student I had Don Lindsay as an instructor, who wrote many *Drosophila* books: he bored me to death because he was always talking about loci which didn't interest me at the time. We did a screen, and we sat down with a bioinformatician picking up all the potential guanine nucleotide exchange factors (GEFs), making double stranded RNA for all of them. We then used S6K as a reporter and started knocking them all down. We have picked up a couple of potential GEFs.

LeRoith: Could you expand on this question of the feedback? In cases of insulin resistance we often get some pathways blocked and others that are not. Draznin has shown that blocking the PI3K up-regulates the MAPK, making it more sensitive to mitogens. His theory is that this may explain why in endothelial cells insulin can potentiate mitogens and cause vascular changes. There is evidence in liver that insulin resistance can cause the lack of insulin-stimulated gene expression or some genes can be affected while gluconeogenesis may not be affected. There is a divergent pathway in insulin-resistant states. In this case, PI3K could be blocked by the nutritional effects. Would you see this as blocking the PI3K pathway and allowing other pathways to remain open? Could this also be an explanation for some of the divergences in insulin resistance where some pathways are still active and others are blocked?

Zick: I would argue that if you block the PI3K pathway you could end up shutting down insulin signalling.

LeRoith: That is, insulin signalling to one mechanism.

Zick: Yes, through the glucose transport mechanism and through other various key pathways. If PI3K is blocked we assume PKB is blocked and all its downstream effectors. This would be a major cause of insulin resistance. On the other hand, in a very minute manner you relieve what we call the feedback loops that emanate downstream of the PI3K. But this is only secondary to the major block of the pathway itself that is basically mediating the insulin resistance. Only when you block PI3K pathway induction of resistance is obvious. I wanted to deviate slightly from your question and get back to data published by Jerry Olefsky, Kanety and others, where they demonstrated that it is possible to induce insulin resistance by activating other growth factors, such as the EGF receptor (Hemi et al 2002). They did studies in endothelial cells in which they stimulated the PI3K pathway, the kinase that phosphorylates elements of the insulin signalling pathway. So you shut down insulin action at the expense of promoting PDGF action at that particular set-up. If I can speculate, this probably applies for any other pathway that impinges on the PI3K pathway, activating downstream kinases that will then feed back and switch off insulin action. The balance of the signalling is therefore shifted from more metabolic effects towards growth-promoting effects.

LeRoith: So the outcome may be similar, but it is basically blocking the metabolic pathway which is maintaining the mitogenic pathway.

Zick: You mentioned in passing that mTor is regulated by nutrition, for example by amino acids and ATP. Could you elaborate on this?

Thomas: A few years ago we showed that ATP and amino acids regulate differentially (Dennis et al 2001). We came up with this idea because ribosome biogenesis in *Escherichia coli* is regulated differentially by amino acids and by energy. If you take away amino acids you block tRNA charging. If you change the ATP:ADP ratio you block the equivalent of the Pol1 rRNA polymerase, which will continue to elongate but can no longer initiate. We showed that if you take away amino acids you shut down S6K. There is no effect on ATP levels. If you lower ATP levels there is no effect on amino acid levels but you still shut down S6K in both cases. It is a nice story. We had pulled out this unusual 389 site in S6K which is present in all the second messenger family protein kinases, including PKB. It is a critical site of regulation. We identified this site a few years ago through a lot of hard slogging, and at the time we didn't believe it because it wasn't thought to be a phosphorylation site, but we found out that it was. We got together with Stuart Schreiber who had just cloned mTOR at the time, we exchanged reagents and neither one of us obtained phosphorylation. Three years later David Sabatini showed that he could get a small effect. Then everyone went back and tried to reproduce this, but they couldn't get it to go. We tried it and found a trivial reaction, so we didn't think it was real. Then the postdoc in my lab tried a new phosphospecific antibody and saw phosphorylation. This suggested to us that potentially it was regulated by ATP. We are being challenged at this level because Yonezawa in Nishizuka's institute in Japan showed in a two-hybrid screen that AMP-dependent kinase was associated with mTOR and used things like AICAR to show that they also regulate S6K activity. He argued that all the ATP effects we were seeing were through the AMP-dependent kinase. We have gone back and re-evaluated these data and found that he did one thing differently to us. He added 2-deoxyglucose and took away glucose, whereas we just added 2-deoxyglucose. When we add 2-deoxyglucose we don't see any effect; we have to take a lot of glucose away. The ATP effects that we see require just a small change in total ATP levels. The K_m we measured is around 2 mM for S6K, and it is similar for other family members. It appears that there might be two levels of regulation, through the AMP-dependent kinase and through direct effects of ATP sensing. In addition, it looks like amino acids and ATP are coming in from the side, not upstream of TSC. These amino acids affect the ability of mTOR to form a complex with Raptor. Raptor is required to interact with the substrates downstream. If you take out amino acids this stops Raptor from associating with mTOR properly.

LeRoith: When Avruch and the others discovered Raptor a few years ago they thought it might be a scaffold protein. Is that still what it is considered to be?

Thomas: In S6K and 4BP1 there is a domain called the TOS domain, which is required for the interaction for Raptor. When Raptor associates with Tor it allows Tor to interact with substrates downstream. It looks like this is what amino acids and ATP are regulating: they are regulating the ability of mTOR to associate with Raptor, which then allows it to signal downstream. All the TSC stuff appears to be on the growth factor side. We did an experiment recently in which we overexpressed Rheb, the small GTPase, and blocked the effects of amino acid deprivation. This would argue against what I just said. But we are thinking we are over-driving the growth pathway by this overexpression, which is driving the growth. We are now at a point where we are using siRNA to take out Rheb and ask whether we block the amino acid response. If we do block it then we have already separated TSC, which suggests there is another GAP or there is a GEF involved.

Kaaks: I have a more general comment. I am fascinated by what you have told us about mTOR. It seems that both insulin and IGF play a very important role in the energy metabolism of the organism and of cells, and in regulating anabolic processes as a function of available energy and nutrients. This concept of nutrient sensing in the cell being needed for mTOR signalling and mitogenesis is fascinating. There is a similar issue in that fatty acid synthesis is usually overexpressed in tumour cells, and this is a pathway that is strongly influenced by insulin. In the cell there seems to be a number of checkpoints between the anabolic pathways and all the machinery that regulates cell proliferation and growth. A recent discovery is that the acetyl-coA carboxylase, which catalyses the first step in fatty acid synthesis from ACoA specifically co-precipitates with the breast cancer 1 protein (BRCA1) product. No one knows exactly what this means, but it suggests a link between these anabolic pathways and cell proliferation. It is a very interesting concept to think about in a broad sense. We have been talking very much about how the signalling of insulin and IGF may lead to cancer promotion. However, it seems that there is more to it: the energy status of the cell itself and the nutrient and energy sensing within the cell that interacts with this. I also wonder whether this might be a fruitful area for research in the future. It might be worth re-doing some energy restriction studies in animals. This is one of most strongly established protective nutritional factors against cancer development. There are similar data on protein restriction. It could be interesting to make transgenic mice or other animals with specific knockouts of some of the elements in pathways that we have just heard about, and to do caloric restriction studies again. This could tell us about the effects at the cellular level of nutrient and energy availability, signalling through IGF and insulin receptors, and tumour development. Likewise, from a more epidemiological perspective, we have tried to do a few studies on a candidate gene basis to see whether there are naturally occurring polymorphisms in genes that would show associations shedding some light on this type of question.

De Meyts: There are recent papers by Paolisso's group showing polymorphisms in the insulin/IGF-1 signalling pathways being associated with centenarians (Barbieri et al 2003).

Ohlsson: We have earlier discussed the link between height and the risk of cancer. I don't know how many of you are familiar with Marcus Pembrey's hypothesis, where he is arguing that increased height during the last century involves epigenetic memory. In other words, if your ancestral generation enjoyed a good nutritional status, there is a higher likelihood of being taller yourself. When one makes this kind of analysis the offspring to parent increase rather than taking the overall height, should be considered.

Clark: Can you argue that the epidemic of obesity will be exaggerated by the same mechanism?

Ohlsson: Perhaps.

Clark: That's not a good thought.

References

Barbieri M, Bonafé M, Franceschi C, Paolisso G 2003 Insulin/IGF-I signalling pathway: an evolutionarily conserved mechanism of longevity from yeast to man. Am J Physiol Endocrinol Metab 285:E1064–E1071

Dennis PB, Jaeschke A, Saitoh M, Fowler B, Kozma SC, Thomas G 2001 Mammalian TOR: a homeostatic ATP sensor. Science 294:1102–1105

Hemi R, Paz K, Wertheim N, Karasik A, Zick Y, Kanety H 2002 Transactivation of ErbB2 and ErbB3 by tumor necrosis factor-alpha and anisomycin leads to impaired insulin signaling through serine/threonine phosphorylation of IRS proteins J Biol Chem 277:8961–8969

Matsuo T, Kubo Y, Watanabe Y, Yamamoto M 2003 *Schizosaccharomyces pombe* AGC family kinase Gad8p forms a conserved signaling module with TOR and PDK1-like kinases. EMBO J 22:3073–3083

Semenza GL 2000 HIF-1 and human disease: one highly involved factor. Genes Devel 14: 1983–1991

Structural biology of insulin and IGF-1 receptors

Pierre De Meyts, Jane Palsgaard, Waseem Sajid, Anne-Mette Theede and Hassan Aladdin

Receptor Biology Laboratory, Hagedorn Research Institute, Niels Steensens Vej 6, DK-2820 Gentofte, Denmark

Abstract. The insulin and IGF-1 receptors are members of the superfamily of receptor tyrosine kinases (RTKs). Many of these have been implicated in human cancers due to amplification, overexpression or somatic mutations of the gene. Congenital mutations of the RTKs are implicated in a growing number of inherited syndromes. Unlike most RTKs that are single-chain monomeric transmembrane polypeptides, the insulin and IGF-1 receptors are dimers made of two extracellular α subunits and two transmembrane β subunits containing the tyrosine kinase domain. The α subunits contain the ligand binding sites, of which at least three subdomains have been mapped by photoaffinity cross-linking, alanine-scanning mutagenesis or minimized receptor constructs. All RTKs are dimeric or oligomeric in the ligand-activated form, a mechanism that allows for transphosphorylation of the kinase domains and triggers the signalling cascade. The residues of insulin involved in receptor binding have been mapped by alanine-scanning mutagenesis. They form at least two major epitopes that partially overlap with the dimer- and hexamer-forming surfaces of the insulin molecule, and we propose that insulin is using those surfaces to cross-link the receptor α subunits. This mechanism provides a structural basis for negative cooperativity in binding, and probably also operates in the IGF–receptor interaction.

2004 Biology of IGF-1: its interaction with insulin in health and malignant states. Wiley, Chichester (Novartis Foundation Symposium 262) p 160–176

The insulin peptide family members and their receptors

Insulin and the insulin-like growth factors (IGF)-1 and -2 belong to a phylogenetically ancient family of peptide hormones and growth factors that play a fundamental role in the control of essential cellular and physiological processes such as the cell cycle, survival or apoptosis, cell migration, proliferation, differentiation, body growth, metabolism, reproduction and longevity (Barbieri et al 2003). These factors in humans comprise ten members, the closely related insulin and insulin-like growth factors (IGF)-1 and -2, and seven peptides related to relaxin (INSL/RLFs). While insulin and the IGFs bind to receptors that are part of the superfamily of receptor tyrosine kinases (RTKs), the relaxin-like peptides were recently shown to bind to leucine-rich repeat-containing G protein-coupled receptors (LGRs) (Hsu 2003), which are involved in the development and physiology of the reproductive tract.

The RTK superfamily comprises ~60 members distributed into ~20 subfamilies depending on the modular architecture of their extracellular domains and the degree of identity in their intracellular tyrosine kinase domains (Fig. 1). The importance of these receptors is demonstrated by the discovery of a growing number of congenital genetic syndromes linked to gain-of-function (constitutive activation) or loss-of-function (inactive or dominant-negative receptor) mutations (Robertson et al 2000).

Some of the RTKs are oncogenes (Blume-Jensen & Hunter 2001) and at least a dozen of the RTK families, including the IGF-1 and insulin receptors (Blume-Jensen & Hunter 2001, Gray et al 2003, and other chapters in this volume) have been implicated in human cancers due to amplification, overexpression, loss of parental imprinting or somatic gene mutations. Consequently, RTKs are much hunted targets for anticancer therapy (Brunelleschi et al 2002, Drevs et al 2003, Levitzki 2002, Zwick et al 2002, Macaulay 2004, this volume).

Structure of insulin and IGF-1 receptors

The insulin and IGF-1 receptors differ from the other receptors in the RTK family (which are single transmembrane polypeptides, Fig. 1) in that they have a covalent dimeric $\alpha_2\beta_2$ structure, although all the RTKs dimerize or oligomerize upon ligand binding (Heldin & Ostman 1996), resulting in activation of the kinase by transphosphorylation.

The insulin receptor gene has a modular structure with 22 exons (Fig. 2) and 21 introns (Seino et al 1989). The receptors are synthesized as a single chain preproreceptor which is cleaved to yield the mature receptor. Exon 11 is alternatively spliced, resulting in two isoforms (A and B) differing by the absence or presence of a 12-residue sequence (717–729) (Seino & Bell 1989). The two isoforms differ slightly in affinity for insulin, but the A isoform has significantly higher affinity for IGF-1 and IGF-2 (Frasca et al 1999).

Insulin and the IGFs bind with low affinity to the non-cognate receptor. In cells expressing both insulin and IGF-1 receptors, heterodimeric hybrid receptors are formed consisting of one half of each, which bind IGF-1 with high affinity and insulin with low affinity (Soos et al 1993). Their physiological role is unknown.

The α-subunit features successively two homologous globular domains L1 and L2 (1–158 and 309–469) separated by a cysteine-rich region. These are followed by three fibronectin type III domains (Fn_{0-2}), the middle one being split by an insert of unknown structure which comprises the C-terminal portion of the α-subunit and the N-terminal portion of the β-subunit (see De Meyts & Whittaker 2002 for review).

The intracellular portion of the β-subunit contains the kinase catalytic domain (980–1255) flanked by two regulatory regions, a juxtamembrane region involved in docking insulin receptor substrates (IRS) 1–4 and Shc as well as in receptor internalization, and a C-terminal tail containing two phosphotyrosine binding sites.

The details of the modular structure and overall organization of the insulin receptor are shown in Fig. 2. The IGF-1 receptor has a very similar organization with sequence homology varying from 41% to 84% depending on the domain, maximal in the kinase domain (see Adams et al 2000 for details).

The three-dimensional (3D) structure of the L1/Cys-rich/L2 (L1-CR-L2) domain fragment (amino acids 1–460) of the IGF-1 receptor (which by itself does not bind the ligand) has been solved (Adams et al 2000, Garrett et al 1998) (Fig. 4). The 3D structures of the tyrosine kinase domain of the insulin receptor, both in the inactive (unphosphorylated) (Hubbard et al 1994) and in the active state (Hubbard 1997) have also been determined (Figs 1 and 3). The structure of the activated IGF-1 receptor kinase has also been solved (Favelyukis et al 2001). The structures have revealed a novel autoinhibition mechanism, described in Fig. 3, whereby an 'activation loop' behaves as a pseudosubstrate that blocks the active site in the basal state (closed configuration) and is stabilized in an open position upon transphosphorylation.

Recent reports by Yip, Ottensmeyer and colleagues (reviewed in Yip & Ottensmeyer 2003) based on cryoelectron microscopy have revealed an overall globular envelope for the insulin receptor complex. The details of a proposed structural fit of the insulin receptor complex within this envelope have been questioned (De Meyts & Whittaker 2002).

Ligand binding properties

The binding of insulin to its receptor is complex (reviewed in De Meyts 1994). Scatchard plots are curvilinear, indicating the coexistence of high and low affinity binding sites. The dissociation rate of prebound ligand is accelerated by the presence of unlabelled ligand even in an 'infinite' dilution, indicating the existence of negative cooperativity between binding sites. Dose–response curves for this accelerated dissociation are bell-shaped (self-antagonism) with a loss of the dissociation acceleration at insulin concentrations over 100 nM. IGF-1 binding to its receptor shows a similar phenomenology, except that the dose–response curve for accelerated dissociation is sigmoid with no loss at high concentration (Christoffersen et al 1994).

The intact insulin receptor (holoreceptor) binds only one insulin molecule with high affinity, but after reduction of the disulfide bridges, each half receptor remains capable of binding insulin, but only with low affinity. Interestingly, a secreted soluble insulin receptor ectodomain binds insulin with low affinity and lack of negative cooperativity, showing a linear Scatchard plot and a stoichiometry of two insulins bound per receptor dimer, unless the two β subunits are fastened by dimeric IgG constant domains, leucine zippers or include the transmembrane domains. These data (reviewed in De Meyts & Whittaker 2002) show that each $\alpha\beta$ half of the receptor contain partial binding sites for insulin, but cooperation between the two receptor halves is required to create one high affinity binding complex.

Valuable information has also been generated by constructing various monomeric or dimeric minimized receptor constructs in which modules from the insulin receptor extracellular domain have been deleted, with the aims of mapping domains essential for ligand binding as well as obtaining minimized receptor structures more amenable to crystallization (see e.g. Brandt et al 2001, Surinya et al 2002, reviewed in De Meyts & Whittaker 2002).

Mapping of the receptor binding sites on insulin and IGF-1

There has been a consensus for many years that a number of surface residues that have been widely conserved during the evolution of vertebrates are involved in receptor binding: Gly A1, Gln A5, Tyr A19, Asn 21, Val B12, Tyr B16, Gly B23, Phe B24, Phe B25, Tyr B26 ('classical binding surface' [Fig. 4], which overlaps with insulin's dimerization interface) (Pullen et al 1976). A subset of residues from this surface (A21, B23–26) is essential for negative cooperativity (De Meyts et al 1978). In addition, Ile A2 and Val A3 (a residue mutated to Leu in a diabetic patient: insulin Wakayama), which are not on the surface of the molecule, probably become exposed and interact with the receptor upon displacement of the B-chain C-terminus during the receptor binding process (Hua et al 1991, Ludvigsen et al 1998).

However, the concept that the invariant classic binding surface contains the main determinants for receptor binding has been challenged by the fact that hagfish insulin, despite absolute conservation of the classical binding surface and a crystal structure very identical to that of human insulin, shows aberrant binding properties when compared to most vertebrate insulins. Hagfish insulin shows a very slow association rate, a slower dissociation rate than human insulin, a reduced negative cooperativity with a sigmoid rather than bell-shaped dose–response curve (like IGF-1), and an enhanced mitogenic/metabolic potency ratio (De Meyts 1994, Holst 2000). These properties are shared by the insulins from hystricomorphs, a sub-order of mammals that have an accepted rate of mutation

50 times higher than other mammals in the insulin molecule. Most of the mutations are outside of the classic binding surface (De Meyts 1994, Piron 1981). In contrast, guinea-pig IGF-1 is strictly identical to human. Altogether, these data strongly suggest that residues outside the classical binding surface must contact the receptor (De Meyts 1994). This concept was validated by the fact that insulin analogues with mutations at two residues in the hexamer-forming surface, Leu A13 to Ser and Leu B17 to Gln, bind to the receptor with characteristics similar to hagfish and hystricomorph insulins (De Meyts 1994, Schäffer 1994).

These findings prompted a reexamination of the structure–function relationship of insulin by alanine scanning mutagenesis. Kristensen et al determined the impact of alanine mutations on the low affinity component of insulin binding to the soluble receptor ectodomain fused to the IgG fusion protein (Kristensen et al 1997) and showed that the residues from the classical binding surface A2, A19, B23 and B24 were most disruptive of binding, as well as B13. Mutations at B6 and B8 were also disruptive, probably due to conformational alterations. Others have shown that mutation of A3 (Nakagawa & Tager 1992; H. Aladdin, P. De Meyts, unpublished data 2003) and B12 (Nakagawa et al 2000) to Ala is also very disruptive. Since only the low affinity which primarily reflects binding of the classical binding surface (Schäffer 1994) was tested, involvement of A13 and B17 was not confirmed in Kristensen et al (1997). This shows that the classic binding surface is sufficient for low affinity binding but not for high affinity binding. We have then used the high affinity cell-bound receptor on IM-9 human lymphocytes to test the affinity of the alanine mutants. We confirmed the importance of the classic binding surface, but also mapped a new binding surface that overlaps with insulin's hexamerization surface and comprises Ser A12, Leu A13, Glu A17, His B10, Glu B13 and Leu B17 (Jensen 2001). Therefore, it appears, not surprisingly for a small compact molecule like insulin, that it uses more or less the same functional surfaces for receptor binding as for self-aggregation.

Moreover, we recently showed by introducing substitutions from hystricomorph (Palsgaard 2003) or hagfish (W. Sajid, A. S. Andersen, P. De Meyts, unpublished data 2003) insulins into human insulin, alone or in combination, that the aberrant behaviour of these species is largely explained by a small number of deleterious mutations in the novel binding surface.

The structure-function relationships of the IGF-1 and -2 molecules have not been as extensively mapped as insulin's (see Van den Brande 1992 and Adams et al 2000 for detailed review). Unlike insulin, the IGFs conserve a permanent C-peptide and feature a D-peptide extension at the C-terminus. 3D structures have been determined (Brzozowski et al 2002, Vajdos et al 2001). Mutagenesis of IGF-1 has shown Ala 8, Asp 12, Phe 23 and Tyr 24 in the B domain, Tyr 31, Arg 36, Arg 37 in the C-peptide and Met 59, Tyr 60 and Ala 62 in the A domain to be important for high affinity binding to the IGF-1 receptor (Fig. 4).

In addition, a patient with a dwarfism phenotype due to a homozygous missense mutation at the highly conserved Val 44 (to Met) has recently been found (Walenkamp et al 2003). This position is homologous to insulin's Val A3 mutated in the diabetic patient with insulin Wakayama, suggesting that this amino acid is critical for receptor binding of both ligands (the affinity of both mutants for their respective receptor is reduced to less than 1%). The phenotype of the IGF-1 mutant patient is comparable to that of a patient with a partial IGF-1 gene deletion (Woods et al 2000).

Removal of the D domain of IGF-1 had no effect on IGF-1 receptor binding. In contrast, the C-peptide plays a major role. Interestingly, a chimeric molecule with the A and B chains of insulin fused to the IGF-1 C-peptide (ICP) binds with high affinity to both insulin and IGF-1 receptors, while proinsulin's C-peptide causes a 20-fold drop in affinity for the insulin receptor (Kristensen et al 1995).

Mapping of the ligand binding sites on the insulin and IGF-1 receptors

Various approaches have been used to map putative ligand contact sites on the insulin receptor: receptor cross-linking with bifunctional and photoreactive ligands, chimeric receptor constructs in which domains of the insulin and IGF-1 receptors have been swapped, minimized receptor constructs with deletion of various modules of the extracellular domain, and alanine-scanning mutagenesis. These data have been reviewed in great detail recently (Adams et al 2000, De Meyts & Whittaker 2002).

Alanine scanning studies of the insulin receptor ectodomain (Fig. 4) have supported the conclusions of affinity labelling studies and chimeric receptor experiments. Two functional epitopes have been identified in the L1 domain (Williams et al 1995). The first of these is composed of Asp 12, Arg 14 and Asn 15; Gln 34, Leu 36 and Leu 37; Phe 64; Glu 97; Glu 120 and Lys 121. The second one comprises Leu 87, Phe 89, Asn 90 and Tyr 91. This epitope had been earlier identified by site-directed mutagenesis of Phe 89 to Leu (De Meyts et al 1990). Alanine scanning mutagenesis of the secreted receptor confirms that the C-terminus of the α subunit, amino acids 704–715 in the Fn_1 insert, identified by photoaffinity cross-linking, is also an essential component of this ligand binding site (Mynarcik et al 1997). A peptide with this sequence will confer binding to the L1-CR-L2 domain, whether fused to it or simply added in the binding assay (Kristensen et al 2002). In the insulin receptor, the cysteine-rich (CR) domain does not appear to be involved in insulin binding. These binding epitopes contain some of the residues that have been found in natural mutations that impair insulin binding in patients with extreme insulin resistance (Taylor et al 1992, see other references in De Meyts & Whittaker 2002). In the insulin receptor, the involvement of the CR domain suggested by affinity cross-linking to be involved in binding (Yip et al 1988) was not supported by alanine scanning studies.

Alanine scanning of the secreted IGF-1 receptor (Whittaker et al 2001) (Fig. 4) indicates that the L1 and CR domains and the C-terminal peptide of the α-subunit (692–702 corresponding to 705–715 of the insulin receptor) are components of the IGF-1 binding site. In L1 the side chains of residues Asp8 and Asn11, Tyr28, His30 and Leu33, Leu56 and Arg59, and Phe 90 appear to form a functional epitope on the base of the domain. Trp79 in the L1 domain and Arg240, Phe241, Glu242 and Phe251 in the CR domain form a second functional epitope. Alanine mutations of all residues in the C-terminal peptide of the α-subunit with the exception of Phe695, Ser699 and Val702 compromised IGF-1 binding.

Assembling the puzzle

The available data as discussed above suggest the presence on the insulin molecule of two binding surfaces overlapping to a large extent with the dimerization and hexamerization surfaces. Affinity cross-linking suggested the presence on the receptor of three binding epitopes, one in the L1 domain, one in the Fn1 insert (CT peptide), and one in the $L2Fn_0$ region (De Meyts & Whittaker 2002).

Schäffer (1994) and De Meyts (1994) attempted to integrate all available topographic and kinetic evidence by proposing models whereby the two ligand binding surfaces contact two different binding epitopes located on each of the receptor α-subunits, thereby creating one high affinity site, and leaving free two lower affinity binding sites (thus explaining the coexistence of high and low affinity sites seen in the Scatchard plot).

De Meyts proposed that all aspects of the negative cooperativity (high and low affinity sites, accelerated dissociation and bell-shaped dose-response curve) could be explained if the receptor binding sites 1 and 2 were disposed in an antiparallel symmetry, allowing alternative cross-linking of both pairs of binding sites (De Meyts 1994, De Meyts & Whittaker 2002) The concept of an antiparallel symmetry was supported by the EM studies of Tulloch et al (1999).

The bivalent cross-linking concept provides a molecular basis, not only for negative cooperativity, but also for activation of the RTK and signalling pathways. The simultaneous interaction of the bivalent ligand with the two half-receptors may approximate the two kinase domains and permit transphosphorylation.

Photoaffinity labelling data suggest that insulin's classical binding surface binds to a receptor site composed of the L1 domain and the CT domain, agreeing with the alanine scanning data. This is consistent with the L1C–CT construct binding insulin with nanomolar affinity (Kristensen et al 1998). This interaction also probably represents the low affinity binding mode of insulin to the IGF-1 receptor (De Meyts 1994, Schäffer 1994).

The second insulin receptor binding site (which binds the newly uncovered insulin binding surface) has not been mapped by alanine scanning yet, but several lines of evidence suggest that it is located within the structures encoded by exons 6–8, i.e. the C-terminal part of L2 and the first FnIII domain (Fn_0) (Christoffersen et al 1994, De Meyts 1994, De Meyts & Whittaker 2002, Fabry et al 1992, Kadowaki et al 1990). This is the site recognized by inhibitory patient autoantibodies and monoclonal antibodies ('major immunogenic region', Zhang & Roth 1991, Fig. 2).

The existence of multiple (although only partially mapped) binding epitopes on the IGF-1 molecule and the occurrence of negative cooperativity in binding suggest that a similar binding mechanism must be operating in the IGF-1 receptor. The lack of a bell-shaped dose-response curve suggests that the association of the ligand to the third free receptor binding epitope is too slow to compete with reassociation of the first cross-link; this is corrected if the L2-Fn_0 domain of the insulin receptor replaces the equivalent portion of the IGF-1 receptor (Christoffersen et al 1994). The IGF-1 C-peptide, absent in insulin, plays a major role in IGF-1 binding; the insulin receptor however has a binding epitope that recognizes it as shown by the high affinity of the ICP peptide (Kristensen et al 1995).

Conclusions and a word of caution

In the absence of a definitive three-dimensional structure of a high-affinity ligand–receptor complex, circumstantial evidence generated by a multitude of biochemical and molecular biological approaches has generated a plausible working model of the insulin and IGF-1 receptor interaction that provides a rational explanation for a variety of complex equilibrium and kinetic properties, including a solution to the three decades-old riddle of the aberrant behaviour of hagfish and hystricomorph insulins. This model has also provided a rational basis for the design of agonist and antagonist mimetic peptides (Pillutla et al 2002, Schäffer et al 2003, reviewed in De Meyts & Whittaker 2002).

The concept described above of a single bivalent ligand sitting in the middle of a head-to-head dimeric receptor complex (which appears to be the rule in the so far determined RTK or cytokine ligand–receptor structures that have been solved), has been challenged by the recently determined structure of the EGF receptor (which has significant structural homology to the insulin and IGF-1 receptors) complexed to EGF or TGFα (reviewed in Jorissen et al 2003). In those structures, two ligand molecules bind to the external surfaces of a back-to-back receptor dimer with a 2:2 stoichiometry rather than the 1:2 we have advocated for the insulin and IGF-1 receptor. This means that we have to remain open to the possibility that insulin and IGF-1 may link the two α-subunit binding epitopes in a *cis*-fashion within the same subunit rather than a *trans*-fashion between two subunits as we have proposed. However, the EGF receptor back-to-back dimer is formed largely through contacts between two protruding β-hairpin arms in the CR domains that are entirely absent from the insulin and IGF-1 receptors, still making it plausible that their dimer structure is closer to the head-to-head structures also seen in the EGF receptor crystal structures, but deemed in that case less likely to be physiological.

Acknowledgements

The Receptor Biology Laboratory at the Hagedorn Research Institute is an independent basic research component of Novo Nordisk A/S. The laboratory is also supported by grants from the Danish Medical Research Council through the Center for Growth and Regeneration, Medicon Valley Academy and Øresund IT Academy BIO+IT programme. Extensive discussions on the ligand binding mechanism with Lauge Schäffer and Jonathan Whittaker, and on insulin structure with Michael A. Weiss, are gratefully acknowledged, as well the collaboration with Asser S. Andersen in making recombinant mutated insulins.

References

Adams TE, EPA VC, Garrett TP, Ward CW 2000 Structure and function of the type 1 insulin-like growth factor receptor. Cell Mol Life Sci 57:1050–1093

Avruch J 2001 Receptor tyrosine kinases. In: De Groot LJ, Jameson JL (eds) Endocrinology. 4th edn. WB Saunders Co, Philadelphia, p 25–47

Baker EN, Blundell TL, Cutfield JF et al 1988 The structure of 2Zn pig insulin at 1.5 Å resolution. Phil Trans R Soc Lond B19:369–456

Barbieri M, Bonafé M, Franceschi C, Paolisso G 2003 Insulin/IGF-I-signaling pathway: an evolutionarily conserved mechanism of longevity from yeast to humans. Am J Physiol Endocrinol Metab 285:E1064–E1071

Blume-Jensen P, Hunter T 2001 Oncogenic kinase signalling. Nature 411:355–365

Brandt J, Andersen AS, Kristensen C 2001 Dimeric fragment of the insulin receptor alpha-subunit binds insulin with full holoreceptor affinity. J Biol Chem 276:12378–12384

Brunelleschi S, Penengo L, Santoro MM, Gandino G 2002 Receptor tyrosine kinases as target for anti-cancer therapy. Curr Pharm Des 8:1959–1972

Brzozowski AM, Dodson EJ, Dodson GG et al 2002 Structural origins of the functional divergence of human insulin-like growth factor-I and insulin. Biochemistry 41:9389–9397

Christoffersen CT, Bornfeldt KE, Rotella CM et al 1994 Negative cooperativity in the insulin-like growth factor-I (IGF-I) receptor and a chimeric IGF-I/insulin receptor. Endocrinology 135:472–475

De Meyts P 1994 The structural basis of insulin and insulin-like growth factor-I (IGF-I) receptor binding and negative cooperativity, and its relevance to mitogenic versus metabolic signaling. Diabetologia 37:S135–S148

De Meyts P, Whittaker J 2002 Structural biology of insulin and IGF1 receptors: implications for drug design. Nat Rev Drug Discov 1:769–783

De Meyts P, Van Obberghen E, Roth J, Brandenburg D, Wollmer A 1978 Mapping of the residues of the receptor binding region of insulin responsible for the negative cooperativity. Nature 273:504–509

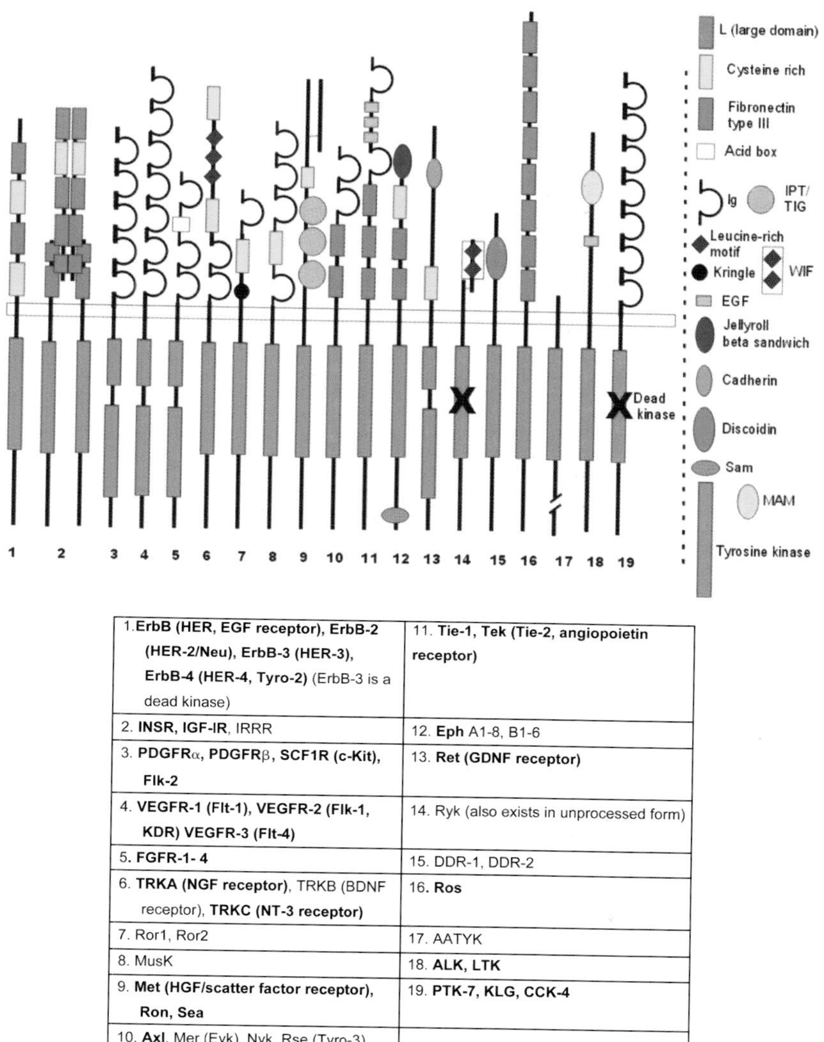

1. **ErbB (HER, EGF receptor), ErbB-2 (HER-2/Neu), ErbB-3 (HER-3), ErbB-4 (HER-4, Tyro-2)** (ErbB-3 is a dead kinase)	11. **Tie-1, Tek (Tie-2, angiopoietin receptor)**
2. **INSR, IGF-IR**, IRRR	12. **Eph** A1-8, B1-6
3. **PDGFRα, PDGFRβ, SCF1R (c-Kit), Flk-2**	13. **Ret (GDNF receptor)**
4. **VEGFR-1 (Flt-1), VEGFR-2 (Flk-1, KDR) VEGFR-3 (Flt-4)**	14. Ryk (also exists in unprocessed form)
5. **FGFR-1- 4**	15. DDR-1, DDR-2
6. **TRKA (NGF receptor)**, TRKB (BDNF receptor), **TRKC (NT-3 receptor)**	16. **Ros**
7. Ror1, Ror2	17. AATYK
8. MusK	18. **ALK, LTK**
9. **Met (HGF/scatter factor receptor), Ron, Sea**	19. **PTK-7, KLG, CCK-4**
10. **Axl**, Mer (Eyk), Nyk, Rse (Tyro-3)	

Plate 1. Modular structure of the receptor tyrosine kinases (RTKs). This figure is adapted from Hubbard & Till (2000), updated with information compiled from various sources (Avruch 2001, Blume-Jensen & Hunter 2001, Loren et al 2003, Robertson et al 2000, Robinson et al 2000) and databases such as Pfam. We found that all published figures on the domain organization of RTKs contain inaccuracies and discrepancies, which we have tried to correct and reconcile. We would be grateful for reports of any remaining error or omission. A 20th RTK, SuRTK106 has been reported from the Sugen database (Blume-Jensen & Hunter 2001), but a number of critical substitutions make it doubtful that it would have kinase activity (T. Hunter, personal communication 2003). The nomenclature of the RTKs is rather complex with alternative names existing besides those shown above (see e.g. Avruch 2001). The RTKs in bold type have been implicated in human malignancies. (Reproduced from Gray et al 2003 with permission.)

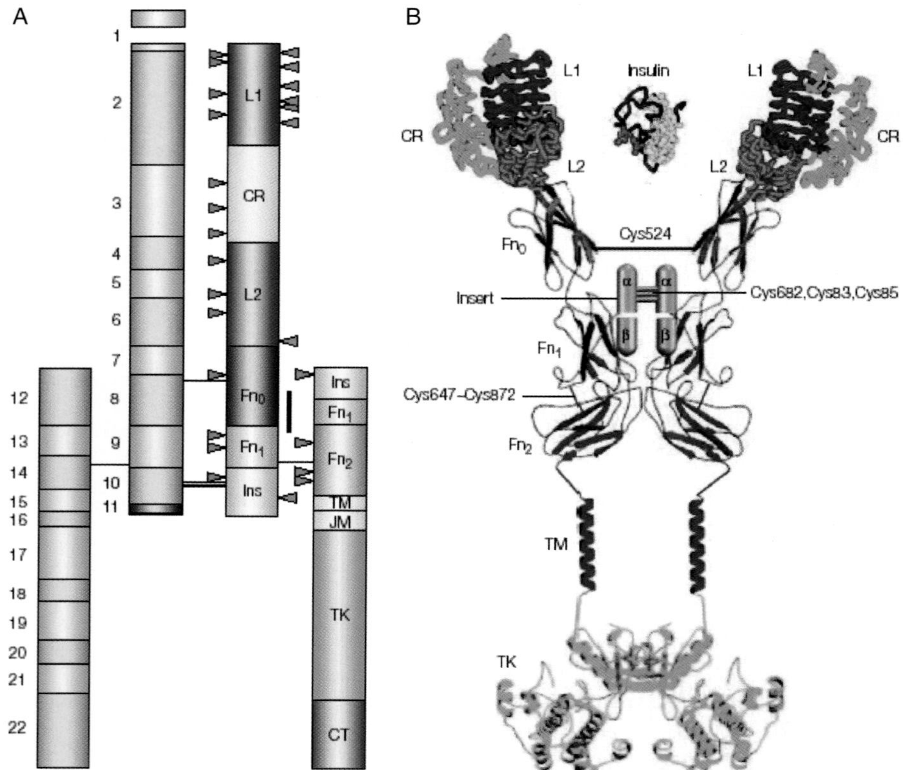

Plate 2. Modular structure of the insulin receptor. (A) cartoon of the $\alpha_2\beta_2$ structure of the insulin receptor, drawn to scale. On the left half of the receptor, spans of the 22 exon-encoded sequences. On the right half, spans of predicted protein modules. Orange arrowheads: *N*-glycosylation sites. Green arrowheads: ligand binding 'hotspots' identified by single amino acid site-directed mutagenesis (see text and De Meyts & Whittaker 2002 for details). (B) Supra-domain organization of the insulin receptor. Stretched-out model of predicted or actual modular structures (L1/CR/L2 and TK domains based on X-ray analysis data; Hubbard et al 1994). The 3D structure of the insulin molecule is also shown. The classical binding surface is shown in yellow as Van der Waals spheres; A13 and B17 Leu in the new binding surface are shown in red. Modelling using DS ViewerLite 5.0 (Accelrys). Reproduced from De Meyts & Whittaker (2002).

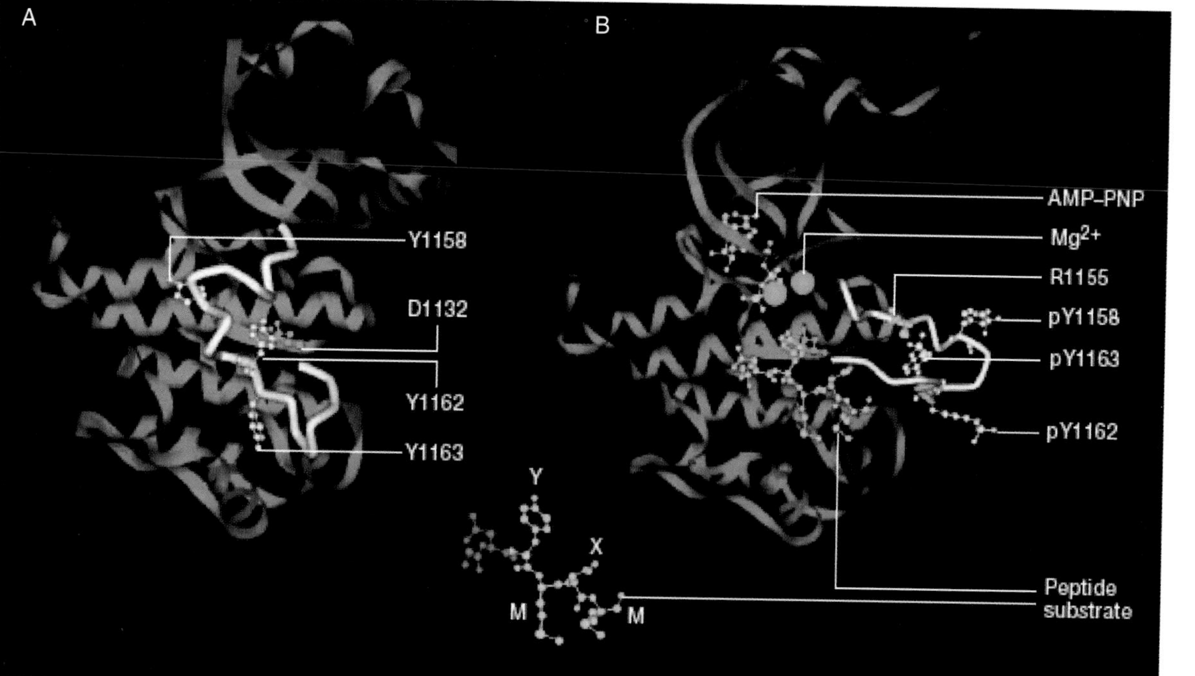

Plate 3. Structures of the inactive insulin receptor kinase (A) and the activated kinase (B). The activated kinase is bound to an ATP analogue (AMP-PNP), peptide substrate and magnesium (Mg^{2+}). This figure illustrates the autoinhibition mechanism whereby Tyr1162, one of the three tyrosines that are autophosphorylated in the activation loop (shown in white) in response to insulin (1158, 1162, 1163) is bound in the active site, hydrogen-bonded to a conserved Asp1132 in the catalytic loop (left). Tyr1162 in effect competes with protein substrates before autophosphorylation. In the activated state (right), the activation loop is tris-phosphorylated and moves out of the active site. Tyr1163 becomes hydrogen-bonded to a conserved Arg1155 in the beginning of the activation loop, which stabilizes the repositioned loop. Also shown is the peptide substrate with the YMXM motif. Adapted from Hubbard & Till (2000), as shown in De Meyts & Whittaker (2002).

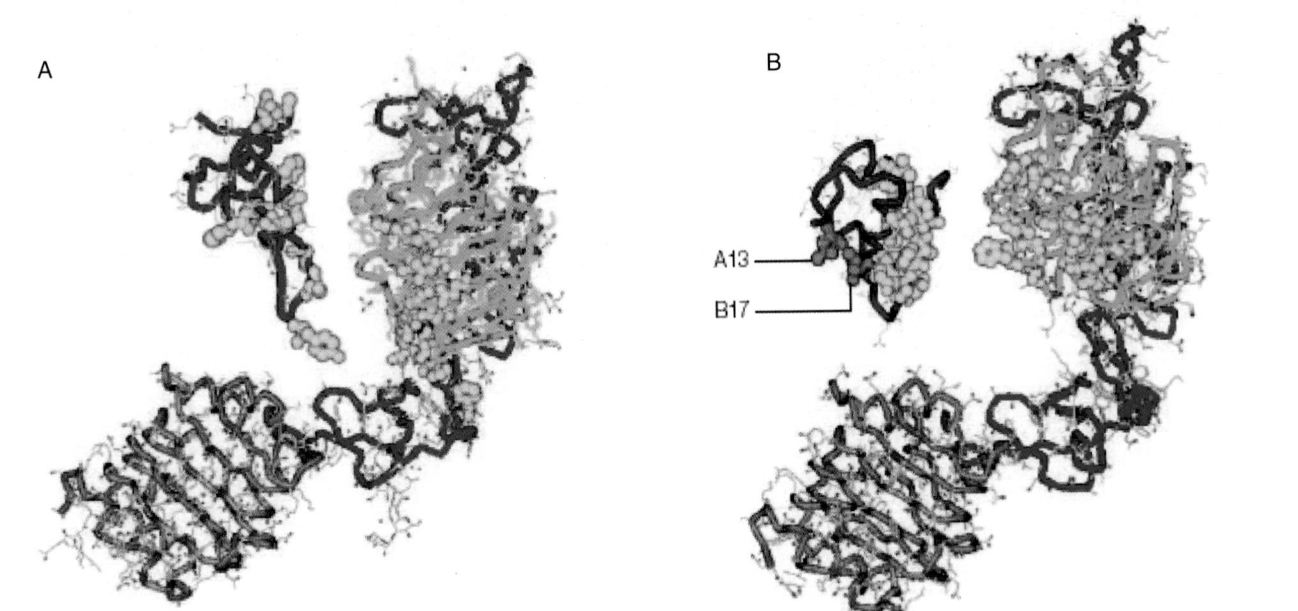

Plate 4. Structures of the insulin and IGF-1 receptors and their ligands. (A) 3D structure of the L1–CR–L2 domain of the IGF-1 receptor determined by X-ray crystallography. The amino acids determined by alanine scanning mutagenesis to be important for ligand binding are shown in yellow as Van der Waals spheres (see text and De Meyts & Whittaker 2002 for details). The 3D structure of the IGF-1 molecule (Brzozowski et al 2002) is shown to scale. The amino acids determined by site-directed mutagenesis to be important for receptor binding are shown in yellow as Van der Waals spheres. Since Arg36 and Arg37 are lacking in the structure, residues 35 and 38 have been highlighted instead to show approximate location in the middle of the C-peptide domain. (B) The insulin receptor L1–CR–L2 domain has been modelled on the IGF-1 corresponding domain coordinates using the program SwissModel. The amino acids determined by site-directed mutagenesis to be important for receptor binding are shown in yellow as Van der Waals spheres (see text and De Meyts & Whittaker 2002 for details). The 3D structure of the insulin molecule (Baker et al 1988) is shown to scale. The classical binding surface is shown in yellow as Van der Waals spheres; A13 and B17 Leu in the new binding surface are shown in red. Modelling using DS ViewerLite 5.0 (Accelrys). From De Meyts & Whittaker (2002).

De Meyts P, Gu JL, Shymko RM, Kaplan BE, Bell GI, Whittaker J 1990 Identification of a ligand-binding region of the human insulin receptor encoded by the second exon of the gene. Mol Endocrinol 4:409–416

Drevs J, Medinger M, Schmidt-Gersbach C, Weber R, Unger C 2003 Receptor tyrosine kinases: the main targets for new anticancer therapy. Curr Drug Targets 4:113–121

Fabry M, Schaefer E, Ellis L, Kojro E, Fahrenholz F, Brandenburg D 1992 Detection of a new hormone contact site within the insulin receptor ectodomain by the use of a novel photoreactive insulin. J Biol Chem 267:8950–8956

Favelyukis S, Till JH, Hubbard SR, Miller WT 2001 Structure and autoregulation of the insulin-like growth factor 1 receptor kinase. Nat Struct Biol 8:1058–1063

Frasca F, Pandini G, Scalia P et al 1999 Insulin receptor isoform A, a newly recognized, high-affinity insulin-like growth factor II receptor in fetal and cancer cells. Mol Cell Biol 19: 3278–3288

Garrett TP, McKern NM, Lou M et al et al 1998 Crystal structure of the first three domains of the type-1 insulin-like growth factor receptor. Nature 394:395–399

Gray SG, Stenfeldt Mathiasen I, De Meyts P 2003 The insulin-like growth factors and insulin-signalling systems: an appealing target for breast cancer therapy? Horm Metab Res 35:857–871

Heldin CH, Ostman A 1996 Ligand-induced dimerization of growth factor receptors: variations on the theme. Cytokine Growth Factor Rev 7:3–10

Holst PA 2000 Interaction of insulin and insulin analogues with the insulin receptor: relationship between structure, binding kinetics and biological function. PhD thesis, Copenhagen University, Copenhagen, Denmark

Hsu SY 2003 New insights into the evolution of the relaxin-LGR signaling system. Trends Endocrinol Metab 14:303–309

Hua XH, Shoelson SE, Kochoyan M, Weiss M 1991 Receptor binding redefined by a structural switch in a mutant human insulin. Nature 354:238–241

Hubbard SR 1997 Crystal structure of the activated insulin receptor tyrosine kinase in complex with peptide substrate and ATP analog. EMBO J 16:5572–5581

Hubbard SR, Till JH 2000 Protein tyrosine kinase structure and function. Ann Rev Biochem 69:373–398

Hubbard SR, Weiss L, Ellis L, Hendrickson WA 1994 Crystal structure of the tyrosine kinase domain of the human insulin receptor. Nature 372:746–754

Jensen AM 2001 Analysis of structure-activity relationships of the insulin molecule by alanine-scanning mutagenesis. Master's thesis, Copenhagen University, Copenhagen, Denmark

Jorissen RN, Walker F, Pouliot N, Garrett TP, Ward CW, Burgess AW 2003 Epidermal growth factor receptor: mechanisms of activation and signalling. Exp Cell Res 284:31–53

Kadowaki H, Kadowaki T, Cama A et al 1990 Mutagenesis of lysine 460 in the insulin receptor. Effects on receptor recycling and cooperative interactions among binding sites. J Biol Chem 265:21285–21296

Kristensen C, Andersen AS, Hach M, Wiberg FC, Schäffer L, Kjeldsen T 1995 A single-chain insulin-like growth factor I/insulin hybrid binds with high affinity to the insulin receptor. Biochem J 305:981–986

Kristensen C, Kjeldsen T, Wiberg FC et al 1997 Alanine scanning mutagenesis of insulin. J Biol Chem 272:12978–12983

Kristensen C, Wiberg FC, Schäffer L, Andersen AS 1998 Expression and characterization of a 70-kDa fragment of the insulin receptor that binds insulin. Minimizing ligand binding domain of the insulin receptor. J Biol Chem 273:17780–17786

Kristensen C, Andersen AS, Ostergaard S, Hansen PH, Brandt J 2002 Functional reconstitution of insulin receptor binding site from non-binding receptor fragments. J Biol Chem 277:18340–18345

Levitzki A 2002 Tyrosine kinases as targets for cancer therapy. Eur J Cancer 38:S11–S18

Loren CE, Englund C, Grabbe C, Hallberg B, Hunter T, Palmer RH 2003 A crucial role for the anaplastic lymphoma kinase receptor tyrosine kinase in gut development in Drosophila melanogaster. EMBO Rep 4:781–786

Ludvigsen S, Olsen HB, Kaarsholm NC 1998 A structural switch in a mutant insulin exposes key residues for receptor binding. J Mol Biol 279:1–7

Macaulay 2004 The IGF receptor as anti-cancer treatment target. In: Biology of IGF-1: its interaction with insulin in health and malignant states (Novartis Found Symp 262). Wiley, Chichester, p 235–246

Mynarcik DC, Williams PF, Schäffer L, Yu GQ, Whittaker J 1997 Analog binding properties of insulin receptor mutants. Identification of amino acids interacting with the COOH terminus of the B chain of the insulin molecule. J Biol Chem 272:2077–2081

Nakagawa SH, Tager HS 1992 Importance of aliphatic side-chain structure at positions 2 and 3 of the insulin A chain in insulin-receptor interactions. Biochemistry 31:3204–3214

Nakagawa SH, Tager HS, Steiner DF 2000 Mutational analysis of invariant valine B12 in insulin: implications for receptor binding. Biochemistry 39:15826–15835

Palsgaard J 2003 Receptor-binding properties of 25 different hystricomorph-like human insulin analogs. Master's thesis, Copenhagen University, Copenhagen, Denmark

Pillutla RC, Hsiao KC, Beasley JR et al 2002 Peptides identify the critical hotspots involved in the biological activation of the insulin receptor. J Biol Chem 277:22590–22594

Piron MA 1981 Etude des relations entre la structure et la fonction de l'insuline chez les Vertébrés. PhD thesis, Catholic University of Louvain, Brussels, Belgium

Pullen RA, Lindsay DG, Wood SP et al 1976 Receptor-binding region of insulin. Nature 259:369–373

Robertson SC, Tynan JA, Donoghue DJ 2000 RTK mutations and human syndromes. When good receptors turn bad. Trends Genet 16:265–271

Robinson DR, Wu YM, Lin SF 2000 The protein tyrosine kinase family of the human genome. Oncogene 19:5548–5557

Schäffer L 1994 A model for insulin binding to the insulin receptor. Eur J Biochem 221: 1127–1132

Schäffer L, Brissette RE, Spetzler JC et al 2003 Assembly of high-affinity insulin receptor agonists and antagonists from peptide building blocks. Proc Natl Acad Sci USA 100: 4435–4439

Seino S, Bell GI 1989 Alternative splicing of human insulin receptor messenger RNA. Biochem Biophys Res Commun 159:312–316

Seino S, Seino M, Nishi S, Bell GI 1989 Structure of the human insulin receptor gene and characterization of its promoter. Proc Natl Acad Sci USA 86:114–118

Soos M, Field CE, Siddle K 1993 Purified hybrid insulin/insulin-like growth factor-i receptors bind insulin-like growth factor-I, but not insulin, with high affinity. Biochem J 290:419–426

Surinya KH, Molina L, Soos MA, Brandt J, Kristensen C, Siddle K 2002 Role of insulin receptor dimerization domains in ligand binding, cooperativity, and modulation by anti-receptor antibodies. J Biol Chem 277:16718–16725

Taylor SI, Cama A, Accili D et al 1992 Mutations in the insulin receptor gene. Endocr Rev 13:566–595

Tulloch PA, Lawrence LJ, McKern NM et al 1999 Single-molecule imaging of human insulin receptor ectodomain and its Fab complexes. J Struct Biol 125:11–18

Vajdos FF, Ultsch M, Schaffer ML et al 2001 Crystal structure of human insulin-like growth factor-1: detergent binding inhibits binding protein interactions. Biochemistry 40: 11022–11029

Van den Brande JL 1992 Structure of human insulin-like growth factors: relationship to function. In insulin-like growth factors. Structure and biological functions. Oxford University Press, Oxford

Walenkamp MJE, Pereira Arias AM, Sluimers C et al 2003 Biochemical features of a 55 year old man with a homozygous missense mutation of IGF-1 and of his heterozygous relatives. Horm Res 60 (suppl 2):15
Whittaker J, Groth AV, Mynarcik DC, Pluzek L, Gadsbøll VL, Whittaker LJ 2001 Alanine scanning mutagenesis of a type 1 insulin-like growth factor receptor ligand binding site. J Biol Chem 276:43980–43986
Williams PF, Mynarcik DC, Yu GQ, Whittaker J 1995 Mapping of an NH2-terminal ligand binding site of the insulin receptor by alanine scanning mutagenesis. J Biol Chem 270:1–5
Woods KA, Camacho-Hubner C, Bergman RN, Barter D, Clark AJ, Savage MO 2000 Effects of insulin-like growth factor I (IGF-I) therapy on body composition and insulin resistance in IGF-I gene deletion. J Clin Endocrinol Metab 85:1407–1411
Yip CC, Hsu H, Patel RG, Hawley DM, Maddux BA, Goldfine ID 1988 Localization of the insulin-binding site to the cysteine-rich region of the insulin receptor alpha-subunit. Biochem Biophys Res Commun 157:321–329
Yip CC, Ottensmeyer P 2003 Three-dimensional structural interactions of insulin and its receptor. J Biol Chem 278:27329–27332
Zhang B, Roth RA 1991 A region of the insulin receptor important for ligand binding (residues 450-601) is recognized by patients autoimmune antibodies and inhibitory monoclonal antibodies. Proc Natl Acad Sci USA 88:9858–9862
Zwick E, Bange J, Ullrich A 2002 Receptor tyrosine kinases as targets for anticancer drugs. Trends Mol Med 8:17–23

DISCUSSION

Roberts: It is interesting that Jerry Olefsky's group and others have put forward the argument that IGF and insulin receptors are actually G protein-coupled receptors (GPCRs), on the basis of the ability of the appropriate inhibitors to prevent IGF or insulin action. Given these data, and that relaxin and relaxin-like peptides do bind directly to GPCRs, do you think that there is another IGF or insulin receptor out there that is GPCR-related, rather than there being an intracellular signalling interaction that explains those data?

De Meyts: We now know pretty much the complete 'kinome' present in the human genome, and what their ligands are, so I don't think there are any hidden RTKs left to be discovered that could be insulin or IGF-1-related receptors. But indeed as you imply there are still many orphan GPCR receptors, and given that some members of the insulin ligand family bind to such receptors (Yu & Hsu 2003), we probably cannot completely exclude that one of these could recognize insulin or IGF-1. I think however that cross-talk between the insulin/IGF-1 receptors and GPCR signalling pathways, as shown by Bob Lefkowitz's group (e.g. Luttrell et al 1995) is a more likely explanation.

Thomas: Tony Hunter made a comment when the human genome was published that all the tyrosine kinases have already been discovered.

De Meyts: That's correct. There are 60 RTKs, I believe.

Pollak: I heard that someone had recently published an anti-IGF-1 antibody which had the property of increasing the biological activity of IGF-1 at the receptor. In a related paradigm, there is always some question of IGF binding proteins occasionally increasing the activity of IGFs. Is there any structural basis for speculating that a change in conformation of the ligand could actually influence the affinity or the interaction of the ligand with the receptor?

De Meyts: I think that is theoretically possible. In order to answer that question we would need a structure of the bound and unbound ligand. Structural data suggest that the end of the B-chain of insulin moves away from the body of the molecule during the binding process. This is why an analogue with a very short cross-link between A1 and B30 has very low potency despite a conserved three-dimensional structure. It is likely that a conformational change in insulin is necessary for achieving the active state, which is blocked by bridging together A1 and B30. It wouldn't be surprising if there were some molecule that could favour or hinder the active conformation. However, considering the fact that insulin is probably pretty much buried inside the receptor dimer after binding (De Meyts & Whittaker 2002), I am not sure if an antibody bound to the ligand would be able to fit in there. In fact, the first project I did with Jesse Roth in the early 1970s, was to try and measure receptor occupancy by using insulin antibodies to measure bound insulin. What I found was that once insulin was bound I could not find any antibody which would bind to the complex on the cells, a result confirmed by others later.

Holly: So your speculation is that once the ligand is in the receptor it is buried, and therefore it is unlikely that something else will get to it. Going on the data of negative and positive cooperativity, is there a possibility that an IGF-binding protein could alter the conformation or still be attached in some way where it binds to one surface and then interferes with either the negative or positive cooperativity, and then is displaced when the other surface binds to the receptor?

De Meyts: We cannot exclude that possibility.

LeRoith: Sticking with our 1970s theme, I'd like to ask you about chicken and turkey insulin, which both have higher affinity, yet biologically they are less active than you'd anticipate.

De Meyts: That's an excellent point. Insulin analogues that differ several hundred-fold in affinity *in vitro*, end up having comparable biological activity *in vivo*. In fact much secreted or injected insulin is cleared on the first passage through the liver. It binds to the liver receptors and perhaps 50% gets cleared by receptor-mediated endocytosis. A high-affinity insulin will then be endocytosed very fast and get out of the circulation. A low-affinity insulin will circulate longer and have an increased half-life that almost exactly compensates for the loss of affinity. This may be why patients with insulin mutations like insulin Wakayama are only mildly diabetic. It has also been shown in pig studies with a number of insulin analogues of varying affinity, that they cluster around the same activity *in vivo* (Ribel et al 1990).

LeRoith: So do you think the reduction in biological activity is just a compensation for the greater receptor affinity?

De Meyts: Yes, this is what several studies seem to indicate.

Yee: Have you examined the interaction of IGF-2 with the IGF receptor?

De Meyts: No. It is difficult to do direct binding studies with IGF-2 due to the prevalence of the IGF-2/mannose-6-phosphate receptor. But we recently got a couple of cell lines devoid of this receptor to do such studies. We also plan to introduce every single mutation in IGF-1 and IGF-2 into the insulin molecule in order to see how we can explain the low affinity of IGF-1 for the insulin receptor. The low affinity of insulin for the IGF receptor is easily explained by the lack of C peptide, but the opposite is not easy to account for. We know that insulin has the binding site for the C peptide. If you put the IGF-1 C peptide on insulin, the chimeric ligand binds very nicely to the insulin as well as the IGF-1 receptor.

Rosenfeld: It would be interesting to see why IGF-2 has a better affinity than IGF-1 for the insulin receptor.

De Meyts: It has been speculated that this is because the C peptide is shorter, but I think we need to do the structural studies to answer that question.

Zick: In your experience of binding interactions between insulin and the receptor, do you have any evidence that the glycosylation state of the receptor affects the binding in any way?

De Meyts: This has been reviewed in detail recently (Adams et al 2000). You can get rid of a number of the glycosylation sites, but there are some that are indispensable for the receptor to be expressed. This unfortunately complicates attempts at crystallization.

Clark: I'd like to raise the Novo data where an insulin analogue that was in the clinic was withdrawn because of toxicology: the analogue induced mammary tumours in rats (Hansen et al 1996). Could you tell us the story?

De Meyts: We understand this much better now. We have done systematic studies of a large number of analogues, and it is very clear that those which turn out to be supermitogenic are those with a longer residence time on the receptor.

Clark: Is this on the insulin receptor?

De Meyts: That is part of the answer. We have one cell line, a T cell lymphoma devoid of IGF-1 receptors, where the Asp B10 insulin is nevertheless supermitogenic. In this cell line, the dissociation rate also correlates with the mitogenic:metabolic ratio. But a second important factor is increased affinity for the IGF-1 receptor, which is also the case for Asp B10 insulin. To explain the increased mitogenicity of Asp B10 insulin, you can pretty much add the free energies due to longer residence time on the insulin receptor and the increased affinity for the IGF-1 receptor.

Clark: So the increased number of mammary tumours in the toxicology study is attributable to binding to the insulin receptor or to the IGF receptor?

De Meyts: The sum of the effect is probably in part due to both, but supermitogenicity could possibly be caused by either one separately.

Clark: Was the effect in the toxicology a change in the phenotype of the mammary tumours or an increased number of mammary tumours in rats?

De Meyts: It was an increased number, I think.

Holly: How does this compare with the IGF-1 toxicology?

Clark: That's what I wanted some detail on.

Yee: Were the increased mammary tumours seen in a model of insulin resistance?

De Meyts: No, they were seen in regular Wistar rats.

Yee: I have always been a little puzzled about hyperinsulinaemia and breast cancer risk. If one makes the assumption that there are defects in the receptor signalling pathway, one would also have to make the assumption that if the insulin is the direct cause, those signalling defects do not exist in mammary gland. I don't know if anyone has ever really looked at this very carefully.

De Meyts: Rudolf Kaaks, didn't you propose there might be a relationship between insulin and breast cancer?

Kaaks: Yes, but this was for completely different reasons, and this complicates the story even further. Insulin also potentially has effects on steroidogenesis, particularly in women who have a tendency to become hyperandrogenic. It might stimulate ovarian androgen synthesis and perhaps also adrenal androgen synthesis. This is perhaps more important for endometrial cancer than for breast cancer. In addition, insulin is a key regulator of sex hormone binding globulin (SHBG). It down-regulates SHBG levels which in turn can lead to higher free sex steroid levels in blood. Through this pathway there may also be an increase in breast cancer risk. It doesn't all have to be explained at the level of the insulin receptor or the IGF receptor in the tissue (e.g., breast or endometrium) where cancer develops. Physiologically, it is very complex.

Laron: You said that when a ligand binds for a longer time, it is probably more mitogenic. This is one hypothesis. Is it known whether the longer acting insulins affect one single pathway, or by their prolonged action are other pathways also activated?

De Meyts: You are confusing two completely different concepts. When we talk about long-acting or basal insulins, we are talking about prolonged *in vivo* half-life. This has nothing to do with an increased residence time on the receptor that I was just discussing. Once a basal insulin reaches the receptor, it has the same residence time as regular insulin.

Holly: Does it apply to all cells, whether the receptors are out on the microvilli or whether they are in caveolae?

De Meyts: That is a good question.

But going back to the previous question as to whether an insulin antibody or IGF binding protein could modulate ligand binding, my answer above was based on our current model that the ligand sits in the middle of the receptor dimer. However, if the EGF receptor model (where the EGF sits on the outside in a crevice in each receptor monomer) turns out to apply to the insulin or IGF-I receptor, one could imagine that a binding protein or antibody could facilitate its fitting into the hole.

LeRoith: Some people would prefer blocking it getting to the hole, as opposed to nicely delivering it to the hole.

Pollak: These aren't mutually exclusive: everything depends on the context. Perhaps the context is defined by stoichiometry. The particular concentrations of binding proteins and the microenvironment of the receptors will have an effect. At the cell biology level there are many observations that binding proteins can either accentuate or diminish the activity of IGF-1 in ways that are not fully understood. There are many models about this, including IGF receptor-independent actions of IGF binding proteins and so on. I wonder whether one understudied area is the detailed kinetics of IGF binding proteins interfering or modulating IGF receptor–IGF-1 binding.

De Meyts: Definitely. Moreover, we have no detailed kinetics on how differently IGF-1 and IGF-2 bind to the IGF receptor. No one has studied this. There are data indicating they may induce different patterns of gene expression.

Laron: If we give one injection the clearance of insulin is relatively fast and the biological activity passes away. For IGF-1 the clearance is a little slower, and still there is an activity over 24 h. What is responsible?

De Meyts: Binding proteins?

Laron: Why doesn't insulin have binding proteins?

De Meyts: There is one in insects, as mentioned earlier. It has been cloned (Andersen 2000) but there is no equivalent in the human genome.

Rosenfeld: I think the difference in kinetics of insulin and IGF is all explainable in terms of binding proteins. Insulin has weak affinity, three orders of magnitude lower, for IGF binding proteins.

Pollak: Evolutionarily you need to modulate your insulin activity more rapidly meal to meal. It would be physiologically not very useful to have a steady state insulin level.

De Meyts: Except now we are trying to make one to give basal treatment to patients. We did this by using a binding protein (human serum albumin).

Rosenfeld: Now that humans have evolved to a point where they eat continuously, this is what we want!

References

Adams TE, Epa VC, Garrett TP, Ward CW 2000 Structure and function of the type 1 insulin-like growth factor receptor. Cell Mol Life 57:1050–1093

Andersen AS, Hertz Hansen P, Schäffer LS, Kristensen C 2000 A new secreted insect protein belonging to the immunoglobulin superfamily binds insulin and related peptides and inhibits their activities. J Biol Chem 275:16948–16953

De Meyts P, Whittaker J 2002 Structural biology of insulin and IGF1 receptors: implications for drug design. Nat Rev Drug Discov 1:769–783

Hansen BF, Danielsen GM, Drejer K et al 1996 Sustained signalling from the insulin receptor after stimulation with insulin analogues exhibiting increased mitogenic potency. Biochem J 315:271–279

Luttrell LM, van Biesen T, Hawes BC, Koch WJ, Touhora K, Lefkowitz RJ 1995 G$\beta\gamma$ subunits mediate mitogen-activated protein kinase activation by the tyrosine kinase insulin-like growth factor 1 receptor. J Biol Chem 270:16495–16498

Ribel U, Hougaard P, Drejer K, Sørensen AR 1990 Equivalent in vivo biological activity of insulin analogues and human insulin despite different in vitro potencies. Diabetes 39: 1033–1039

Yu S, Hsu T 2003 New insights into the evolution of the relaxin-LGR signalling system. Trends Endocrinol Metab 7:303–309

Genetic blockade of the insulin-like growth factor 1 receptor for human malignancy

Yasushi Adachi, Choon-Taek Lee* and David P. Carbone†[1]

*First Department of Internal Medicine, Sapporo Medical University, Sapporo, 060-8543, Japan, *Division of Pulmonary and Critical Care Medicine, Department of Internal Medicine, Lung Institute of Medical Research Center, Seoul National University College of Medicine, Seoul 110-799, Korea, and †Vanderbilt-Ingram Cancer Center and Departments of Medicine and Cell Biology, Vanderbilt University, Nashville, TN 37232-6838, USA*

Abstract. Growth factor receptor signals, including insulin-like growth factor (IGF)-1 receptor (IGF-1R), are required for carcinogenesis and tumour progression in many human malignancies. The concept of targeting specific tumorigenic receptors has been validated by successful clinical application of multiple new drugs, including trastuzumab and gefitinib. In this paper, we review strategies of the genetic blockade of IGF-1/IGF-1R that validate this receptor as a promising anticancer target. Adenoviruses efficiently transduce malignant epithelial cells in culture and are useful for such target validation and potentially also as clinical therapeutics. To block IGF-1R signalling, we constructed adenoviruses expressing antisense IGF-1R and two truncated IGF-1R (482 and 950 amino acids long, IGF-1R/482st and IGF-1R/950st, respectively) that function as dominant negative inhibitors (IGF-1R/dn). The truncated receptors were also cloned into tetracycline regulated expression vectors to study the effects of modulating this pathway without the use of viral vectors. Blocking for IGF-1R suppressed tumorigenicity both *in vitro* and *in vivo* and effectively blocked both IGF-1 and IGF-2-induced activation of Akt-1. IGF-1R/dn expression increased radiation- and chemotherapy-induced apoptosis and these combination therapies with chemotherapy were very effective against tumours in mice. In an intraperitoneal dissemination mouse model, blockade of IGF-1R reduced dissemination and prolonged survival times. IGF-1R/482st was more effective than IGF-1R/950st due to its bystander effect. These studies confirm the validity of IGF-1R as a therapeutic target and genetic blockade as a potential strategy for several malignancies, including lung, colon and pancreatic carcinoma.

2004 Biology of IGF-1: its interaction with insulin in health and malignant states. Wiley, Chichester (Novartis Foundation Symposium 262) p 177–192

[1]This paper was presented at the symposium by David P. Carbone to whom correspondence should be addressed.

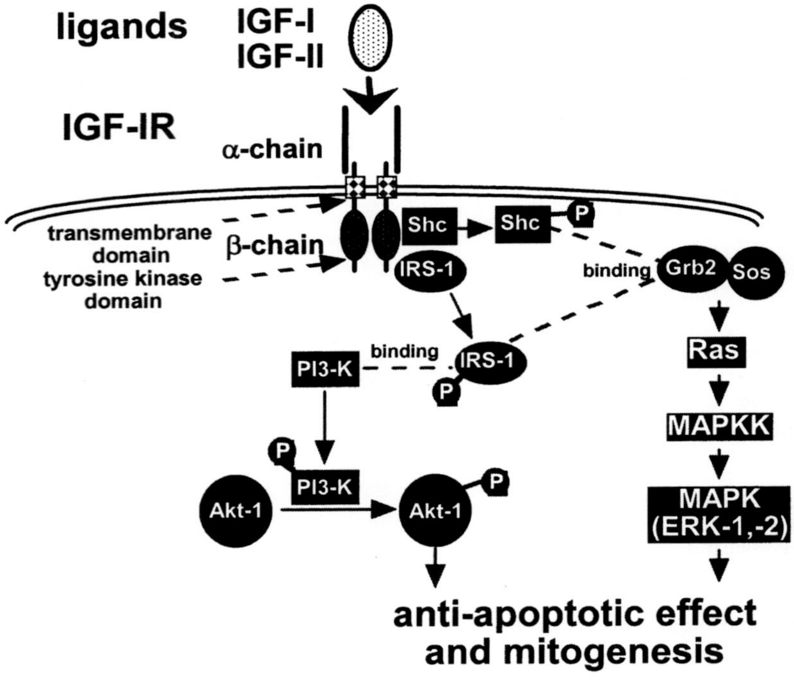

FIG. 1. IGF-1R is constructed with an α chain (extracellular domain) and a β chain (transmembrane and tyrosine kinase domains). After binding to the ligands (IGF-1 and IGF-2), IGF-1R turns on its signal transduction results in anti-apoptotic effect and mitogenesis.

Insulin-like growth factor 1 receptor in human tumours

A variety of growth factor signals are required for carcinogenesis and tumour progression in human malignancies (Baserga 1994). Signals from these receptors alter regulation of the cell cycle, induction of apoptosis, and interactions of tumour cells with their environment that affect the continuous growth potential of tumour cells (Baserga 1994). Insulin-like growth factor (IGF)-1 receptor (IGF-1R) signalling is able to potently stimulate cellular proliferation and induce cellular differentiation (Sara & Hall 1990).

IGF-1R is synthesized as a single precursor peptide of 1367 amino acid residues and then is cleaved at residue 706 into an α subunit (containing extracellular domain) and β subunit (having transmembrane and tyrosine kinase domains) (Fig. 1) (Ullrich et al 1986). Binding of the ligands, IGF-1 and IGF-2, to IGF-1R, which is a heterotetramer of two α and two β chains, causes receptor autophosphorylation and activation of tyrosine kinase activity, which subsequently phosphorylates a host of intracellular substrates, including insulin receptor substrate 1 (IRS-1) and Shc. These early events activate multiple signalling pathways, including the mitogen-activated protein kinase (MAPK; also called extracellular signal-regulated kinase [ERK]) and phosphatidylinositide 3-kinase (PI3K)/Akt-1 (protein kinase B) pathways (Baserga 1995, Yu & Rohan 2000). In certain systems, the IGF-1R appears to be essential for malignant transformation (Baserga 1995, Sell et al 1993). IGF-1R is also important for the maintenance as well as the initiation of the malignancy (Baserga 1995). Reduction of IGF-1R has been shown to induce apoptosis in tumours, but produce only growth arrest in untransformed cells (Baserga 1994), implying that receptor blockade may have a greater therapeutic index than strategies targeting fundamental cell mechanisms such as DNA synthesis or the cell cycle. In support of this, IGF-1R knockout mice are viable (though physically much smaller than wild-type) indicating that relatively normal tissue development and differentiation can occur in its absence (Liu et al 1993).

Strategies for the blockade of IGF-1R signalling

Several possible approaches to blocking IGF-1R signalling have been studied and reported, which are summarized and reviewed by Sumacz (2003) as follows:

- Blocking IGF-1R transcription (with triple helix) or translation (with antisense oligodeoxynucleotides, antisense RNA constructs, and siRNA) can bring elimination or reduction of IGF-1R protein expression.
- Binding of inactivating antibodies to the receptor can abolish its function (prevents ligand binding and induces receptor degradation).
- Small-molecule inhibitors can reduce IGF-1R tyrosine kinase activity.
- IGF mimetic peptides can compete with natural ligands, IGF-1 and IGF-2, and their binding inactivates the receptor.
- Defective IGF-1R with mutated or lacking tyrosine kinase domain can act as dominant negative (dn) receptors.
- Expression of myristylated IGF-1R C-terminus, which is a domain with intrinsic proapoptotic activity, can down-regulate survival signals.
- Excess IGF binding proteins or inhibition of ligand expression (on the transcriptional or post-transcriptional level) can reduce its ligands.

In our own experiments, we first constructed adenoviral vectors to deliver antisense IGF-1R (Lee et al 1996). A variety of mutant receptors have been constructed and demonstrated to function in a dominant negative (dn) fashion, so we then constructed adenovirus vectors with dn receptor constructs for IGF-1R which can inhibit the function rather than the expression of the naturally expressed receptor. There are two major ways to construct dn inhibitors for IGF-1R. One approach is to generate receptors having either a mutant or deleted intracellular tyrosine kinase domain (containing transmembrane domain) (Burgaud et al 1995, Li et al 1996, Prager et al 1994). Another is to use truncated receptors constructed with portions of the extracellular domain only (without the transmembrane domain) (D'Ambrosio et al 1996, Dunn et al 1998). We generated two different truncated IGF-1R constructs (950 and 482 amino acid residue IGF-1Rs, IGF-1R/950st and IGF-1R/482st, respectively) (Adachi et al 2002). The former produces an intact α subunit and defective β subunit lacking the tyrosine kinase domain and is thought to remain on the membrane of the transduced cells and to form non-functional heterodimers. The latter is a defective α chain of IGF-1R (lacking the β chain) and thus should generate a secreted soluble form of the receptor that may affect signal transduction in adjacent cells in addition to the transduced cells. In addition to the construction of adenoviruses expressing two IGF-1R/dns, we developed a tetracycline (tet) repressible vector expressing IGF-1R/482st to study the acute effects of pathway modulation in a single cell, without the potential problems that accompany the use of adenoviruses.

Adenovirus expressing antisense IGF-1R

An established strategy for blocking growth factor signalling is to reduce receptor expression directly using antisense cDNA vectors. Stable transfection of antisense plasmids expressing the first 300 bp of IGF-1R reduced the tumorigenicity of a variety of tumour cell lines and has been reported to induce systemic antitumour effects against established tumours in animal models (Long et al 1995, Resnicoff et al 1994). In order to develop these observations into a clinical therapeutic approach, we made an adenovirus expressing an antisense cDNA of IGF-1R (IGF-1R/as) containing 321 bp of the IGF-1R open reading frame including ATG initiation codon (Ad-IGF-1R/as) (Lee et al 1996). A single transduction by Ad-IGF-1R/as (at a multiplicity of infection of 10) decreased the IGF-1R number by about 50% in human lung cancer cell lines NCI-H460 and SCC5, as measured by an ^{125}I-labelled IGF-1 competitive binding assay. This modest reduction of IGF-1R number in NCI-H460 cells by an Ad-IGF-1R/as induced marked suppression of colony formation in a soft agar clonogenic assay (an 84% decrease compared to the cells infected with a control virus). Intraperitoneal (i.p.) treatment with Ad-IGF-1R/as in nude mice bearing established i.p. NCI-H460 cells resulted in significantly prolonged survival compared to nude mice treated with a control virus.

These studies demonstrating a therapeutic effect of ad-IGF-1R/as on *in vitro* tumorigenicity and on established human lung cancer xenografts provided additional support for the potential effectiveness of targeting this receptor.

Tetracycline-regulated dominant negative IGF-1R

We then investigated more potent strategy of dn receptors for IGF-1R. To characterize and assess efficacy of IGF-1R/482st, we first constructed in tetracycline (tet)-repressive expression vector (Adachi et al 2002). We reasoned that the tet-repressible system may be a valuable tool to study the isolated effects of regulated IGF-1R signalling blockade in a single clonal cell line. The ability to switch IGF-1R-mediated signalling on and off in a single clone of tumour cells eliminates artefacts induced by the selection of paired clones of cells stably expressing dominant inhibitors and comparison to cloned vector controls used in previous studies. The tet repressible IGF-1R/482st construct was stably transfected into the human colon cancer cell line HT29 and referred to as HT29dn. IGF-1R/482st was detected in the culture medium after withdrawal of tet, but not in media containing tet. Soft agar assays showed that the number of colonies of HT29dn was suppressed by two to three orders of magnitude when IGF-1R/482st was expressed (without tet) compared to the same cells with suppressed expression of the dn receptor (with tet).

In order to assess the mechanism of tumour inhibition, HT29dn cells with or without dn receptor expression were additionally stressed by chemotherapy, serum starvation (over 24 h) or heat shock (42 °C for 30 min) and were evaluated by Annexin-V assay and TUNEL assay. Although neither starvation nor heat are efficient inducers of apoptosis for HT29dn, IGF-1R/482st increased apoptosis two- to fourfold compared to tet(+) controls (Fig. 2). When HT29dn cells were treated with chemotherapy agents (10 M cisplatin or 260 M 5-fluorouracil [5-FU]), chemotherapy-induced apoptosis was significantly up-regulated in the presence of IGF-1R/482st.

Wortmannin, an inhibitor of PI3K, increased 5-FU-induced apoptosis in HT29dn cultured with tet, but the MEK1 inhibitor PD98059 did not affect apoptosis. Conversely, the increased apoptosis observed in IGF-1R/dn expressing cells was reduced to baseline by dominant active Akt expression. IRS-1 phosphorylation was reduced in IGF-1R/482st expressing HT29dn compared to the cells cultured with tet. Akt-1 phosphorylation was eliminated in the presence of IGF-1R/dn, while phosphorylation of ERK was not influenced very much. IGF-induced Akt activity was effectively blocked by the expression of IGF-1R/dn assessed by Akt kinase assays. These results indicate that IGF-1R/482st blocks IGF-1R signalling mainly by modulating PI3-K/Akt pathway in these cells.

In addition, as predicted by the structure of the product, IGF-1R/482st has a pronounced bystander effect, which was confirmed using a double chamber system and Western blot assays.

Subcutaneous (SC) tumours in mice derived from HT29dn cells were dramatically suppressed when IGF-1R/dn expression was turned on at the time

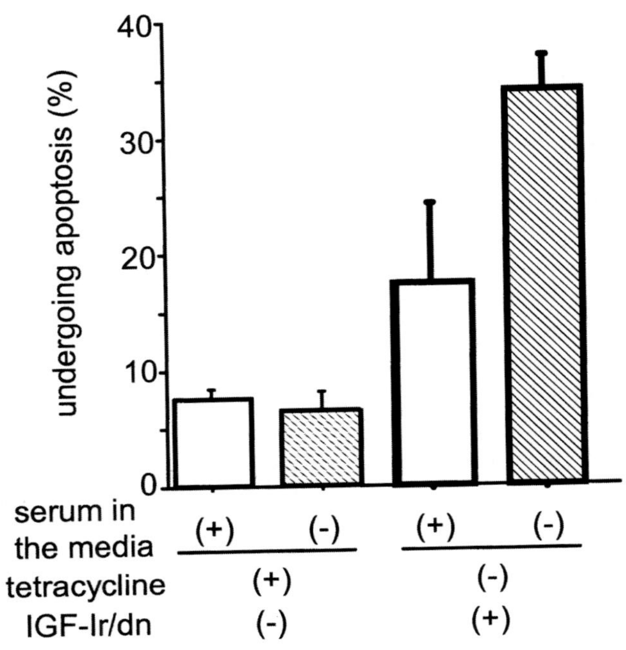

FIG. 2. In the presence of IGF-1R/482st, serum starvation-inducing apoptosis was up-regulated in colon cancer cell HT-29dn, evaluated by Annexin-V assay.

of injection compared to those in which it was suppressed, indicating that IGF-1R/482st effectively reduced tumorigenicity *in vivo*. More strikingly, when HT29dn cells with repressed dn receptor expression were inoculated into nude mice and allowed to form evident tumours in the presence of tet, induction of IGF-1R/482st by removal of tet from the drinking water resulted in rapid shrinkage of these pre-existing tumours. This indicates that IGF-1R blockade might be an effective therapeutic strategy for clinically evident tumours. The effect of combined IGF blockade with chemotherapy was then assessed. For both groups of mice fed water with and without tet, the size of tumours was smaller in mice treated with 5-FU than in control mice (Fig. 3a). The combination therapy of IGF-1R/482st and 5-FU maximally suppressed SC tumour growth. The number of apoptotic cells was significantly increased in IGF-1R/dn expressing HT29dn tumours by TUNEL assay.

These results suggest that IGF-1R/482st has significant potential for both prevention and treatment of human cancer cells.

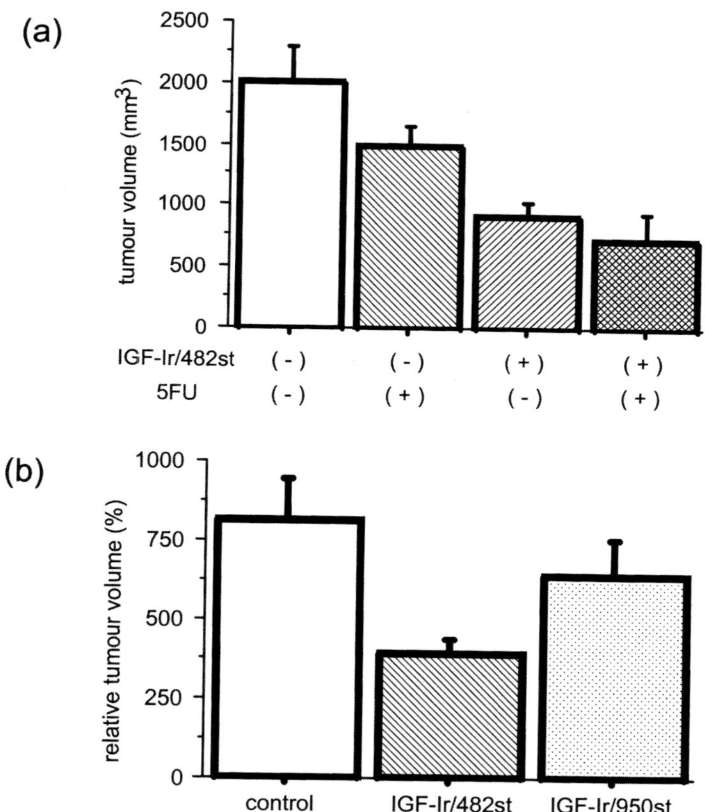

FIG. 3. (a) Both 5-FU (i.p.) and IGF-1R/482st (intratumour expression) reduced growth of HT-29dn SC tumour on nude mice. The combination therapy was most effective among four groups. (b) Both Ad-IGF-Ir/dn suppressed HT-29 SC tumour growth in mice. Ad-IGF-1R/482st was more effective than Ad-IGF-1R/950st.

Adenovirus expressing IGF-1R/dn, *in vitro* effects

Previous studies using stable transfectants showed that IGF-1R/482st can reduce both tumorigenicity and tumour progression, but stable transfection of *in situ* human tumours is not a clinically achievable goal. To facilitate the potential application of dominant negative blockade of IGF-1R into clinical practice, we constructed two adenoviruses expressing IGF-1R/dns, Ad-IGF-1R/482st and Ad-IGF-1R/950st (Adachi et al 2002, Lee et al 2003, Min et al 2003). Both Ad-IGF-1R/dns can induce truncated receptors in a dose-dependent fashion roughly proportional to the dose of adenovirus in colon, pancreas, and lung cancer cell

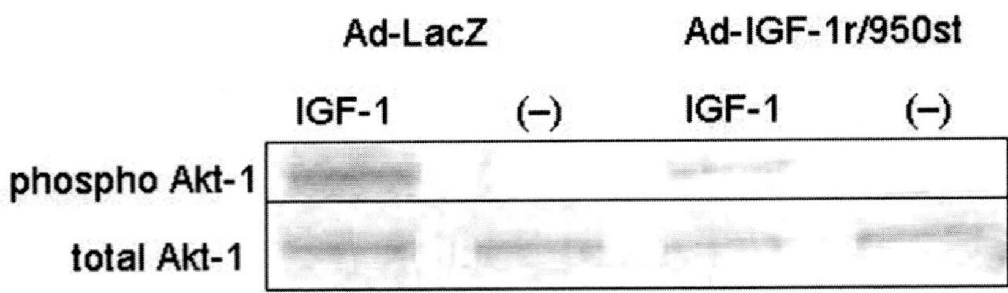

FIG. 4. Ad-IGF-Ir/950st blocked IGF-1-induced phosphorylation of Akt-1 in NCI-H460 cells evaluated by Western blot assay.

lines, confirmed by FACS and Western blotting. As expected, in these experiments IGF-1R/950st is detected on the cell surface and IGF-1R/482st is secreted.

Blockade of IGF-1 signalling by ad-IGF-1R/dns effectively blocked IGF-1 induced DNA synthesis, an index of mitogenesis. This finding suggested that the truncated IGF-1Rs are competing with normal IGF-1R for the ligands. Both Ad-IGF-1R/dns induced marked suppression of NCI-H460 colony formation in a soft agar assay, indicating that Ad-IGF-1R/dn transduction reduces *in vitro* tumorigenicity. Although control cells transduced with Ad-LacZ continued to grow, three pancreatic cancer cells (PANC-1, BxPC-3, and AsPC-1) infected with Ad-IGF-1R/482st decreased the number of viable cells significantly, as detected by trypan blue dye exclusion assays.

Ad-IGF-1R/dns up-regulated chemotherapy and stressor (serum starvation and 5% ethanol) induced apoptosis in two pancreatic cancer cells (BxPC-3 and AsPC-1) as analysed by caspase 3 colorimetric protease assay and DNA fragmentation assay. Ad-IGF-1R/dn also enhanced chemotherapy (5-FU)- and radiation-induced apoptosis in both pancreatic and colon cancer cells (BxPC-3 and HT29).

IGF-induced phosphorylated Akt was reduced by infection with both Ad-IGF-1R/dns in all of the colon, pancreatic, and lung cancer cells analysed, as assessed by Western blotting and Akt-kinase assays (Fig. 4). In both AsPC-1 and BxPC-3 cells, Ad-IGF-1R/dn also blocked IGF-1 induced phosphorylation of p38 MAPK but did not influence those of ERK-1 and -2 significantly. IGF-1R/482st blocked des(1-3)IGF-1-induced phosphorylation of Akt in both pancreatic cancer cells. des(1-3)IGF-1 is a mutant of IGF-1 that does not bind to IGF binding proteins (IGFBPs), suggesting that the effects of IGF-1R/dn we are observing are not likely mediated by changes in binding by the IGFBPs in these models.

In order to investigate signal pathways downstream from IGF-1R, we used three inhibitors with BxPC-3 cells. Both the PI3K inhibitor wortmannin and the MEK1 inhibitor PD98059 suppressed the *in vitro* cell growth of both AsPC-1 and

BxPC-3 cells (as well as Ad-IGF-1R/482st), but the p38 inhibitor SB203580 did not. Combined with the fact that IGF-1R/dn blocked IGF-induced phosphorylation of both Akt and p38 but not that of ERK, these data suggest that the anti-mitogenic effect of IGF-1R/dn is mediated by the inhibition of PI3K/Akt in pancreatic cancer cells. Both wortmannin and SB203580 up-regulated ethanol-induced apoptosis, but PD98059 did not. In total, these data suggest that both the PI3K/Akt pathway and the p38 pathway appear to mediate the anti-apoptotic effect of the IGFs in BxPC-3 cells.

As IGF-1R/482st is secreted protein, we tried to confirm whether Ad-IGF-1R/482st has a bystander effect. BxPC-3 cells were infected with Ad-IGF-1R/482st or Ad-LacZ, after being washed, and subsequently cultured with complete medium. These conditioned media were then transferred to untreated cultures of BxPC-3 cells. Conditioned media from cells infected with Ad-IGF-1R/482st suppressed cell growth significantly by trypan blue assay and resulted in increased ethanol-induced apoptosis by a caspase-3 assay. These results suggest that a gene therapeutic strategy using IGF-1R/482st should have enhanced antitumour effects by virtue of its bystander effect.

Adenovirus expressing IGF-1R/dn, *in vivo* effects

As Ad-IGF-1R/dns have a marked potential to reduce mitogenesis and to induce apoptosis *in vitro*, then we investigated their *in vivo* efficacy using mouse tumour models (Adachi et al 2002, Lee et al 2003, Min et al 2003).

The growth of SC tumours derived from the BxPC-3 cells infected with Ad-IGF-1R/dn was diminished significantly compared to those infected with a control virus. Moreover, tumours derived from IGF-1R/dn expressing cells had much more limited invasion to the underlying muscle. These results indicate that IGF-1R/482st effectively down-regulates *in vivo* tumorigenicity and invasiveness.

Intratumoural injection of Ad-IGF-1R/dn resulted in growth retardation or shrinkage of established tumours of HT29, BxPC-3 and NCI-H460. The tumour suppressive effect of Ad-IGF-1R/482st was more apparent than that of Ad-IGF-1R/950st, undoubtedly due to the bystander effect of IGF-1R/482st (Fig. 3b). Tumour invasiveness was also suppressed by IGF-1R/dn. The results suggest that IGF-1R/482st can both effectively treat pre-existing *in vivo* tumours and reduce their local invasiveness. Again in this model, the number of apoptotic cells was significantly increased in tumours injected with Ad-IGF-1R/482st compared to controls, evaluated by TUNEL assay.

The combination therapy of Ad-IGF-1R/482st with chemotherapy for SC BxPC-3 tumours in mice was then assessed. Adenovirus was injected intratumourally and 5-FU was injected intraperitoneally. This combination therapy of Ad-IGF-1R/482st and 5-FU was more effective than ad-IGF-1R/482st alone or 5-FU alone, and one-third of tumours in the mice treated with this combination were cured, while none were cured with either agent alone. This indicates that Ad-IGF-1R/482st has potential to enhance the effectiveness of standard cancer therapies.

In addition, AsPC-1 cells forms lymph node and distant metastases after i.p. transplantation. To assess the effect of IGF-1Rdn on metastasis, AsPC-1 bearing mice were treated by the i.p. administration of Ad-IGF-1R/482st or control virus. Ad-IGF-1R/482st reduced the number of lymph node metastases and metastatic liver nodules and, moreover, resulted in a significant prolongation of survival in these mice. The data indicate that Ad-IGF-1R/482st may have additional efficacy in reducing both peritoneal dissemination and metastasis.

Discussion

IGF-mediated growth responsiveness is found in most cancer cells of epithelial origin, including lung, colon and pancreas (Bergmann et al 1995, Freier et al 1999, Nakanishi et al 1988). Recent studies have shown that elevation of serum IGF-1 increases the risk of developing several cancers, e.g. colon, prostate and breast (Chan et al 1998, Hankinson et al 1998, Ma et al 1999). Many studies have reported that IGFs/IGF-1R signals affect tumour development in ways other than mitogenic or anti-apoptotic effects. Overexpressed IGF-1R signals are thus also important in tumour dissemination through the control of adhesion, migration and metastasis.

For lung cancer, the IGFs and their receptors are very important in lung development and the growth of cells in the respiratory system (Stiles & D'Ercole 1990). Many human lung cancer cell lines produce both the ligand and the receptor, indicating that in this tumour IGF-1 and IGF-1R can mediate autocrine proliferation (Ankrapp & Bevan 1993, Nakanishi et al 1988). In human colorectal carcinomas, exogenous IGFs stimulate the proliferation of cancer cells, whereas blocking IGF-1R inhibits tumour growth (Lahm et al 1994, Remacle-Bonnet et al 1992). Intestinal fibroblast-derived IGF-2 has been shown to stimulate proliferation of intestinal epithelial cells in a paracrine manner (Simmons et al 1999). Both IGF-2 and IGF-1R messages are increased in colon cancers (Freier et al 1999). Moreover, high levels of circulating IGF-1 and low levels of IGF-binding protein 3 are related to an increased risk of colorectal cancer (Ma et al 1999). In pancreatic cancer, aberrant activation of IGF-1R by paracrine and autocrine mechanisms has been suggested because IGF-1 expression is increased in cancer tissue (Bergmann et al 1995). The functional importance of IGF-1R in pancreatic cancer was demonstrated by the fact that introduction of antisense IGF-1R decreased both basal and IGF-1-stimulated cell proliferation of AsPC-1. IGF-1 has also been shown to antagonize the antiproliferative effects of cyclooxygenase 2 inhibitors on BxPC-3 cells (Levitt & Pollak 2002). The IGF/IGF-1R system has also been reported to be important in haematological tumours, e.g. multiple myeloma (Tai et al 2003). Thus, these approaches for blocking for IGF-1R might have potency in a wide range of malignancies other than carcinomas in the three organs presented here (lung, colon and pancreas).

In some cancers, IGF-2 is more important for tumour progression than IGF-1, and an IGF-2/IGF-1R autocrine loop has been reported (Freier et al 1999, Simmons et al 1999). We have shown that Ad-IGF-1R/dn can block not only IGF-1 but also IGF-2 stimulation of cancer cells, broadening the potential activity of IGF-1R/dn as an antitumour therapeutic.

We and others have found that most of the anticancer effects of IGF signalling blockade seen in the cancer models tested is mediated through inhibition of Akt-1 activation. Akt-1 has in fact been shown to up-regulate IGF-1R expression and increase tumour invasiveness (Tanno et al 2001).

We have constructed two truncated IGF-1Rs and in our *in vivo* studies IGF-1R/482st is more potent than IGF-1R/950st. The main functional difference between these two dn receptors is the demonstrable bystander effect observed with IGF-1R/482st, and this property may be important for practical application to human malignancies. IGF-1R/dn significantly enhances chemotherapy- and radiation-induced apoptosis *in vitro* and chemotherapeutic efficacy *in vivo*, suggesting the testing of combinations with standard therapies.

While adenovirus delivery of receptor mutants has been an effective way to validate the IGF-1R as a therapeutic target, there are drawbacks to this approach as well, primarily as a consequence of the viral vector chosen. The advantages of adenovirus include that it is highly infective for actively dividing, slowly dividing and non-dividing tumour cells that often coexist in solid tumours, and it causes the expression of high levels of the transduced gene (Tang et al 1994). However, clinical results from adenoviral gene therapy approaches are less successful than expectations from *in vitro* data, at least partly as a consequence of the low observed clinical gene transfer rate. In a human tumour mass, it is very difficult to transfer the therapeutic gene to even the majority of tumour cells with currently available gene transfer vectors. The intratumoural dispersion of replication-defective viral vectors is usually confined to the injection site, resulting in impractical and ineffective schemes requiring dozens of injections into tumours in clinical trials. In addition, a few side effects have been reported from gene therapy using adenovirus vectors. Thus although an adenoviral vector has huge advantages compared to stable transfection, there are some unsolved hurdles in its practical application. Recombinant receptor fragment peptides, tyrosine kinase inhibitors, interfering RNA or one of the recently reported IGF-1-specific antibodies (Maloney et al 2003) may be more practical.

In summary, these studies have shown that blockade of IGF-1R signals suppresses tumorigenicity of human lung, colon and pancreatic cancer cells both *in vitro* and *in vivo*. It increases chemotherapy and stressor-induced apoptosis in these cancer cells, both *in vitro* and *in vivo*, and IGF-1R/482st has a clear bystander effect. IGF-1R/dn exerts its anticancer effects mainly via inhibition of Akt-1. The blockade for IGF-1R signals also reduces peritoneal dissemination and prolongs survival in peritoneal models. These data suggest that the blockade of IGF/IGF-1R signalling by IGF-1R/dn may be a useful therapeutic strategy for human malignancies, including lung, colon and pancreatic cancer.

References

Adachi Y, Lee CT, Coffee K et al 2002 Effects of genetic blockade of the insulin-like growth factor receptor in human colon cancer cell lines. Gastroenterology 123:1191–1204

Ankrapp DP, Bevan DR 1993 Insulin-like growth factor-I and human lung fibroblast-derived insulin-like growth factor-I stimulate the proliferation of human lung carcinoma cells *in vitro*. Cancer Res 53:3399–3404

Baserga R 1994 Oncogenes and the strategy of growth factors. Cell 79:927–930

Baserga R 1995 The insulin-like growth factor I receptor: a key to tumor growth? Cancer Res 55:249–252

Bergmann U, Funatomi H, Yokoyama M, Beger HG, Korc M 1995 Insulin-like growth factor I overexpression in human pancreatic cancer: evidence for autocrine and paracrine roles. Cancer Res 55:2007–2011

Burgaud JL, Resnicoff M, Baserga R 1995 Mutant IGF-1 receptors as dominant negatives for growth and transformation. Biochem Biophys Res Commun 214:475–481

Chan JM, Stampfer MJ, Giovannucci E et al 1998 Plasma insulin-like growth factor-I and prostate cancer risk: a prospective study. Science 279:563–566

D'Ambrosio C, Ferber A, Resnicoff M, Baserga R 1996 A soluble insulin-like growth factor I receptor that induces apoptosis of tumor cells in vivo and inhibits tumorigenesis. Cancer Res 56:4013–4020

Dunn SE, Ehrlich M, Sharp NJ et al 1998 A dominant negative mutant of the insulin-like growth factor-I receptor inhibits the adhesion, invasion, and metastasis of breast cancer. Cancer Res 58:3353–3361

Freier S, Weiss O, Eran M et al 1999 Expression of the insulin-like growth factors and their receptors in adenocarcinoma of the colon. Gut 44:704–708

Hankinson SE, Willett WC, Colditz GA et al 1998 Circulating concentrations of insulin-like growth factor-I and risk of breast cancer. Lancet 351:1393–1396

Hannon GJ 2002 RNA interference. Nature 418:244–251

Lahm H, Amstad P, Wyniger J et al 1994 Blockade of the insulin-like growth-factor-I receptor inhibits growth of human colorectal cancer cells: evidence of a functional IGF-II-mediated autocrine loop. Int J Cancer 58:452–459

Lee CT, Wu S, Gabrilovich D et al 1996 Antitumor effects of an adenovirus expressing antisense insulin-like growth factor I receptor on human lung cancer cell lines. Cancer Res 56:3038–3041

Lee CT, Park KH, Adachi Y et al 2003 Recombinant adenoviruses expressing dominant negative insulin-like growth factor-I receptor demonstrate antitumor effects on lung cancer. Cancer Gene Ther 10:57–63

Levitt RJ, Pollak M 2002 Insulin-like growth factor-I antagonizes the antiproliferative effects of cyclooxygenase-2 inhibitors on BxPC-3 pancreatic cancer cells. Cancer Res 62:7372–7376

Li S, Resnicoff M, Baserga R 1996 Effect of mutations at serines 1280–1283 on the mitogenic and transforming activities of the insulin-like growth factor I receptor. J Biol Chem 271: 12254–12260

Liu JP, Baker J, Perkins AS, Robertson EJ, Efstratiadis A 1993 Mice carrying null mutations of the genes encoding insulin-like growth factor I (Igf-1) and type 1 IGF receptor (Igf1r). Cell 75:59–72

Long L, Rubin R, Baserga R, Brodt P 1995 Loss of the metastatic phenotype in murine carcinoma cells expressing an antisense RNA to the insulin-like growth factor receptor. Cancer Res 55:1006–1009

Ma J, Pollak MN, Giovannucci E et al 1999 Prospective study of colorectal cancer risk in men and plasma levels of insulin-like growth factor (IGF)-I and IGF-binding protein-3. J Natl Cancer Inst 91:620–625

Maloney EK, McLaughlin JL, Dagdigian NE et al 2003 An anti-insulin-like growth factor I receptor antibody that is a potent inhibitor of cancer cell proliferation. Cancer Res 63: 5073–5083

Min Y, Adachi Y, Yamamoto H et al 2003 Genetic blockade of the insulin-like growth factor-I receptor: a promising strategy for human pancreatic cancer. Cancer Res 63:6432–6441

Nakanishi Y, Mulshine JL, Kasprzyk PG et al 1988 Insulin-like growth factor-I can mediate autocrine proliferation of human small cell lung cancer cell lines *in vitro*. J Clin Invest 82:354–359

Prager D, Li HL, Asa S, Melmed S 1994 Dominant negative inhibition of tumorigenesis *in vivo* by human insulin-like growth factor I receptor mutant. Proc Natl Acad Sci USA 91: 2181–2185

Remacle-Bonnet M, Garrouste F, el Atiq F, Roccabianca M, Marvaldi J, Pommier G 1992 des-(1-3)-IGF-I, an insulin-like growth factor analog used to mimic a potential IGF-II autocrine loop, promotes the differentiation of human colon-carcinoma cells. Int J Cancer 52:910–917

Resnicoff M, Coppola D, Sell C, Rubin R, Ferrone S, Baserga R 1994 Growth inhibition of human melanoma cells in nude mice by antisense strategies to the type 1 insulin-like growth factor receptor. Cancer Res 54:4848–4850

Sara VR, Hall K 1990 Insulin-like growth factors and their binding proteins. Physiol Rev 70:591–614

Sell C, Rubini M, Rubin R, Liu JP, Efstratiadis A, Baserga R 1993 Simian virus 40 large tumor antigen is unable to transform mouse embryonic fibroblasts lacking type 1 insulin-like growth factor receptor. Proc Natl Acad Sci USA 90:11217–11221

Simmons JG, Pucilowska JB, Lund PK 1999 Autocrine and paracrine actions of intestinal fibroblast-derived insulin-like growth factors. Am J Physiol 276:G817–827

Stiles AD, D'Ercole AJ 1990 The insulin-like growth factors and the lung. Am J Respir Cell Mol Biol 3:93–100

Tai YT, Podar K, Catley L et al 2003 Insulin-like growth factor-1 induces adhesion and migration in human multiple myeloma cells via activation of beta1-integrin and phosphatidylinositol 3′-kinase/AKT signaling. Cancer Res 63:5850–5858

Tang DC, Johnston SA, Carbone DP 1994 Butyrate-inducible and tumor-restricted gene expression by adenovirus vectors. Cancer Gene Ther 1:15–20

Tanno S, Mitsuuchi Y, Altomare DA, Xiao GH, Testa JR 2001 AKT activation up-regulates insulin-like growth factor I receptor expression and promotes invasiveness of human pancreatic cancer cells. Cancer Res 61:589–593

Ullrich A, Gray A, Tam AW et al 1986 Insulin-like growth factor I receptor primary structure: comparison with insulin receptor suggests structural determinants that define functional specificity. EMBO J 5:2503–2512

Yu H, Rohan T 2000 Role of the insulin-like growth factor family in cancer development and progression. J Natl Cancer Inst 92:1472–1489

DISCUSSION

LeRoith: My understanding was that adenoviruses are losing favour compared with lentiviruses and others as vectors of gene therapy.

Carbone: Other viruses such as lentiviruses have the ability to stably transduce cells, but in cancer the goal is to kill the cell, not to result in perpetual gene expression. Adenoviruses may be better for this because they tend to have a high transduction efficiency, especially the new re-targeted vectors. They are also useful as a molecular probe of the pathway. Until you have your TKI to block a receptor you can use the virus to put in a dominant negative and test the result of blocking the pathway. We did all of these experiments before siRNA was described. Even siRNA has some limitations, including non-target effects. Adenoviruses can be generated pretty readily, and are very easy to propagate. If you want to treat an animal with an adenovirus you just grow it up in tissue culture and it takes a few days, whereas making therapeutic quantities of siRNA is much more difficult and expensive.

Ohlsson: The tumour formation was not totally inhibited.

Carbone: In some cases it was: we had several cured animals with some of the more effective recombinants.

Ohlsson: What was the reason for incomplete cure in many cases? Is it because some tumours were not using the IGF-1R pathway initially, or did you adapt these cells during treatment?

Carbone: This was one of my concerns with the stable transfection experiments. In order to grow out a colony of tumour cells that stably express the dominant negative, you are selecting for cells that are tolerant to that perturbation. I thought this was not an effective model for a cancer therapy. This is why we used recombinant adenoviruses and the tet-regulated model. The question could be answered differently in two different settings. In the tet-regulated clone we did not see any cures. We always saw outgrowth of escape variants. I am not sure what the physiology of these were. The tet is never that good a regulator and it is possible that there was clonal outgrowth of non-producing variants. I also suspect that in the adenovirus experiments the problem was the inefficiency of transduction. You can imagine poking a needle into a tumour and not achieving a homogeneous distribution of virus expression. Our greatest number of cures occurred when we combined the ad-IGF with a conditionally replicated virus and we could then cure most of those animals with palpable tumours.

Pollak: Given the results you showed, particularly with the precedent for the delivery system with p53 and your evidence that another package to deliver by the same technology is 10–100-fold stronger, and given that bronchoalveolar cancer is basically a fatal untreatable disease, what are your plans? Do you plan a clinical trial with this approach in bronchoalveolar cancer?

Carbone: It is difficult to make a clinically approvable virus product. The only reason I used that p53 is because a company made it and they gave it to me. No one makes the Ad-dns that I know of. It would take a couple of hundred thousand dollars to produce this, and it is a side project in my lab so we can't afford this. I have been interested in trying to get some of the TKIs to use in phase I studies in patients. But I think that in certain situations, such as bronchoalveolar cancer, I would like to try it.

Jenkins: Have you looked at the expression of any of the IGF-1 axis members in lung cancer?

Carbone: No, we haven't started to look at this. We have been looking more at doing molecular predictive pattern analysis with the proteomics and trying to define lymph node involvement patterns or survival patterns.

Yee: Have you looked at Iressa (gefitinib) resistance and sensitivity patterns in the bronchoalveolar carcinoma line?

Carbone: We have a pattern in cell lines. These are *de novo* patterns: they are not cell lines that have been induced to be resistant to gefitinib. The ideal experiment would require fresh human tumour tissue from a statistically significant number of people who respond to gefitinib. Because only 10% of patients respond to gefitinib and it is approved for metastatic disease where you don't get surgical tissue samples, this ideal is very difficult to accomplish.

Yee: I thought the response rate in bronchoalveolar carcinoma was higher.

Carbone: One report was around 30%, but this has not yet been published. I have one patient who has sustained a complete response for over three years, but the majority don't respond at all.

Macaulay: Your 482 soluble receptor was more effective *in vivo* than the 950 dominant negative. Was it a smaller construct, or did you have the full-length cDNA with a truncating mutation?

Carbone: It was a stop mutant construct expressing only an extracellular fragment of the receptor.

Macaulay: Do you think part of the increased efficacy *in vivo* might be because it was smaller and the efficiency of transduction was better?

Carbone: I don't think so. The virus is 30 kb. We are talking small differences. We have shown in a lot of experiments that there is a true bystander effect with that construct that doesn't exist with the others. A bystander effect is the most plausible explanation.

Macaulay: I thought your clinical study was very interesting. Was that in non-small cell patients?

Carbone: It was non-small cell patients but they had to have a bronchoalveolar carcinoma component. These weren't all pure bronchoalveolar carcinomas. This was primarily a safety study: people didn't realize that you could fill up a third of the lung in a patient who already has pulmonary compromise from bronchoalveolar carcinoma with 10^{12} recombinant adenoviruses and that they would still be alive.

Macaulay: Was that a single administration?

Carbone: The study is designed to have two administrations two weeks apart, but individual patients received more than a dozen treatments.

Macaulay: Did you see any immune responses?

Carbone: Yes, huge serum antibody levels developed in these patients. But some of them had as many as 15 injections with no clear adverse effects associated with these antibody responses. We allowed them to continue treatments if they perceived benefit. We saw some transient increased dyspnoea and low-grade fever, but no really significant side effects.

Macaulay: Do you have any way of assessing whether there was an attenuation of clinical benefit in patients who had an immune response?

Carbone: It is difficult to assess. These tumours are hard to measure.

Macaulay: The one you showed appeared to be an objective partial response.

Carbone: The portion of the tumour that responded was the non-solid part, which is what you would expect. This is the part that causes the patient's symptoms. You can live with a basketball-sized tumour in your chest but it is the infiltrative complement that blocks the alveolae and causes you to suffocate to death.

Macaulay: There is a large body of data now to support the concept that the IGF-1R plays an important role in invasion. We referred earlier to the work of Hanahan in which pancreatic tumours develop in Rip-Tag mice that express SV40 T antigen from the rat insulin promoter. Concurrent overexpression of the IGF receptor causes these tumours to become invasive and spontaneously metastatic (Lopez & Hanahan 2002).

Carbone: We saw the same effect in our model: tumours implanted on the peritoneal surface didn't invade as effectively in the presence of the dominant negative receptor.

Reference

Lopez T, Hanahan D 2002 Elevated levels of IGF-1 receptor convey invasive and metastatic capability in a mouse model of pancreatic islet tumorigenesis. Cancer Cell 1:339–353

IGF-1 and prostate cancer

Charles T. Roberts Jr

Department of Pediatrics, NRC5, 3181 SW Sam Jackson Park Road, Portland, OR 97239, USA

Abstract. By virtue of their potent proliferative and anti-apoptotic effects, the insulin-like growth factors (IGFs) have been the subject of long-term scrutiny for their role in tumorigenesis. With regard to prostate cancer in particular, IGF-1 has been shown to stimulate the proliferation of human prostate epithelial cells in culture and to be necessary for normal growth and development of the rat and mouse prostate. Epidemiological studies have established a link between high circulating serum IGF-1 levels and the risk of later developing advanced prostate cancer, and overexpression of IGF-1 in the prostate basal epithelial layer of transgenic mice results in prostate adenocarcinoma that is similar to human disease. Thus, IGF-1 action appears to be important for prostate cancer initiation. On the other hand, decreased IGF action, subsequent to the down-regulation of IGF-1 receptor expression, is associated with advanced, metastatic disease. This decrease in IGF-1 receptor may confer a survival advantage to prostate cancer cells that have entered the circulation by making them resistant to the differentiative effects of IGF-1 at metastatic sites such as bone. The molecular mechanisms that effect IGF-1 receptor down-regulation appear to involve novel oncogenic functions of the Wilms' tumour suppressor, as well as novel actions of the androgen receptor.

2004 Biology of IGF-1: its interaction with insulin in health and malignant states. Wiley, Chichester (Novartis Foundation Symposium 262) p 193–204

An important aspect of the IGF system in postnatal human physiology is its involvement in tumorigenesis. This was to be expected, given the demonstrated role of IGF-1, in particular, as a potent growth regulator in many cell types and tissues. Evidence accumulated over the last several years of a strong association of circulating IGF-1 levels with the risk of developing a number of important human cancers, as well as the ongoing studies of the molecular mechanisms of IGF action in cancer cells, have renewed interest in the therapeutic and diagnostic possibilities of the IGF system in cancer therapy. The sections below summarize these molecular and epidemiological data with respect to prostate cancer.

IGF-1 action in prostate growth and development

A significant amount of data has been accumulated that suggests that the IGF system plays an important role in the normal growth and development of the prostate. Prostatic stromal cells and epithelial cells in primary culture secrete IGF binding proteins (IGFBPs) and stromal cells produce IGF-2, and both stromal and epithelial cells express the IGF-1 receptor (IGF-1R) and are responsive to IGF-1 with respect to proliferation (Peehl et al 1994, Cohen et al 1994, Boudon et al 1996). Prostate epithelial cells respond to locally produced IGF-2 as well as circulating IGF-1 through both paracrine and endocrine mechanisms. The prostate epithelial cell component comprises luminal and basal cell populations, and the latter is thought to contain a presumptive stem cell-like component that is likely to constitute the likely precursors of prostatic intraepithelial neoplasia and prostatic adenocarcinoma. Additional support for an important role for IGF action in prostate growth came from studies showing that systemic administration of IGF-1 increases rat prostate growth (Torring et al 1997), that modulation of rat ventral prostate weight by the 5α-reductase inhibitor finasteride was correlated with altered levels of IGF-1 receptor and IGFBP3 gene expression (Huynh et al 1998), and that IGF-1-deficient mice exhibit decreased prostate size and complexity of prostate architecture (Ruan et al 1999).

IGF-1 and the IGF-1R in prostate cancer-molecular studies

The most direct evidence for a role for IGF-1 in prostate cancer development is based on the phenotype of transgenic mice with targeted expression of IGF-1 in the basal prostatic epithelium (DiGiovanni et al 2000). The increased local production of IGF-1 resulted in the appearance of hyperplastic lesions that resembled prostatic intraepithelial neoplasia by 6 months of age, and prostatic adenocarcinomas or small cell carcinomas were eventually seen in 50% of the transgenic animals. Thus, overexpression of IGF-1 and the constitutive activation of IGF-1 receptors in basal epithelial cells resulted in tumour development and progression similar to that seen in human disease.

A number of studies reported over the last 10–15 years have described overexpression of the IGF-1R in breast, prostate and other tumour types. For the most part, however, these are analysed tissue homogenates or established cancer cell lines for which appropriate normal controls do not exist. The apparent IGF-1R content of homogenates, in particular, can be affected by contamination with stroma, which would dilute the IGF-1R content of normal epithelium or small tumours. Studies of IGF-1R expression in breast and prostate samples employing immunohistochemistry, or of matched cell lines corresponding to normal and tumour tissue, revealed that normal epithelium and early-stage tumours both express abundant IGF-1R, while IGF-1R expression was significantly reduced in advanced, metastatic prostate and breast cancer (Tennant et al 1996, Happerfield et al 1997, Chott et al 1999, Damon et al 2001). Decreased IGF-1R expression is also seen in metastases in the TRAMP prostate cancer model

(Kaplan et al 1999). Additionally, Plymate et al (1997) have reported that re-expression of the IGF-1R in metastatic prostate epithelial cells reversed their malignant phenotype and increased sensitivity to apoptosis. These studies support the novel hypothesis that reduced IGF-1R action is necessary for prostate cancer progression. The activation of the IGF-1R present in normal epithelium by elevated circulating levels of IGF-1 may explain the epidemiological data described in more detail below, whereas the subsequent decrease in IGF-1R expression (if substantiated by additional studies) may represent an attempt by established cancer cells to avoid the potential differentiating effects of IGF-1 at sites of metastasis. Alternatively, decreased expression of the IGF-1R may protect metastasizing cells from a novel, non-apoptotic form of programmed cell death that has been recently described as being triggered by the unliganded IGF-1R (Sperandio et al 2000).

In contrast to the reports of IGF-1R down-regulation in prostate cancer progression cited above, Hellawell et al (2002) have reported that IGF-1R expression is decreased in some metastatic prostate cancer samples as compared to benign or carcinoma tissue, but is increased in a majority of samples studied (eight out of 12). In this study, however, IGF-1R immunostaining with a single β-subunit antibody was diffusely cytoplasmic in most samples, in contrast to the expected membrane localization reported by Chott et al (1999), using two different α-subunit antibodies. In a separate study, Nickerson et al (2001) found a three- to fourfold increase in IGF-1R (and IGF-1) gene expression during progression to androgen dependence in LNCaP and LAPC-9 xenografts, but a 10-fold decrease in IGF-1R expression in the LAPC-4 xenograft model. From these studies, it is clear that the extent and prevalence of IGF-1R over- or underexpression in prostate cancer progression remains controversial.

In tissue culture models in which IGF-1R expression is down-regulated in metastatic vs. non-metastatic cells, two potential mechanisms have been proposed that may explain decreased IGF-1R gene expression. The WT1 Wilms' tumour suppressor gene product is a potent repressor of IGF-1R gene expression (Werner et al 1994) and its expression is increased in prostate cancer (Ng et al 1996). Introduction of WT1 into immortalized prostate epithelial cells reduces endogenous IGF-1R promoter activity and expression (Damon et al 2001). Based on these data, it is possible that one component of IGF-1R down-regulation in metastatic prostate cancer is the increased action of WT1. Another potential mode of IGF-1R down-regulation involves the androgen receptor. Re-expression of the androgen receptor in androgen receptor-deficient prostate cancer cells that express low levels of the IGF-1R increases IGF-1R expression and reduces tumorigenicity in nude mouse xenografts (Plymate et al 2004). Thus, the alteration of androgen receptor action seen in the conversion to androgen-independent disease may result in the loss of IGF-1R expression.

Apparently contradictory reports have also been published on the effect of altered IGF-1R expression on prostate cancer cell behaviour. In addition to the reports cited above on the anti-tumorigenic effects of IGF-1R re-expression (Plymate et al 1997), there are other reports that antisense inhibition of IGF-1R gene expression (Burfeind et al 1996) or expression of a dominant-negative IGF-1R in prostate cancer cells can also inhibit tumorigenicity. These conflicting findings can be reconciled if there exist different levels or 'set points' of IGF-1R activity (determined by changes in IGF-1R gene expression, intrinsic receptor activity, or the activity of signal transduction pathways), and that deviation from this set point in either direction modulates cellular phenotype. This concept is supported by the earlier studies of Rubini et al (1997) demonstrating that small changes in IGF-1R levels in the physiological range modulate the mitogenic and transforming phenotype of mouse embryo cells.

IGF-1 and prostate cancer: epidemiological studies

The potent mitogenic activity of IGF-1 in cell culture made it an obvious candidate risk factor in cancer development, but it was not until 1998 that several prospective studies suggested that high circulating levels of IGF-1 were associated with an increased risk of prostate cancer (Mantzoros et al 1997, Wolk et al 1998, Cohen 1998). The association between IGF-1 levels and prostate cancer risk was questioned in subsequent cross-sectional studies (Cutting et al 1999, Kurek et al 2000), while Djavan et al (1999), in a prospective study, found that the IGF-1/prostate-specific antigen (PSA) ratio was superior to IGF-1 or PSA measurements alone for predicting prostate cancer risk. A meta-analysis of the data available in 2000 (Shaneyfelt et al 2000) concluded that high circulating IGF-1 levels (although still within normal limits) posed a risk equivalent to that associated with high testosterone. In a screening trial, Finne et al (2000) did not find an association between serum IGF-1 levels and prostate cancer risk, while Baffa et al (2000) found that circulating IGF-1 levels were actually lower in a group of patients undergoing radical prostatectomy as compared to age-matched controls. In additional prospective studies, however, Harman et al (2000) and Stattin et al (2000) found that IGF-1 levels were associated with prostate cancer risk, and that this association was especially evident in younger men. A second meta-analysis of 14 case-controlled studies (Shi et al 2001) concluded that high normal circulating IGF-1 levels were associated with prostate cancer risk. In a subsequent cross-sectional study, Latif et al (2002) did not find a correlation between levels of IGF-1 or IGFBP3 and prostate cancer stage, while, in the latest prospective study (Chan et al 2002), circulating IGF-1 levels appeared to be most predictive of advanced prostate cancer.

While the conclusions of this extensive series of studies are contradictory, there is some consistency. Prospective studies have consistently demonstrated an association between high circulating IGF-1 levels and prostate cancer risk, while cross-sectional studies have generated variable results. These data suggest that high serum IGF-1 levels in younger men predict the occurrence of advanced prostate cancer years later, while IGF-1 levels at the time of diagnosis may be less informative. Specifically, long-term exposure of prostate epithelial cells to high levels of serum-derived IGF-1 may increase the probability of initiating hyperplasia in these cellular precursors of prostatic intraepithelial neoplasia and subsequent prostate adenocarcinoma.

Summary

From the studies described above, it is clear that IGF-1 action is important in normal prostate growth and development as well as prostate cancer initiation and progression. The action of the IGF system in prostate tumorigenesis includes both expected and unanticipated effects of this complicated signalling mechanism. Specifically, the effects of IGF-1 on prostate growth and tumour development in mice and the association of high circulating IGF-1 concentrations with increased prostate cancer risk in humans are consistent with the well-characterized mitogenic properties of IGF-1, while the counter-intuitive decrease in IGF-1R expression seen in advanced human and murine prostate cancer and cell lines derived from prostate metastases may necessitate a re-evaluation of the assumptions that underlie our current understanding of IGF system function in growth and development in general. In any case, the data that continue to accumulate regarding the role of IGF-1 action in prostate cancer consistently support the appropriateness of IGF-1 and IGF-1 signalling as a target for diagnosis and therapy of this important disease.

References

Baffa R, Reiss K, El-Gabry EA et al 2000 Low serum insulin-like growth factor 1 (IGF-1): a significant association with prostate cancer. Tech Urol 6:236–239

Boudon C, Rodier G, Lechevallier E, Mottet N, Barenton B, Sultan C 1996 Secretion of insulin-like growth factors and their binding proteins by human normal and hyperplastic prostatic cells in primary culture. J Clin Endocrinol Metab 81:612–617

Burfeind P, Chernicky CL, Rininsland F, Ilan J, Ilan J 1996 Antisense RNA to the type I insulin-like growth factor receptor suppresses tumor growth and prevents invasion by rat prostate cancer cells *in vivo*. Proc Natl Acad Sci USA 93:7263–7268

Chan JM, Stampfer MJ, Ma J et al 2002 Insulin-like growth factor-I (IGF-I) and IGF binding protein-3 as predictors of advanced-stage prostate cancer. J Natl Cancer Inst 94:1099–1106

Chott A, Sun Z, Morganstern D et al 1999 Tyrosine kinases expressed *in vivo* by human prostate cancer bone marrow metastases and loss of type 1 insulin-like growth factor receptor. Am J Pathol 155:1271–1279

Cohen P 1998 Serum insulin-like growth factor I levels and prostate cancer risk — interpreting the evidence. J Natl Cancer Inst 90:876–876

Cohen P, Peehl DM, Rosenfeld RG 1994 The IGF axis in the prostate. Horm Metab Res 26: 81–84

Cutting CW, Hunt C, Nisbet JA, Bland JM, Dalgleish AG, Kirby RS 1999 Serum insulin-like growth factor-1 is not a useful marker of prostate cancer. BJU Int 83:996–999

Damon SE, Plymate SR, Carroll JM et al 2001 Transcriptional regulation of insulin-like growth factor-I receptor gene expression in prostate cancer cells. Endocrinology 142:21–27

DiGiovanni J, Kiguchi K, Frijhoff A et al 2000 Deregulated expression of insulin-like growth factor 1 in prostate epithelium leads to neoplasia in transgenic mice. Proc Natl Acad Sci USA 97:3455–3460

Djavan G, Bursa B, Seitz C et al 1999 Insulin-like growth factor 1 (IGF-1), IGF-1 density, and IGF-1/PSA ratio for prostate cancer detection. Urology 54:603–606

Finne P, Auvinen A, Koistinen H et al 2000 Insulin-like growth factor I is not a useful marker of prostate cancer in men with elevated levels of prostate-specific antigen. J Clin Endocrinol Metab 85:2744–2747

Happerfield LC, Miles DW, Barnes DM, Thomsen LL, Smith P, Hanby AM 1997 The localization of the insulin-like growth factor receptor 1 (IGFR-1) in benign and malignant breast tissue. J Pathol 183:412–417

Harman SM, Metter EJ, Blackman MR, Landis PK, Carter HB 2000 Serum levels of insulin-like growth factor I (IGF-I), IGF-II, IGF-binding protein-3, and prostate-specific antigen as predictor of clinical prostate cancer J Clin Endocrinol Metab 85: 4258–4265

Hellawell GO, Turner GD, Davies DR, Poulsom R, Brewster SF, Macaulay VM 2002 Expression of the type 1 insulin-like growth factor receptor is up-regulated in primary prostate cancer and commonly persists in metastatic disease. Cancer Res 62: 2942–2950

Huynh H, Seyam RM, Brock GB 1998 Reduction of ventral prostate weight by finasteride is associated with suppression of insulin-like growth factor I (IGF-I) and IGF-I receptor genes and with an increase in IGF binding protein 3. Cancer Res 58:215–218

Kaplan PJ, Mohan S, Cohen P, Foster BA, Greenberg NM 1999 The insulin-like growth factor axis and prostate cancer: lessons from the transgenic adenocarcinoma of mouse prostate (TRAMP) model. Cancer Res 59:2203–2209

Kurek R, Tunn UW, Eckart O, Aumuller G, Wong J, Renneberg H 2000 The significance of serum levels of insulin-like growth factor-1 in patients with prostate cancer. BJU Int 85: 125–129

Latif Z, McMillan DC, Wallace AM et al 2002 The relationship of circulating insulin-like growth factor 1, its binding protein-3, prostate-specific antigen and C-reactive protein with disease stage in prostate cancer. BJU Int 89:396–399

Mantzoros CS, Tzonou A, Signorello LB, Stampfer M, Trichopoulos D, Adami HO 1997 Insulin-like growth factor 1 in relation to prostate cancer and benign prostatic hyperplasia. Br J Cancer 76:1115–1118

Ng YK, Teng SP, Bales W, Rodeck U, Veltri RW 1996 Increased expression of Wilms' tumor protein (WT1) in prostate cancer. In: 87th Annual Meeting of the American Association of Cancer Research, Washington DC, p 599

Nickerson T, Chang F, Lorimer D, Smeekens SP, Sawyers C, Pollak M 2001 *In vivo* progression of LAPC-9 and LNCaP prostate cancer models to androgen independence is associated with increased expression of insulin-like growth factor I (IGF-I) and IGF-I receptor (IGF-IR). Cancer Res 61:6276–6280

Peehl DM, Cohen P, Rosenfeld RG 1994 The insulin-like growth factor system in the prostate. World J Urol 13:306–311

Plymate S, Bae VL, Maddison L, Quinn LS, Ware JL 1997 Reexpression of the type 1 insulin-like growth factor receptor inhibits the malignant phenotype of simian virus 40 T antigen immortalized human prostate epithelial cells. Endocrinology 138:1728–1735

Plymate SR, Tennant MK, Culp SH et al 2004 Androgen receptor (AR) expression in AR-negative prostate cancer cells results in differential effects of DHT and IGF-1 on proliferation and AR activity between localized and metastatic tumors. Prostate, in press

Ruan W, Powell-Braxton L, Kopchick JJ, Kleinberg DL 1999 Evidence that insulin-like growth factor I and growth hormone are required for prostate gland development. Endocrinology 140:1984–1989

Rubini M, Hongo A, D'Ambrosio C, Baserga R 1997 The IGF-I receptor in mitogenesis and transformation of mouse embryo cells: role of receptor number. Exp Cell Res 230:284–292

Shaneyfelt T, Husein R, Bubley G, Mantzoros CS 2000 Hormonal predictors of prostate cancer: a meta-analysis. J Clin Oncol 18:847–853

Shi R, Berkel HJ, Yu H 2001 Insulin-like growth factor-I and prostate cancer: a meta-analysis. Br J Cancer 85:991–996

Sperandio S, de Belle I, Bredesen DE 2000 An alternative, nonapoptotic form of programmed cell death. Proc Natl Acad Sci USA 97:14376–14381

Stattin P, Bylund A, Rinaldi S et al 2000 Plasma insulin-like growth factor-I, insulin-like growth factor-binding proteins, and prostate cancer risk: a prospective study. J Natl Cancer Inst 92:1910–1917

Tennant MK, Thrasher JB, Twomey PA, Drivdahl RH, Birnbaum RS, Plymate S 1996 Protein and mRNA for the type 1 insulin-like growth factor (IGF) receptor is decreased and IGF-II mRNA is increased in human prostate carcinoma compared to benign prostate epithelium. J Clin Endocrinol Metab 81:3774–3782

Torring N, Vinter-Jensen L, Pederson SB, Sorensen FB, Flyvbjerg A, Nexo E 1997 Systemic Administration of insulin-like growth factor I (IGF-I) causes growth of the rat prostate. J Urol 158:222–227

Werner H, Rauscher FJ 3rd, Sukhatme VP, Drummond IA, Roberts CT Jr, LeRoith D 1994 Transcriptional repression of the insulin-like growth factor I receptor (IGF-I-R) gene by the tumor suppressor WT1 involves binding to sequences both upstream and downstream of the IGF-IR gene transcription start site J Biol Chem 269:12577–12582

Wolk A, Mantzoros CS, Andersson SO et al 1998 Insulin-like growth factor 1 and prostate cancer risk: a population-based, case-control study. J Natl Cancer Inst 90:911–915

DISCUSSION

Holly: I was fascinated with the situation in the metastatic and advanced cells where you have low levels of the IGF-1R and you see constitutively high activity of MAP kinase. In one experiment you were looking at the interaction with the androgen receptor. If I understood correctly, then you added the MAP kinase inhibitor with the androgen receptor (AR) agonist and got opposite effects depending on whether you had IGF-1R or not. This suggests that MAP kinase without IGF-1 is having the opposite effects in synergy with the androgen. What do think is causing that activation of MAP kinase without the IGF-1R, and how does that impact on the cell's response to all the other ligands that activate pathways which use MAP kinase? Do the cells become less responsive to everything else that uses MAP kinase?

Roberts: We haven't addressed this directly. We can't raise the elevated level of ERK activation any further by IGF-1 unless we put the IGF-1R back in. The re-expression of the IGF-1R drops to basal so that IGF-1 now can activate ERK above a low basal level. What we haven't asked is whether with EGF or PDGF it is possible to raise that basal even higher. The level of activation of ERK that we see in M12 cells without IGF activation is as high as you can get it if you put IGF receptor back in and use maximal doses of IGF-1. It is still hard for me to imagine how with a different growth factor with it maximally activated you could bring it up even more.

Holly: The consequence of activation of MAP kinase depends on where it is in the cell. Have you looked to see where this active MAP kinase is?

Roberts: We are doing this now by confocal microscopy. We have some separate work in myocytes for a different project. With certain ligands that activate the MAP kinase pathway, we see nuclear translocation. With certain others we get equivalent ERK phosphorylation but it stays in the cytoplasm.

Holly: Are Ras and Raf, which are upstream of MAP kinase, also on?

Roberts: We haven't looked.

LeRoith: Conceptually, I am wondering whether when you up- or down-regulate the IGF-1 receptor the cells have a compensation that takes over in either direction. This could explain some of your results. Would microarrays pull out some changes in genes here?

Roberts: We have switched to the M12 metastatic cell line where there is a progression in the gradual decrease in IGF-1R expression from primary epithelial cells to the immortalized cells to the metastatic ones. At low levels the IGF-1R is still doing something, because at the lowest level it is inhibiting AR transcriptional activity. At the same time, insulin receptor (IR) expression, which in the non-tumorigenic cells is extremely low, is increased significantly in the M12 cells. It is principally the IR-A variant. For whatever reason, for a cell to become successfully metastatic it needs to down-regulate the IGF-1R, perhaps to escape some of the differentiating effects of IGF-1. But they still need some sort of IGF-like signalling. The way they do this is to up-regulate the IGF-2 binding version of the insulin receptor because these advanced tumorigenic cells also make IGF-2.

Holly: Is that sustaining activation of MAP kinase.

Roberts: Perhaps, yes. But not PI3K, interestingly enough.

Yee: When you express the IGF receptor in those cells, is the down-regulation of constitutively phosphorylated MAP kinase independent of adding IGF-1 to those culture conditions?

Roberts: Yes, and then you can bring it back by adding IGF-1.

Yee: Is it possible that putting in the IGF-1 receptor is taking away something else? For example, it could be taking Grb2 away from the EGF receptor.

Roberts: That's a possibility. The effects of AR on IGF-1 receptor expression are pretty big. But when we add the receptor back to the M12 cells we are going from about 3500 to 20 000 — it's only a five- or sixfold change. This may be enough to titrate out IRS-1 or IRS-2, but it isn't likely that the huge change we see could be working simply by squelching something out.

Yee: If you block that with αIR3 do you restore the tumorigenicity?

Roberts: We haven't tried this because αIR3 is kind of messy. Now we have the Imclone antibody which looks like it is a clean blocker without activating, so we can try that.

Werner: Are there are any differences in IGF-2 expression between the prostate cancer-derived P69 and M12 cell lines? Is it possible that the decrease in IGF-1R expression that is seen in M12 compared with P69 cells is due to an increase in IGF-2 levels?

Roberts: The M12 cells do make IGF-2 whereas the earlier ones make little or none. You are asking whether the increased IGF-2 is enough to induce ligand-mediated receptor down-regulation. It is possible, but there isn't any evidence that IGF-2 regulates IGF-1R transcription, and we clearly see transcriptional down-regulation for a lot of this. In the greater scheme of things what is happening is that in metastatic disease there is some transcriptional down-regulation. In androgen-independent disease it may be a different mechanism whereby rather than down-regulating gene expression at the transcriptional level, you are losing the ability of AR to maintain the translational level.

LeRoith: I know translational regulation is sexy, but have you done the simple experiment of using a lysosomal or proteosomal inhibitor to see whether those pathways are involved?

Roberts: We haven't done that.

Holly: If IGF-2 expression is increased, if you reinstall the receptor does this knock down IGF-2 expression?

Roberts: We haven't looked at IGF-2 expression in the IGF receptor re-expressing cells.

Ohlsson: What happens to the IGF-1 receptor if you do WT1 antisense?

Roberts: It does go back up, but not as much as we might expect. The reason is as follows. WT1 is subject to alternative splicing. At this point there are 32 different versions, all from the same gene. Most cells express some complicated version of WT1. If we put in a certain version of WT1 and show down-regulation we are putting in one version. When we use the antisense we are knocking out all those versions. We did see some up-regulation but not as much as we'd expect.

Ohlsson: Could it be that a very small population of your cells, that expressed the IGF-1R, were co-selected? Is this possible?

Roberts: In this case I don't think so. We have recently done the same thing by doing retroviral transfection of AR. We don't have time to select this sort of rare variant.

Macaulay: Your story sounds very consistent, and I hesitate to mention in this context that in a clinical study we got results that were different (Hellawell et al 2002). We did *in situ* hybridization and immunostaining for the receptor in primary tumours and showed clear evidence of IGF-1R up-regulation compared with benign prostatic epithelium. We also obtained paired biopsies: a diagnostic prostate biopsy in a patient with androgen-responsive disease, and a bone biopsy in the same patient after development of androgen resistance. This was only 12 pairs, but it is difficult to obtain these paired biopsies. Three of the cases had staining differences that were compatible with the changes that you are describing. They had significant reduction in IGF receptor levels and IRS-1. Interestingly, those three also lost expression of PTEN. These changes are consistent with the hypothesis that prostate cancer cells may lose expression of IRS-1 in order to disrupt E-cadherin function and therefore metastasis, achieving reactivation of the Akt pathway by PTEN mutation. In this context, IGF receptor down-regulation may be necessary to avoid Shc-mediated terminal differentiation (Reiss et al 2000). However in the majority of cases in our series (nine of 12), IGF receptor levels in the metastases were maintained at levels comparable with those in the primary (Hellawell et al 2002). The IGF receptor staining we detected in fixed tissues was granular cytoplasmic staining. In formalin-fixed pellets of R+ cells we saw the expected pattern of membrane staining. Others have described the same pattern of granular cytoplasmic staining in tissues, and suggest that tissue fixation can disrupt membrane staining (Turner et al 1997, Tennant et al 1996). However, your staining is on the membrane and is very convincing. I had a couple of questions about the concept of the tumour 'wanting' to down-regulate the IGF receptor: actually that's a daft way of putting it because these mutations are purely random. Can you test this concept of down-regulating the receptor to avoid terminal differentiation or apoptosis? If you overexpress the receptor in your cells and treat them with IGF-1 do you see changes compatible with differentiation or apoptosis?

Roberts: The cell has to go into the circulation to metastasize. Perhaps a quick way to do this is to ask whether or not cells with a low level of receptor, or a higher level, or a very high level exhibit differential survival in 100% male serum. This is what they are going to see when they are trying to be metastatic. We are going to do this in a three-dimensional culture system, trying to reflect what potentially an extravasated cell would have to do to get to a metastatic site. The group that suggested that unliganded receptor induces this novel form of programmed cell death had an idea that when cells are under optimal or insufficient trophic support, the IGF-1 receptor is anti-apoptotic, but if cells are subjected to excess trophic support, the IGF-1 receptor can induce programmed cell death. Potentially, a cell exposed to complete human serum would be receiving excess trophic support and in those situations IGF-1 receptor function may be deleterious. This is why we asked whether lower receptor levels enhance survival in 100% serum. To my knowledge, no one has done this, but this is what they see when they are potentially going to become metastatic. This is a quick and easy experiment to do, and may give us some guidance as to what may be going on.

Macaulay: Do your cells have PTEN mutation? The fact that they showed a fairly low level of basal Akt phosphorylation, with increase after stimulation, suggests that they are probably wild-type.

Pollak: To support what Val Macaulay is saying, I think the definitive experiment here for proof of concept would be to take IGF-1 receptor tyrosine kinase inhibitor and see whether you can find any circumstance in which this stimulates the growth of the cells. There are two problems here that stop us figuring out what is really going on. One is that Steve Plymate's model system is based on SV40. We don't know whether the whole action of the signalling pathways is different in a system that has been SV40 immortalized. What everything hinges on are the actual measurements of the receptor levels in the clinical specimens. Val has results in one direction; you have results in another direction. Also, we have results with Charles Sawyer's LA PC series which may be more in tune with Val's.

Roberts: The LA PC9 was one way, the LA PC4 was this way.

Pollak: All of these clinical observations are still incomplete. We need activated receptor levels on the clinical specimens.

Roberts: I agree. Until we get good consistent, believable clinical data we are beating around the bush.

Laron: We know that the treatment of choice for prostatic cancer is GnRH analogue to suppress sex hormones. You said that there are some sex hormone-resistant cells. On the other hand, the question is whether the IGF-1 receptors are high or low. Would this be a sufficient indication to say that before you treat you should do a biopsy and test for androgen sensitivity as well as for the degree of IGF-1R binding, or is this premature?

Roberts: We would like to suggest that there is a cross-talk between IGF receptor and androgen receptor signalling. Here we see an effect of IGF receptor expression level on androgen action, and the effect of IGF-1 on androgen action. Other groups have shown at a biochemical level that the androgen receptor function can modulate IGF receptor function and vice versa. There is a lot of interplay. I think it is too soon to say that we can predict the level of androgen dependence from the IGF receptor level.

References

Hellawell GO, Turner GD, Davies DR, Poulsom R, Brewster SF, Macaulay VM 2002 Expression of the type 1 insulin-like growth factor receptor is up-regulated in primary prostate cancer and commonly persists in metastatic disease. Cancer Res 62:2942–2950

Reiss K, Wang JY, Romano G et al 2000 IGF-I receptor signaling in a prostatic cancer cell line with a PTEN mutation. Oncogene 19:2687–2694

Tennant MK, Thrasher JB, Twomey PA, Drivdahl RH, Birnbaum RS, Plymate SR 1996 Protein and messenger ribonucleic acid (mRNA) for the type 1 insulin-like growth factor (IGF) receptor is decreased and IGF-II mRNA is increased in human prostate carcinoma compared to benign prostate epithelium. J Clin Endocrinol Metab 81:3774–3782

Turner BC, Haffty BG, Narayanan L et al 1997 Insulin-like growth factor-I receptor overexpression mediates cellular radioresistance and local breast cancer recurrence after lumpectomy and radiation. Cancer Res 57:3079–3083

IGF-1 and breast cancer

Per Eystein Lønning and Svein Inge Helle

Section of Oncology, Institute of Medicine, Haukeland University Hospital, N-5021, Bergen, Norway

Abstract. While there have been significant improvements in breast cancer therapy over the last few decades, the fact that metastatic breast cancer remains incurable as well as the finding that adjuvant therapy reduces the breast cancer death hazard ratio by about 30% only underlines the need for novel therapeutic strategies. Currently, there is much interest in 'targeting therapy' for different malignancies. The majority of breast cancers harbour the insulin-like growth factor (IGF)-1 receptor, and IGF-1 has been found to be one of the most potent mitogens to breast cancer cells *in vitro*. Recent findings that the level of IGF-1 predicts subsequent risk of breast cancer in premenopausal patients further underlines the potential biological importance of this growth factor to the disease. While endocrine treatment with anti-oestrogens as well as progestins have been found to interact with the IGF system *in vivo*, the extent of these effects on antitumour action remains poorly understood. This paper discusses current strategies and results aiming at targeting IGF-1 as therapy for breast cancer.

2004 Biology of IGF-1: its interaction with insulin in health and malignant states. Wiley, Chichester (Novartis Foundation Symposium 262) p 205–214

Breast cancer is the most frequent malignancy among females in developed countries. Despite improvement with respect to early diagnosis as well as adjuvant therapy, the fact that more than one-third of all females achieving a diagnosis of breast cancer will subsequently die from the disease underlines the needs of developing novel therapeutic strategies.

While trials with different 'targeting therapeutics' have revealed a mixed picture, some of the experiences, like the effects of trastuzumab in HER-2-positive breast cancer and imatinib in c-KIT-positive tumours has substantiated the concept that 'targeted' strategies may have antitumour effects in selected tumours. Considering the insulin-like growth factor (IGF) system, *in vitro* experiments revealing pro-mitotic and anti-apoptotic effects of different components of the IGF system as well as the findings that the majority of human breast cancers express the IGF-1 receptor (IGF-1R) suggests that the IGF system may be a suitable therapeutic target in breast cancer.

In vitro data

IGF-1 has been found to be one of the most potent mitogens to breast cancer cells *in vitro* (Karey & Sirbasku 1988). In addition, IGF-1 has been found to rescue MCF-7 breast cancer cells treated with doxorubicin as well as paclitaxel, suggesting an anti-apoptotic role of IGF-1 in addition to its mitogenic effects (Gooch et al 1999). These effects all seem to be mediated by the IGF-1R. Further, stimulation of the IGF-1R has been shown to attenuate the growth inhibitory effects of trastuzumab in breast cancer cell lines (Lu et al 2001).

A controversial issue is the ligand-independent action of the IGF binding proteins (IGFBPs) in cancer cells. While *in vitro* evidence clearly has shown IGFBP-3 to have growth inhibitory as well as pro-apoptotic effects independent of IGF-1 (Schedlich & Graham 2002), the importance of these effects *in vivo* remains poorly understood. Further, *in vitro* studies have revealed a complex interaction between the IGF system and the growth stimulatory action of oestrogen hormones in oestrogen receptor (ER)-positive breast cancer cell lines (Daly et al 1991, Zhang & Yee 2000).

The IGF system in breast cancer patients

While some studies have reported elevated levels of IGF-1 in breast cancer patients, the findings are not consistent (Barni et al 1994, Bruning et al 1995, Ng et al 1998, Peyrat et al 1993).

IGF-1R is found to be expressed in the majority of breast cancers. While some studies suggested receptor expression to predict a good prognosis, others have reported opposite results (Bonneterre et al 1990, Foekens et al 1989, Railo et al 1994). Notably, any correlation between expression of a single biological parameter and outcome may not necessarily suggest a particular biological role of that factor, in as much as it may just be a co-variate to other factors linked to, for example, histological differentiation (Lønning 2003).

An interesting observation is a different expression of IGFBPs between ER-negative and ER-positive tumours, with higher expression of mRNA for IGFBP-3 in receptor-negative compared to receptor-positive tumours (Shao et al 1992) while the levels of mRNA for IGFBP-4 were reported to correlate to expression of ER as well as the progesterone receptor (PgR) (McGuire et al 1994).

Epidemiological evidence linking the IGF system to breast cancer development

High levels of total IGF-1 have been reported to be a risk factor for breast cancer among premenopausal women (Hankinson et al 1998). In another study, Byrne et al (2000) reported mammographic density, a surrogate parameter strongly linked to subsequent breast cancer development, to be positively correlated to IGF-1 levels but inversely related to the levels of IGFBP-3. A recent study found no correlation between either plasma levels of IGF-1 or its binding proteins to subsequent breast cancer risk in postmenopausal women (Keinan-Boker et al 2003).

The IGF system as a therapeutic target

As mentioned above, conflicting evidence has suggested elevated levels of IGF-1 in breast cancer patients. However, a substantial number of patients suffering from advanced breast cancer express elevated protease activity for IGFBP-3 (Frost et al 1996), a finding reported in patients suffering from diverse critical illnesses. Whether the observed elevation of IGFBP-3 protease activity represents a non-specific phenomenon or may have some kind of cancer-specific cause remains unclear. One possibility is that capillary leakage of proteolytic enzymes or their activators may represent a source of IGFBP-3 protease; another is interactions with enzyme inhibitors (Maile et al 2000). In theory, elevated levels of IGFBP-3 protease activity may be anticipated to be detrimental to the tumour disease, and possibly to enhance delivery of IGF-1 to the tumour tissue.

A proposed model outlining a 'vicious circle' based on activation of the IGFBP-3 protease system is illustrated in Fig. 1. It is well known that tumours developing over slow time periods may suddenly go into an 'accelerated phase', and the possibility exists that activation of the IGF system through enhanced IGFBP-3 protease activity could play a detrimental role in this respect.

The known effects of endocrine agents currently or previously used for breast cancer therapy on different components of the IGF-system are outlined in Table 1. Thus, several reports have shown anti-oestrogens like tamoxifen and droloxifene to suppress plasma levels of total IGF-1 but also to elevate IGFBP-1 (Colletti et al 1989, Helle et al 1996a, Lønning et al 1992, Pollak et al 1990). Most likely, these findings represent oestrogen agonistic effects of these compounds on the liver, as anti-oestrogens have been shown to modulate a number of other globulins secreted by the liver in an oestrogen-agonistic fashion (Lønning & Lien 1995).

A different effect is seen during treatment with progestins in high doses. Thus, treatment with medroxyprogesterone acetate or megestrol acetate in doses of 1000 mg or 160 mg daily, respectively, have been shown to be effective antitumour agents in breast cancer (Lønning & Lien 1995). In two studies, we found treatment with megestrol acetate to significantly reduce the IGFBP-3 protease activity in plasma (Frost et al 1996, Helle et al 1999). This may be a glucocorticoid agonistic effect of megestrol acetate and not an effect mediated through the progesterone receptor; thus, glucocorticoids have been found to reduce 'bioavailable' IGF-1 while leaving total plasma levels unaffected

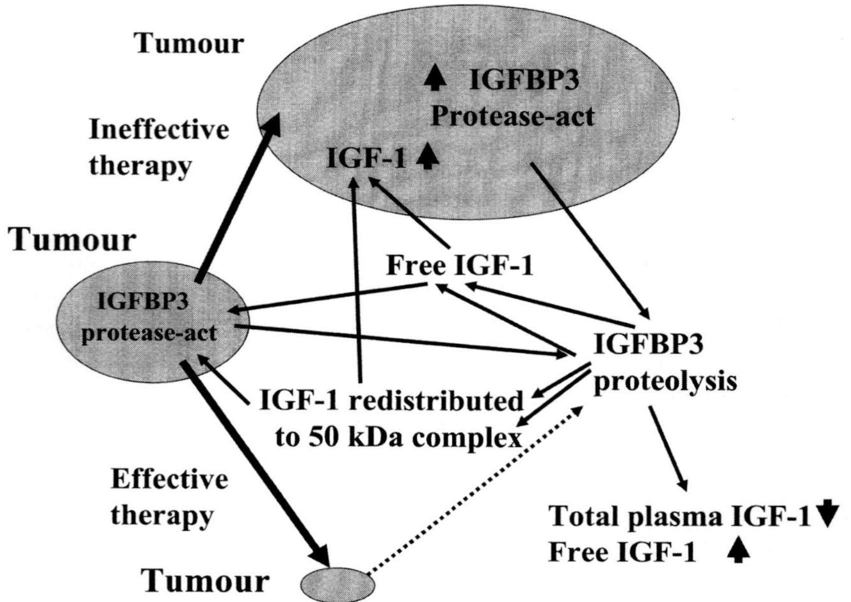

FIG. 1. Proposed mechanism behind the increased IGFBP-3 protease activity and a potential vicious circle enhancing tumour growth in patients with advanced cancer. Increased IGFBP-3 protease activity causes a redistribution of IGF-1 to lower molecular weight complexes and increases the free fraction which are more readily available to the tissues and in particular tumour tissue which has increased capillary permeability and may potentially extract a relatively higher amount of growth factor. This may potentially stimulate tumour growth while plasma stores levels are subsequently depleted despite compensatory increased synthesis. This situation can be reversed through effective antitumour therapy or by treatment with megestrol acetate which acts through decreasing capillary permeability (independent of tumour response).

Table 1. Effects of different endocrine therapies on different parameters of the IGF-system in plasma (approximate percentage change) based on previous studies

	IGF-1	*free-IGF-1*	*IGFBP-1*	*IGFBP-3*	*IGFBP-3 protease*
Diethylstilboestrol	−40%	−70%	+70%	−30%	−20%
Tamoxifen	−30%	no data	+80%	no change	no change
Droloxifene	−40%	no data	+70%	no change	no data
Megestrol acetate	+90%	+40%	no change	+20%	−50%
Aminoglutethimide	+30%	no data	no change	no change	no change
Octreotide	−50%	no data	+50%	−15%	no change

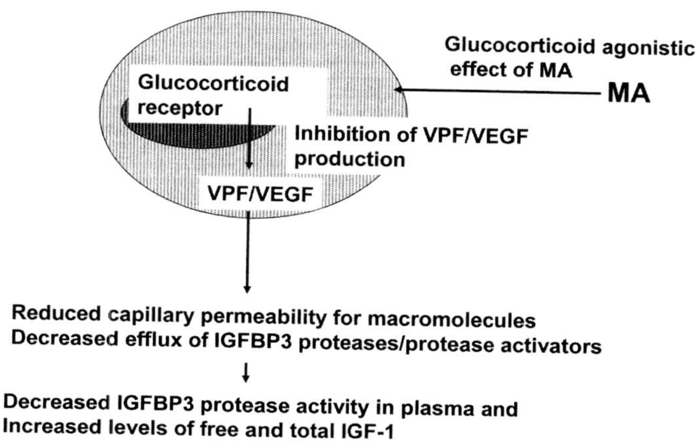

FIG. 2. Proposed mechanism for the effect of megestrol acetate (MA) and glucocorticoid on IGFBP-3 protease activation in malignant disease.

(Gourmelen et al 1982). Based on the findings of Heiss et al (Heiss et al 1996), Fig. 2 outlines a proposed mechanism by which glucocorticoids and their agonists may influence tissue permeability for macromolecules and, thereby, factors involved in IGFBP-3 proteolysis. Interestingly, while we found alterations in the IGFBP-3 protease activity in patients treated with tamoxifen for metastatic breast cancer (Helle et al 1996b), this was obviously related to tumour burden, with an increased activity during progressive disease but a drop in activity in relation to tumour shrinkage. In contrast, the effects seen with megestrol acetate developed shortly after implementing therapy and were reversible upon terminating the drug.

Considering treatment with aromatase inhibitors, we found aminoglutethimide to increase plasma IGF-1 by a mean of about 25% (Lien et al 1992). While others have reported modest elevations in IGF-1 during treatment with other aromatase inhibitors (Ferrari et al 1994, 2002), we found no change in plasma levels of any of the IGF parameters during treatment with the steroidal aromatase inactivator formestane (Lien et al 1992). Notably, aminoglutethimide has several biochemical effects in addition to acting as an aromatase inhibitor (Lønning & Kvinnsland 1988). Whether any alterations in plasma levels of IGF-1 may occur during treatment with different aromatase inhibitors the change seems to be of a small magnitude and not likely to play a significant role in influencing the antitumour effects of these compounds.

Somatostatin analogues are known to suppress plasma levels of IGF-1 due to inhibition of growth hormone secretion; such compounds have now become more convenient for clinical use due to the development of long-acting depot formulations like OncoLAR (Helle et al 1998). Based on preclinical studies revealing beneficial effects of somatostatin analogues as antitumour agents in breast cancer (Weckbecker et al 1994), two recent studies have compared tamoxifen monotherapy to tamoxifen and the somatostatin analogue sandostatin administered either as its short-acting or depot formulation (Ingle et al 1999). Experimental data suggest the two compounds may act in concert suppressing plasma IGF-1 (Huynh & Pollak 1994). Preliminary data suggest addition of sandostatin did not improve clinical outcome. In the second of these studies, we have analysed plasma levels of IGF-1 and IGF-2 together with their binding proteins and the IGFBP-3 protease activity; the results will be reported in the near future.

Future aspects

In summary, alterations in plasma levels of IGF-1 may occur during treatment with several agents shown to be effective in endocrine responsive tumours. While the decrease in IGF-1 during treatment with tamoxifen may be of benefit and the increase during treatment with AG has the opposite effect, the clinical efficacy of these drugs is fairly similar. Thus, clinical data do not suggest that moderate alterations in plasma levels of IGF-1 affect clinical outcome in patients with metastatic disease. Whether a more powerful suppression of plasma IGF-1 levels or interference with the IGF-1R may be of clinical benefit remains to be shown.

While the results from epidemiological studies suggesting a role for IGF-1 as a risk factor for breast cancer development, and the (so far) lack of evidence suggesting a therapeutic benefit from suppressing IGF-1 in advanced breast cancer at first glance may be at conflict, this may not necessarily be the case. Looking at oestrogens and breast cancer, there is now substantial evidence linking variation in plasma oestrogen levels within the physiological range to subsequent breast cancer risk in postmenopausal women (Key et al 2003). On the contrary, profound suppression of plasma oestrogen levels are required to achieve optimal antitumour effects (Lønning 2002). Making a parallel to the IGF system, it may well be that aggravated suppression of IGF-1 or receptor blockade may cause dramatic antitumour effects in breast cancer. Strategies aiming at effectively blocking the effects of IGF-1 on breast cancers should be evaluated in breast cancer therapy.

References

Barni S, Lissoni P, Brivio F et al 1994 Serum levels of insulin-like growth factor-I in operable breast cancer in relation to the main prognostic variables and their perioperative changes in relation to those of prolactin. Tumori 80:212–215

Bonneterre J, Peyrat JP, Beuscart R, Demaille A 1990 Prognostic significance of insulin-like growth factor I receptors in human breast cancer. Cancer Res 50:6931–6935

Bruning PF, Doorn JV, Bonfrèr JMG et al 1995 Insulin-like growth-factor-binding protein 3 is decreased in early-stage operable pre-menopausal breast cancer. Int J Cancer 62:266–270

Byrne C, Colditz GA, Willett WC et al 2000 Plasma insulin-like growth factor (IGF) I, IGF-binding protein 3, and mammographic density. Cancer Res 60:3744–3748

Colletti RB, Roberts JD, Devlin JT, Copeland KC 1989 Effect of tamoxifen on plasma insulin-like growth factor I in patients with breast cancer. Cancer Res 49:1882–1884

Daly RJ, Harris WH, Wang DY, Darbre PD 1991 Autocrine production of insulin-like growth factor II using an inducible expression system results in reduced estrogen sensitivity of MCF-7 human breast cancer cells. Cell Growth Differ 2:457–464

Ferrari L, Zilembo N, Bajetta E et al 1994 Effect of two 4-hydroxyandrostenedione doses on serum insulin-like growth factor I levels in advanced breast cancer. Breast Cancer Res Treat 30:127–132

Ferrari L, Martinetti, A, Zilembo, N et al 2002 Short-term effects of anastrozole treatment on insulin-like growth factor system in postmenopausal advanced breast cancer patients. J Steroid Biochem Mol Biol 80:411–418

Foekens JA, Portengen H, Putten WLJ et al 1989 Prognostic value of receptors for insulin-like growth factor I, somatostatin, and epidermal growth factor in human breast cancer. Cancer Res 49:7002–7009

Frost VJ, Helle SI, Lønning PE, Stappen JWJ, Holly JMP 1996 Effects of treatment with megestrol acetate, aminoglutethimide, or formestane on insulin-like growth factor (IGF) I and II, IGF-binding proteins (IGFBPs), and IGFBP-3 protease status in patients with advanced breast cancer. J Clin Endocrinol Metab 81:2216–2221

Gooch JL, Van Den Berg CL, Yee D 1999 Insulin-like growth factor (IGF)-I rescues breast cancer cells from chemotherapy-induced cell death—proliferative and anti-apoptotic effects. Breast Cancer Res Treat 56:1–10

Gourmelen M, Girard F, Binoux M 1982 Serum somatomedin/insulin-like growth factor (IGF) and IGF carrier levels in patients with Cushing's syndrome or receiving glucocorticoid therapy. J Clin Endocrinol Metab 54:885–892

Hankinson SE, Willett WC, Colditz GA et al 1998 Circulating concentrations of insulin-like growth factor-I and risk of breast cancer. Lancet 351:1393–1396

Heiss JD, Papavassiliou E, Merrill MJ et al 1996 Mechanism of dexamethasone suppression of brain tumor-associated vascular permeability in rats. Involvement of the glucocorticoid receptor and vascular permeability factor. J Clin Invest 98:1400–1408

Helle SI, Anker G, Tally M, Hall K, Lønning PE 1996a Influence of droloxifene on plasma levels of insulin-like growth factor (IGF)-I, pro-IGF-1IE, insulin-like growth factor binding protein (IGFBP)-1 and IGFBP-3 in breast cancer patients. J Steroid Biochem Mol Biol 57:167–171

Helle SI, Holly JMP, Tally M, Hall K, Van der Stappen J, Lønning PE 1996b Influence of treatment with tamoxifen and change in tumor burden on the IGF-system in breast cancer patients. Int J Cancer (Pred Oncol) 69:335–339

Helle SI, Geisler, J, Poulsen JP et al 1998 Microencapsulated octreotide pamoate in advanced breast cancer: a phase I study. Br J Cancer 78:14–20

Helle SI, Lundgren S, Geisler S et al 1999 Effects of treatment with megestrol acetate on the insulin-like growth factor system: time and dose dependency. Eur J Cancer 35:1070–1075

Huynh H, Pollak M 1994 Enhancement of tamoxifen-induced suppression of insulin-like growth factor I gene expression and serum level by a somatostatin analogue. Biochem Biophys Res Com 203:253–259

Ingle JN, Suman VJ, Kardinal CG et al 1999 A randomized trial of tamoxifen alone or combined with octreotide in the treatment of women with metastatic breast carcinoma. Cancer 85:1284–1292

Karey KP, Sirbasku DA 1988 Differential responsiveness of human breast cancer cell lines MCF-7 and T47D to growth factors and 17β estradiol. Cancer Res 48:4083–4092
Keinan-Boker L, de Mesquita HBB, Kaaks R et al 2003 Circulating levels of insulin-like growth factor I, its binding proteins-1,-2, -3, C-peptide and risk of postmenopausal breast cancer. Int J Cancer 106:90–95
Key TJ, Appleby, PN, Reeves, GK et al 2003 Body mass index, serum sex hormones, and breast cancer risk in postmenopausal women. J Natl Cancer Inst 95:1218–1226
Lien EA, Johannessen DC, Aakvaag A, Lønning PE 1992 Influence of tamoxifen, aminoglutethimide and goserelin on human plasma IGF-I levels in breast cancer patients. J Steroid Biochem Mol Biol 41:541–543
Lønning PE 2002 Aromatase inhibitors and inactivators for breast cancer therapy. Drug Aging 19:277–298
Lønning P 2003 Study of suboptimum treatment response: lessons from breast cancer. Lancet Oncology 4:177–185
Lønning PE, Lien E 1995 Mechanisms of action of endocrine treatment in breast cancer. Crit Rev Oncol Haematol 21:158–193
Lønning PE, Kvinnsland S 1988 Mechanisms of action of aminoglutethimide as endocrine therapy of breast cancer. Drugs 35:685–710
Lønning PE, Hall K, Aakvaag A, Lien EA 1992 Influence of tamoxifen on the plasma levels of insulin-like growth factor I and insulin-like growth factor binding protein I in breast cancer patients. Cancer Res 52:4719–4723
Lu YH, Zi XL, Zhao YH, Mascarenhas D, Pollak M 2001 Insulin-like growth factor-I receptor signaling and resistance to trastuzumab (Herceptin). J Natl Cancer Inst 93:1852–1857
Maile LA, Whellams EJ, Holly JMP 2000 Endogenous IGFBP-3 is protected from inducible IGFBP-3 protease activity in normal adult serum. Growth Horm IGF Res 10:71–77
McGuire SE, Hilsenbeck SG, Figueroa JA, Jackson JG, Yee D 1994 Detection of insulin-like growth factor binding proteins (IGFBPs) by ligand blotting in breast cancer tissues. Cancer Lett 77:25–32
Ng EH, Ji CY, Tan PH et al 1998 Altered serum levels of insulin-like growth-factor binding proteins in breast cancer patients. Ann Surg Oncol 5:194–201
Peyrat JP, Bonneterre J, Hequet B et al 1993 Plasma insulin-like growth factor-1 (IGF-1) concentrations in human breast cancer. Eur J Cancer 29A:492–497
Pollak M, Constantino J, Polychronakos C et al 1990 Effect of tamoxifen on serum insulin-like growth factor I levels in stage I breast cancer patients. J Natl Cancer Inst 82:1693–1697
Railo MJ, Smitten KV, Pekonen F 1994 The prognostic value of insulin-like growth factor-I in breast cancer patients. Results of a follow up study on 126 patients. Eur J Cancer 30A:307–311
Schedlich LJ, Graham LD 2002 Role of insulin-like growth factor binding protein-3 in breast cancer cell growth. Microsc Res Tech 59:12–22
Shao Z-M, Sheikh MS, Ordonez JV et al 1992 IGFBP-3 gene expression and estrogen receptor status in human breast carcinoma. Cancer Res 52:5100–5103
Weckbecker G, Tolcsvai L, Stolz B, Pollak M, Bruns C 1994 Somatostatin analogue octreotide enhances the antineoplastic effects of tamoxifen and ovariectomy on 7,12-dimethylbenz(*a*)anthracene-induced rat mammary carcinomas. Cancer Res 54:6334–6337
Zhang XH, Yee D 2000 Tyrosine kinase signalling in breast cancer — insulin-like growth factors and their receptors in breast cancer. Breast Cancer Res 2:170–175

DISCUSSION

Jenkins: I agree with your conclusions. In the somatostatin analogue trials, the IGF-1 suppression was only down to about 50% of normal. What is intriguing is that the preliminary studies with the GH receptor antagonist pegvisomant, which reduces IGF-1 levels down to about 10% of normal in animal models of breast cancer, have shown a marked inhibitory effect.

Lønning: My guess is that we can see exactly the same thing as with oestrogens. Also, if we go back 40 years, glucocorticoids were used for breast cancer therapy. This results in an incomplete suppression of oestrogen levels and a very low response rate.

Jenkins: Also, if we go back 40–50 years, hypophysectomy used to be quite a good treatment for metastatic breast disease, even in oopherectomized women.

Lønning: That is true, but adrenalectomy and hypophosectomy were both much better than glucocorticoids. We have to be a little careful here, because hypophosectomy is a multi-hormonal manipulation. Growth hormone (GH) goes at the same time.

Yee: Given your experience with sandostatin, do you have any enthusiasm for doing a pegvisomant trial in breast cancer? If I remember correctly, Michael Pollak's data in animals suggest that somatostatin analogues and tamoxifen are effective. This might not always translate into humans, but this is the same place where we are now with pegvisomant. There are some animal model data suggesting that it may be effective.

Pollak: Early on, one of the first ways to manipulate the system was the use of somatostatin analogues. This is why we did some of these trials. But we still have an ongoing trial in Canada with randomization of tamoxifen versus tamoxifen plus a somatastatin analogue in the adjuvant setting. The early impression from the 600 patients is that after a while people develop tolerance to chronic octreotide therapy with respect to the suppression of IGF-1. If you think about this, the actual potency of a somatostatin analogue reducing an acromegalic level to a normal level is very strong compared with asking the drug to go from a normal level to a sub-normal level. In the latter situation you are going to invoke counter-regulatory hormones because you are creating a deficiency state. For example, if you give more octreotide, your pituitary is going to make more GH-releasing hormone (GHRH) in an effort to restore normality. The early unpublished results from the chronic octreotide study would suggest that the suppression of IGF levels — the endeavour to create IGF deficiency by chronic octreotide — is achieved for the first few months, but after a while the IGF levels rise again. Consequently, we never really get to test the hypothesis in a chronic situation. I am not sure that we can manipulate IGF production currently anywhere as near as well as we can inhibit oestrogen production by the use of aromatase inhibitors.

Rosenfeld: As a paediatric endocrinologist, I don't understand the rationale in 2003 for using somatostatin analogues in studies. If you believe that IGF-1 has a tumour-promoting role, there are so many more effective means of getting at it, for example by using the GH receptor antagonists. How can you justify using somatostatin analogues?

Pollak: I can't. This trial was initiated in the 1980s and it is now in the follow-up period. None of these patients are being treated. I fully agree: it is a historical note. If one is seriously interested in these hypotheses now, the tyrosine kinase inhibitors are the way to go, or possibly the antibodies. Manipulating the ligand levels is of more historical interest than current experimental therapeutics. This is in contrast to the oestrogen side of things, where the aromatase inhibitors have proven to be very successful.

Lønning: The story with the aromatase inhibitors versus receptor blockade tells us that you can't give the answer before you have put it to the test.

Rosenfeld: You have to have a reasonable rationale.

Lønning: I am not talking about somatostatin analogues. I am talking about suppression versus receptor blockage: which is most effective? I want to emphasize the importance of differentiating between the three test situations. We have three scenarios: metastatic disease, the adjuvant or early setting, and we have prevention. The story we learned from oestrogen suppression is that there really is a difference between risk, or prevention and therapy of cancer. Modest changes of oestrogen levels influence the risk but don't influence therapy. When you look at metastatic breast cancer as compared with adjuvant disease, the lessons that we have learned from all types of endocrine therapy and chemotherapy are that you will escalate the benefits from the metastatic disease into the adjuvant setting. We are able to cure patients in the adjuvant setting with a therapy that doesn't cure them in metastatic disease. However, there is no report of any compound that has worked in the adjuvant setting that did not also work to some extent in metastatic disease. As long as this is negative in metastatic disease, it would be highly unlikely that it would provide any benefit in the adjuvant setting.

Laron: What is known concerning IGF-1 in mammary cancer in males? It is rarer than in females but it occurs.

Lønning: Very little, because it is such a rare disease. One male gets breast cancer for every 200 females. One thing we can say is that in endocrine therapy as well as chemotherapy, all these compounds seem to work as well in male breast cancer as in the female.

Laron: Ron Rosenfeld just proposed using the new antagonists. They cost US$80 000–100 000 for therapy per year. It is a theoretical issue.

Rosenfeld: It is a marketing decision.

LeRoith: I am not sure they are that expensive.

Jenkins: It is conceivable that they will be judging by the doses used in some of the preliminary studies. The oncological doses were in the region of 80–100 mg a day plus a large loading dose. It is intriguing in colon cancer, because the most impressive data are for a rat model with human implants of colonic cancer, in combination with irinotecan, almost completely obliterated hepatic metastases compared with either treatment alone.

IGFBPs and cancer

Peng Fang, Vivian Hwa and Ron Rosenfeld[1]*†

*Department of Pediatrics, Oregon Health & Science University, Portland, OR 97239-3098, *Lucile Packard Foundation for Children's Health, 770 Welch Road, Suite 350, Palo Alto, CA 94304, and †Department of Pediatrics, Stanford University, Stanford, CA 94305, USA*

Abstract. The proposed insulin-like growth factor binding protein (IGFBP) superfamily are a group of secreted proteins that are structurally, functionally and evolutionarily related, and include six IGFBPs and over 10 IGFBP-related proteins. The IGFBPs have high affinities for insulin-like growth factors (IGFs), thereby modulating the mitogenic, anti-apoptotic and metabolic actions of IGFs. In addition, IGFBPs, particularly IGFBP-3, also have IGF-independent, anti-proliferative and pro-apoptotic functions. The IGFBPs are, in turn, modulated by proteolysis. Epidemiological data correlating serum IGF/IGFBP levels with the risk of several human cancers suggest a possible protective role for IGFBP-3. *In vitro* studies suggest that the potential protective effects of IGFBP-3 involve both IGF-dependent and IGF-independent mechanisms. Further studies are necessary to demonstrate whether the ability of IGFBPs to inhibit the proliferation of cancer cells under *in vitro* conditions has significant clinical implications.

2004 Biology of IGF-1: its interaction with insulin in health and malignant states. Wiley, Chichester (Novartis Foundation Symposium 262) p 215–234

Insulin-like growth factors (IGF-1 and IGF-2) are small peptides that act as endocrine, paracrine and autocrine hormones to exert mitogenic and anti-apoptotic effects on diverse cell types including normal and tumour cells. The mitogenic effects of IGFs are mediated predominantly through the type 1 receptor (IGF-1R), a transmembrane tyrosine kinase. IGFs also interact with specific binding proteins (IGFBPs), a family of six secreted proteins that share high structural homology. IGFBPs have higher affinities for IGFs than does the IGF-1R, thus, *via* sequestration of IGFs, the IGFBPs modulate the bioavailability and actions of IGFs. In addition to these IGF-dependent actions, IGFBPs also have actions independent of modulating IGF availability, including anti-proliferative and pro-apoptotic functions on cancer cells. Support for the IGF-independent functions of IGFBPs came from the identification of a group of

[1]This paper was presented at the symposium by Ron Rosenfeld, to whom correspondence should be addressed.

proteins that share structural similarity with the N-terminal domains of IGFBPs, but have considerably lower affinities for IGFs. The expression of these IGFBP-related proteins, along with IGFBPs, is altered in tumorigenesis and their role(s) in cancer progression have been under intensive investigations. The focus of this review will be on our current understanding of the mechanisms by which IGFBPs exert their effects on cancer cells. We will also summarize recent epidemiological data correlating serum IGF/IGFBP levels with the risk of several human cancers, and attempt to provide general concepts and perspectives on IGFBP protective actions and their role in human cancers.

Characteristics of IGFBPs

The IGFBP superfamily

The concept of the IGFBP superfamily was proposed to acknowledge the identification of proteins that are related structurally, functionally and evolutionarily to the IGFBPs (Hwa et al 1999). The six IGFBPs and over 10 IGFBP-related proteins are cysteine-rich, modular proteins, which share a common N-terminal domain (Fig. 1). This conserved N-terminal domain is encoded within one exon for all members of the IGFBP superfamily (Hwa et al 1999), and is critical for the binding of IGFs.

IGFBPs. IGFBPs bind IGFs with high affinity (K_d ~0.1 nM). The six IGFBPs share high similarity in their primary amino acid sequence (36% overall homology for mammalian IGFBPs), and possess the same structural organization: a conserved N-terminal region containing 10–12 cysteines, a non-conserved mid-region, and a conserved C-terminal region containing 6 cysteines. High affinity binding of IGFs requires both N-terminal and C-terminal domains (Hwa et al 1999). Mutations generated within these two regions have resulted in IGFBPs that have lost their high affinity binding to IGFs, and have served as valuable tools for discriminating the IGF-dependent and IGF-independent roles of IGFBPs (see below).

IGFBP related proteins. The IGFBP related proteins consist of a diverse group of cysteine-rich proteins that have in common the conserved N-terminal domain of the IGFBPs. These include the Mac25/IGFBP-rP1, the CCN family of proteins, L56, and ESM-1 (Fig. 1). *In vitro* binding assays indicated that, for those tested, the IGFBP-related proteins bind IGF with very low affinity (summarized in Hwa et al 1999), suggesting that binding is mediated through the conserved N-terminal domain. Furthermore, the data indicate that the main biological function(s) of these IGFBP related proteins is not the sequestration of IGFs, but is

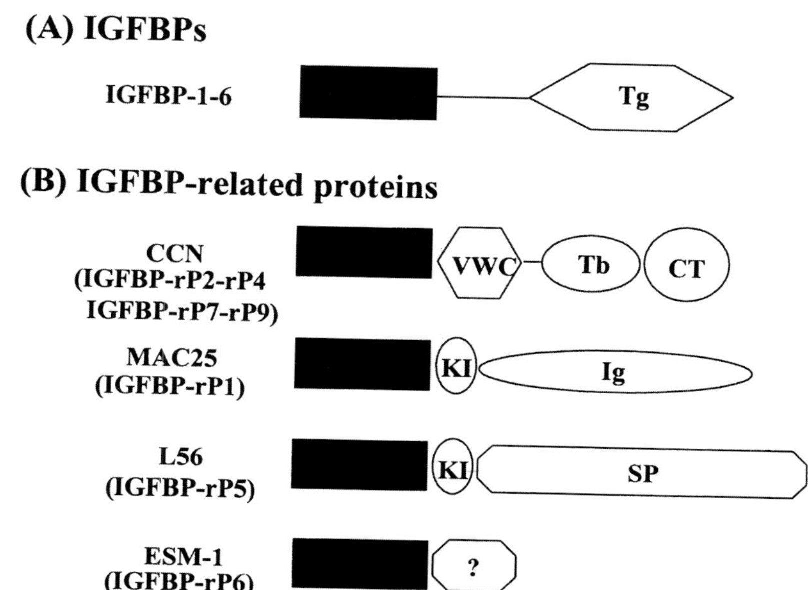

FIG. 1. Modular architecture of protein domains in the IGFBP superfamily. The IGFBP superfamily is subgrouped into (A) IGFBPs (IGFBP-1 to 6); and (B) IGFBP-rPs (as indicated). The N-terminal module is shown as a solid *black box*. The other modules are as indicated and are abbreviated as follows: Tg, thyroglobulin-type I domain; VWC, von Willebrand factor type C repeat; Tb, thrombospondin type I repeat; CT, C-terminal domain; KI, Kazal-type serine proteinase inhibitor; Ig, immunoglobulin-like domain; SP, serine protease. The "?" indicates no obvious similarity to known domains or protein motifs (from Hwa et al 1999).

IGF-independent. The characteristics of members in the IGFBP superfamily are summarized in Table 1.

Distribution of IGFBPs

The IGFBPs and related proteins are found ubiquitously, and expression is often dysregulated in cancers (Lopez-Bermejo et al 2000). In serum, IGFBP-3 sequesters about 75% of circulating IGFs in 150 kDa complexes consisting of IGF-1/2, IGFBP-3 and acid-labile subunit (ALS) (Collett-Solberg & Cohen 2000, Mohan & Baylink 2002); a smaller 130 kDa complex, consisting of IGFBP-5, IGFs and ALS has also been reported (Twigg & Baxter 1998). The formation of these complexes prolongs the half-life of IGFs and allows the complexes to serve as reservoirs for IGFs, since the complexes cannot cross the vascular endothelium.

TABLE 1 Characteristics of IGFBP superfamily

Protein	*Molecular weight (kDa)*	*No. of mino acids*	*No. of cysteines*	*Chromosomal location*	*Gene size (kb)*	*mRNA size (kb)*	*No. of exons*
IGFBP, high affinity IGF binder							
IGFBP-1	25.3	234	18	7p12–7p14	5.2	1.6	4
IGFBP-2	31.4	289	18	2q31–2q34	32.0	1.5	4
IGFBP-3	28.7	264	18	7p12–7p14	8.9	2.4	5
IGFBP-4	26.0	237	20	17q12–17q21	15.3	1.7	4
IGFBP-5	28.6	252	18	2q31–2q34	33.0	1.7, 6.0	4
IGFBP-6	22.8	216	16	12q13	4.7	1.1	4
IGFBP-rp, low-affinity IGF binder							
IGFBP-rp1 (Mac25)	26.4	256	18	4q12–4q13	>30	1.1	5
IGFBP-rp2 (CTGF)	35.5	323	38	6q23.1	nd	2.4	5
IGFBP-rp3 (novH)	36.0	329	38	8q24.1	7	2.4	5
IGFBP-rp4 (Cyr61)	39.5	358	38	1p22.3	nd	2.5, 4.0	nd
IGFBP-rp5 (L56)	49.0	458	16	nd	nd	2.3	nd
IGFBP-rp6 (ESM-1)	18.1	165	18	nd	nd	2.2	nd
IGFBP-rp7 (WISP-2)	24.4	228	28	20q12–13	nd	nd	nd
IGFBP-rp8 (WISP-1)	38.0	345	38	8q24.1–24.3	nd	nd	nd
IGFBP-rp9 (WISP-3)	37.1	334	34	6q23.1	nd	nd	nd

About 20∼25% of circulating IGFs are bound by other IGFBPs to form small complexes of 40–50 kDa, which are able to penetrate the vascular endothelium and thus make IGF available to local tissues (Baxter 2000, Mohan & Baylink 2002).

IGFBPs are also produced locally by a variety of tissues, and by different cell types (Jones & Clemmons 1995, Kelley et al 1996, Collett-Solberg & Cohen 2000, Mohan & Baylink 2002). The IGFBPs function both to inhibit, as well as to potentiate, IGF actions, dependent on cell type (Collett-Solberg & Cohen 2000, Mohan & Baylink 2002). The exception appears to be IGFBP4, which is consistently reported to only have inhibitory effects (reviewed recently in Zhou et al 2003); for example, overexpression of IGFBP4 could delay the formation of human prostate cancers (Damon et al 1998). The abnormal levels of IGFBPs in some tissues have been associated with pathological conditions, as discussed below.

IGFBPs in human cancer

Alterations in concentrations of IGFBPs and their potential roles in human cancer development and progression have been intensively investigated by epidemiological studies, clinical studies and investigations with *in vitro* cell model systems (for recent review see Cohen et al 2000, Khandwala et al 2000, Yu & Rohan 2000). Most of these studies have revealed a significant correlation between IGFBPs and the carcinogenesis process. For example, IGFBP-1, 3 and 4 are down-regulated in patients with hepatocarcinoma (reviewed in Scharf et al 2001), while IGFBP2 is highly expressed in many, but not all, cancers, such as tumours of the central nervous system (CNS) (Zumkeller & Westphal 2001). Epidemiological studies, including both retrospective and case–control investigations, have focused on cancer risk in association with the serum/plasma levels of IGFs, IGFBP-3, or the combination of the two.

Prospective epidemiological studies have, on the whole, suggested strong correlations between altered serum IGFs and IGFBP-3 concentrations and the detection (if not pathogenesis) of cancer. Statistical analyses from several large population-based prospective studies have consistently indicated that high serum (or plasma) IGF-1, or a high IGF-1/IGFBP-3 ratio, is associated with an increased risk of breast cancer in premenopausal women, as well as in prostate and colorectal cancers (Table 2). The level of IGFBP-3 by itself was less predictive of cancer risk, although the majority of the studies suggest that high IGFBP-3 concentrations are associated with reduced risks of prostate, lung, colorectal cancers and breast cancer in premenopausal women (Table 2). High levels of other IGFBPs are also associated with the reduced risks of cancers, as seen in two studies where high levels of IGFBP-2 are associated with a reduced risk of breast cancer in postmenopausal women, and a high level of IGFBP-1 is associated with a reduced risk of lung cancer in women (Table 2).

Mechanisms for protective effects of IGFBPs

The protective effects of IGFBPs could be mediated by inhibiting the mitogenic effect of IGF through regulating the amount of available IGFs both in serum and in local tissues. Similarly, reduced expression of IGFBPs could promote dysregulated IGF actions and lead to uncontrolled cell proliferation and tumorigenesis. In addition, some of the IGFBPs have been shown to have anti-proliferative and pro-apoptotic actions in human cancer cells, which are IGF-independent (reviewed in Firth & Baxter 2002, Mohan & Baylink 2002, Collett-Solberg & Cohen 2000, Hwa et al 1999).

TABLE 2 Epidemiological studies of IGF-1, IGFBP-3 and cancer risk

Cancer	*Subject (nested case–control in cohort)*	*High risk*	*Possible protective role of IGFBP*	*Ref.*
Breast	32 826 women in the Nurses'Health Study cohort, 76 cases/105 controls premenopausal, 305 cases/483 controls postmenopausal	In premenopausal women age <50, high plasma IGF-1 and high IGF-1/ IGFBP-3	Yes	a
	95 000 women enrolled in the Kaiser Permanente Medical Care Program, 66 cases/controls premenopausal,	In premenopausal women, high serum IGF-1, high serum IGFBP-3	No	b
	60 cases/controls postmenopausal	In postmenopausal women, low serum IGFBP-2	Yes	
Colon and rectum	14 916 men in Physician Health, 193 cases/ 318 controls	High plasma IGF-1, low plasma IGFBP-3	Yes	c
	32 826 women in the Nurses' Health Study cohort, 79 case/158 control for adenocarcinoma of the colon or rectum; 90 cases/ 90 controls of intermediate/late-stage adenoma, and 107 cases/ 107 controls of early-stage adenoma	For large or tubulovillous/ villous colorectal adenoma and cancer: High plasma IGF-1, and particularly low plasma IGFBP-3	Yes	d
	14 275 women in New York, 102 cases/ 200 controls	High serum IGF-1, high serum IGFBP-3, low serum IGFBP-1	Yes/No	e
	18 244 men in Shanghai, 135 cases/661 controls	High serum IGFBP-2 and IGFBP-3	No	f

(*Continued*)

Modulation of IGF action by inhibitory IGFBPs (IGF-dependent actions of IGFBPs)

Inhibitory effects of IGFBPs on IGF action. The mitogenic effect of IGF is mediated by its transmembrane kinase receptor, IGF-1R. IGFBPs have higher affinity for IGFs (~0.1 nM) than for the IGF-1R (~1 nM). The IGFBPs, therefore, restrict IGF

TABLE 2 *(Continued)*

Cancer	*Subject (nested case–control in cohort)*	*High risk*	*Possible protective role of IGFBP*	*Ref.*
Colon and rectum	35 674 men, 100 924 women in Northern Sweden Health and Disease cohort, 110 colon cancer cases, 58 rectum caner cases/ 336 controls	For colon cancer High plasma IGF-1 and IGFBP-3 For rectal cancer: Low plasma IGF-1 and low plasma IGFBP-3	No Yes	g
Lung	18 244 men in Shanghai, 230 cases/740 controls	Low serum IGFBP-3	Yes	h
	14 254 men and women smokers and 4060 male asbestos workers, 159 cases/257 controls	Current smokers and more recent quitters: high serum IGFBP-3 (?)	No	i
	14 275 women in New York, 93 cases/ 186 controls	Serum IGF-1, IGFBP-1, IGFBP-2 and IGFBP-3 are not associated with risk	No evidence	j
Prostate	14 916 men in Physician Health, 152 case/ 152 control	High plasma IGF-1, low plasma IGFBP-3	Yes	k
	14 916 men in Physician Health, 140 case advanced cancer, 325 case early cancer, 534 control	For advanced stage cancer: high plasma IGF-1, low plasma IGFBP-3	Yes	l
	29 133 men in Finland, 100 cases/400 controls	Serum IGF-1 and IGFBP-3 are not associated with risk	No evidence	m

a. Hankinson et al 1998. b. Krajcik et al 2002. c. Ma et al 1999. d. Giovannucci et al 2000. e. Kaaks et al 2000. f. Probst-Hensch et al 2001. g. Palmqvist et al 2002. h. London et al 2002. i. Spitz et al 2002. j. Lukanova et al 2001. k. Chan et al 1998. l. Chan et al 2002. m. Woodson et al 2003.

access to IGF-1R, and thus inhibit the bioactivity of IGFs. The high-affinity IGF binding of IGFBPs involves both the conserved N- and C-terminal domains of IGFBPs (Yamanaka et al 1997, Hwa et al 1999, Firth & Baxter 2002, Clemmons 2001). Evidence includes recent studies employing two-dimensional nuclear magnetic resonance spectroscopy (Kalus et al 1998) and crystal structural analyses using IGFBP-5 fragments (Zeslawski et al 2001), as well as mutagenesis studies. Specifically, site specific mutations within the conserved N-terminus of IGFBP-3 reduced the affinity of IGFBP-3 for IGF 80–1000-fold (Buckway et al 2001, Hong et al 2002).

The inhibitory effects of IGFBPs on IGF action have been observed in various cell types, including cancer cells. For example, IGFBP-3 inhibited the growth of non-small cell lung cancer and potentiated apoptosis *via* sequestration of IGF-1 (Lee et al 2002), and IGFBP-6 inhibited neuroblastoma cell proliferation and tumour development *via* blocking the action of IGF-2 (Seurin et al 2002).

Regulation of IGFBP inhibitory effects. A number of mechanisms have been demonstrated to modulate the IGF-binding affinity of IGFBPs (Firth & Baxter 2002). The main mechanism being limited proteolytic degradation of the IGFBPs (reviewed recently in Bunn & Fowlkes 2003). The proteolysis of IGFBPs generates protein fragments that have no affinity, or significantly less affinity, for IGFs, thus releasing IGFs from ternary or binary complexes, and thereby promoting IGF action.

A number of IGFBP proteases, as well as their specific proteolytic sites, have been characterized (Maile & Holly 1999, Mohan & Baylink 2002, Firth & Baxter 2002). These proteases are either specific or non-specific proteases for the IGFBPs (Bunn & Fowlkes 2003). Several proteases have been known to associate with human cancers. Matrix metalloproteinases (MMPs), which are frequently overexpressed in human tumours, are known to proteolyse IGFBPs (Bunn & Fowlkes 2003). The marker for prostate cancer, prostate specific antigen (PSA) is also a serine protease that specifically proteolyses IGFBP-3 (Cohen et al 1992).

Alterations in IGFBP proteolysis have been observed in pathological conditions (Muller et al 1994), including some human cancers. For example, increase in plasma IGFBP-3 proteolysis was observed in primary breast cancer (Helle et al 2001). The activity of IGFBP proteases may in turn be regulated by protease activators or inhibitors (Conover et al 2001). The acute regulation of IGFBP proteolysis thus modulates availability of IGFs, and, under conditions of increased IGFBP protease activity, increased amounts of mitogenic IGF peptides may become available to local receptors.

In addition to these classical functions, the proteolysis of IGFBPs may also activate other biological functions, as was demonstrated by the observations that the N-terminal fragment of IGFBP-3 is able to bind insulin (Yamanaka et al 1997). The role(s) of IGFBP fragments in cancer has yet to be fully elucidated. Clearly, IGFBP proteolysis not only is one of the major mechanisms for modulating IGF bioavailability, but may also result in gain-of-function for the proteolysed fragments.

IGF-independent effects of IGFBPs

In addition to their growth inhibitory effects *via* modulation of IGF actions, IGFBPs can exert growth inhibitory effects in the absence of any direct interactions with IGFs. The IGF-independent actions of IGFBPs have been observed in a variety of cell types, especially in human cancer cells, and are involved in the processes of cell migration, cell growth and apoptosis (reviewed recently in Firth & Baxter 2002, Mohan & Baylink 2002).

The IGF-independent actions of IGFBP-3 on cancer cells are well documented. First reported in Hs578T, a human breast cancer cell line (Oh et al 1993a) that does not respond to exogenous IGFs (Oh et al 1992), it was demonstrated that the exogenous addition of IGFBP-3 causes growth inhibition. This inhibitory effect was specific for IGFBP-3 since addition of IGFBP-1 has no effect. IGF-1 and IGF-2 analogues with low affinity for IGFBP-3, but retaining high affinity for IGF receptors, did not block IGFBP-3 action, indicating the action of IGFBP-3 is not mediated by inhibition of IGF access to IGF-1R. Instead, the action of IGFBP-3 was likely to be mediated through its own membrane receptors (Oh et al 1993a and see below).

The concept of IGF-independent, anti-proliferative effects of IGFBP-3 in human breast cancer cell lines was further supported by evidence that IGFBP-3 mediates the antiproliferative actions of several growth inhibitors, including transforming growth factor β (TGFβ (Oh et al 1995), retinoic acid (Gucev et al 1996) and anti-oestrogen (Huynh et al 1996). As shown in these studies, treatment of breast cancer cells with these cell growth inhibitors stimulated both the mRNA and the protein expression of IGFBP-3. Blocking the induced expression of IGFBP-3 with IGFBP-3 antisense oligodeoxynucleotide, or preventing the secreted IGFBP-3 from binding to the cell surface by sequestration of IGFBP-3 with high affinity analogues of IGFs, diminished the antiproliferative effects of these growth inhibitors (Oh et al 1995, Gucev et al 1996, Huynh et al 1996). Altogether, these results strongly argue for IGFBP-3 having a direct growth inhibitory effect on breast cancer cells, and suggest that this action is likely to be mediated by its own cell surface receptor (discussed below).

The antiproliferative actions of IGFBPs appear to be through inducing apoptosis. In the human prostate cancer cell line PC-3 the addition of exogenous IGFBP-3 induced dose-dependent apoptosis of the cells (Rajah et al 1997); the stable overexpression of IGFBP-3 in M12 human prostate cancer cells (Devi et al 2002) also induced apoptosis. Apoptosis was only partially inhibited by exogenous IGF and was not inhibited by IGF analogues that do not bind to IGFBPs, suggesting an IGF-independent mechanism for the IGFBP-3 effect (Rajah et al 1997). Corroborating these reports, it was shown that IGFBP-3 could enhance apoptosis induced by ceramide in Hs578T cells in an IGF-independent manner

(Gill et al 1997, Perks et al 2000), and could increase apoptosis induced by ionizing radiation in MCF-7 human breast cancer cells (Butt et al 2000).

Definitive support for the IGF-independent, antiproliferative and proapoptotic actions of IGFBP-3 came from studies employing IGFBP-3 variants characterized by reduced affinity for IGFs. An IGFBP-3 mutant (I56G, L80G, and L81G) with a 1000-fold less affinity for IGF (Buckway et al 2001), when added exogenously, could inhibit the proliferation of chondroprogenitors and early differentiated chondrocytes in a dose-dependent manner (Spagnoli et al 2001). Exogenous addition or overexpression *via* transient expression of this IGFBP-3 mutant could also induce apoptosis in these cells (Longobardi et al 2003). Another IGFBP-3 variant that bears mutations in the same N-terminal region (I56A, Y57A, R75A, L77A, L80A and L81A) displayed an 80-fold reduced affinity for IGFs, and also induced apoptosis in PC-3 cancer cells (Hong et al 2002). These studies clearly demonstrate that IGFBP-3 is capable of exerting IGF-independent, antiproliferative and proapoptotic effects, and thus could play a much wider role in antitumorigenesis.

Potential mechanisms for IGF-independent actions

Several potential mechanisms by which IGFBPs exert their IGF-independent effects have been proposed: IGFBP may either bind specifically to cell surface receptors and activate associated cellular signalling pathways, and/or translocate to the nucleus and serve as transcriptional factors to regulate the expressions of the target genes (Firth & Baxter 2002, Mohan & Baylink 2002).

Cell surface receptor for IGFBPs. IGFBPs have been shown to be able to interact with several cell surface molecules, presumably due to their highly basic sequences in the C-terminal domains (Firth & Baxter 2002). Evidence for a cell membrane receptor specific for IGFBP-3 was demonstrated in Hs578T human breast cancer cells (Oh et al 1993b and references therein). The receptor was detected by affinity cross-linking of cell monolayers and of cell lysates with ^{125}I-labelled *Escherichia coli* recombinant IGFBP-3 ([^{125}I]IGFBP-3$^{E.coli}$). The binding of [^{125}I]IGFBP-3$^{E.coli}$ was competitively inhibited by unlabelled IGFBP-3$^{E.coli}$ or IGFs, but not by low affinity IGF analogues, suggesting IGFBP-3 bound to putative receptors with high affinity and specificity. Partial purification of these putative receptor(s) indicated proteins of 20, 26 and 50 kDa. Further characterization of the IGFBP-3–receptor interaction indicated that the mid-region of IGFBP-3 is responsible for this interaction (Yamanaka et al 1999). In addition to these putative receptors, IGFBP-3 appears to also interact with a 400 kDa type V TGFβ receptor in mink lung epithelial cells (Leal et al 1997), although the physiological significance of this latter interaction is uncertain.

IGFBP-3-induced signalling pathways. Several lines of evidence have indicated that the IGFBP-3-independent actions may be associated with their own signalling pathways, possibly following binding to IGFBP-3's cell surface receptors. In human breast cancer cells, it was shown that interaction of IGFBP-3 with an unknown receptor(s) resulted in a rapid and transient increase of intracellular free calcium (Ricort et al 2002). IGFBP-3 may also activate Smad2/Smad3 in the TGFβ pathway in breast cancer cells (Fanayan et al 2002 and references therein), or activate a phosphotyrosine phosphatase that may interfere with the IGF-1R pathway (Ricort & Binoux 2002). In mesenchymal chondroprogenitors, IGFBP-3 exerts its antiproliferative effect *via* the induction of STAT-1 protein (Spagnoli et al 2001).

Nuclear localization and transcriptional regulation. It is known that IGFBP-3 and IGFBP-5 contain nuclear localization signals (NLS) in their C-terminal domain and nuclear localization appears to be *via* the importin β (Radulescu 1994). The biological functions of nuclear localization of IGFBPs have only just begun to be elucidated. In a recent study, IGFBP-3 was shown to be able to interact with nuclear receptor retinoid X receptor α (RXRα) *via* its C-terminal heparin-binding domain, and IGFBP-3 could bind to the RXRα and RXR response element DNA complexes (Liu et al 2000). The biological consequence of this interaction was enhanced apoptosis in prostate cancer cells (Liu et al 2000). In contrast, nuclear IGFBP-3 did not appear to be involved in the IGFBP-3-induced apoptosis in breast cancer cells (Butt et al 2002). IGFBP-5 was shown to be able to interact with a zinc finger transcriptional activator, FHL2, although the biological function of this interaction is unknown yet (Amaar et al 2002). The mechanism(s) by which IGFBPs are transported into cytoplasm from the extracellular milieu, and subsequently translocated into the nucleus has yet to be fully determined. In one study, transferrin was identified from a yeast two-hybrid screen and was suggested to be a transporter mobilizing secreted IGFBP-3 from the extracellular space into the cytoplasm (Weinzimer et al 2001).

Conclusions

The identification of an IGFBP superfamily and the discoveries of IGF-independent actions of IGFBPs have indicated that the members of the IGFBP superfamily are multifunctional proteins, and are involved in diverse biological processes, especially in the control of cell proliferation, differentiation, programmed cell death and malignant transformation. The epidemiological data, although far from conclusive, have indicated a possible protective role for IGFBPs, particularly for IGFBP-3. This observation is corroborated by the results from a number of *in vitro* studies demonstrating that IGFBP-3 possesses

IGF-independent, antiproliferative and pro-apoptotic activities. However, these *in vitro* activities have yet to be demonstrated *in vivo*.

Although much of the research in this area has concentrated on the actions and role(s) of IGFBP-3, it is important to note that the effects of IGFBP-3 on cell growth or apoptosis are, typically, not dramatic when IGFBP-3 acts on its own, and the effect is usually not immediate. This suggests that the growth inhibitory process is multi-factorial, with IGFBP-3 perhaps acting as an enhancer or collaborator in the process. Nevertheless, a thorough understanding of the role(s) IGFBP-3 plays is necessary for optimization of its pro-apoptotic effects against cancer cells.

In contrast to IGFBP-3, limited information is available about the roles of other IGFBPs in cancer cells. In particular, abnormally high serum levels of IGFBP-2 have been observed in several cancers, but the mechanism(s) for its dysregulation, and its functions, remain a mystery. Furthermore, the observation that IGFBPs could both potentiate and inhibit cancer cell growth, and can associate with different putative cell surface receptors initiating a number of plausible signalling pathways, indicates that IGFBPs may act *via* different mechanisms depending on the environment and cell types. Further studies will be necessary to demonstrate whether the extraordinary ability of these 'cancer proteins' to inhibit the proliferation of cancer cells under *in vitro* conditions has significant clinical implications.

Acknowledgements

The work done in this lab is supported by the grants from NIH and US Army.

References

Amaar YG, Thompson GR, Linkhart TA et al 2002 Insulin-like growth factor-binding protein 5 (IGFBP-5) interacts with a four and a half LIM protein 2 (FHL2). J Biol Chem 277:12053–12060

Baxter RC 2000 Insulin-like growth factor (IGF)-binding proteins: interactions with IGFs and intrinsic bioactivities. Am J Physiol Endocrinol Metab 278:E967–976

Buckway CK, Wilson EM, Ahlsen M et al 2001 Mutation of three critical amino acids of the N-terminal domain of IGF-binding protein-3 essential for high affinity IGF binding. J Clin Endocrinol Metab 86:4943–4950

Bunn RC, Fowlkes JL 2003 Insulin-like growth factor binding protein proteolysis. Trends Endocrinol Metab 14:176–181

Butt AJ, Firth SM, King MA, Baxter RC 2000 Insulin-like growth factor-binding protein-3 modulates expression of Bax and Bcl-2 and potentiates p53-independent radiation-induced apoptosis in human breast cancer cells. J Biol Chem 275:39174–39181

Butt AJ, Fraley KA, Firth SM, Baxter RC 2002 IGF-binding protein-3-induced growth inhibition and apoptosis do not require cell surface binding and nuclear translocation in human breast cancer cells. Endocrinology 143:2693–2699

Clemmons DR 2001 Use of mutagenesis to probe IGF-binding protein structure/function relationships. Endocr Rev 22:800–817

Chan JM, Stampfer MJ, Giovannucci E et al 1998 Plasma insulin-like growth factor-I and prostate cancer risk: a prospective study. Science 279:563–566

Chan JM, Stampfer MJ, Ma J et al 2002 Insulin-like growth factor-I (IGF-I) and IGF binding protein-3 as predictors of advanced-stage prostate cancer. J Natl Cancer Inst 94:1099–1106

Cohen P, Clemmons DR, Rosenfeld RG 2000 Does the GH-IGF axis play a role in cancer pathogenesis? Growth Horm IGF Res 10:297–305

Cohen P, Graves HC, Peehl DM et al 1992 Prostate-specific antigen (PSA) is an insulin-like growth factor binding protein-3 protease found in seminal plasma. J Clin Endocrinol Metab 75:1046–1053

Collett-Solberg PF, Cohen P 2000 Genetics, chemistry, and function of the IGF/IGFBP system. Endocrine 12:121–136

Conover CA, Faessen GF, Ilg KE et al 2001 Pregnancy-associated plasma protein-a is the insulin-like growth factor binding protein-4 protease secreted by human ovarian granulosa cells and is a marker of dominant follicle selection and the corpus luteum. Endocrinology 142:2155

Damon SE, Maddison L, Ware JL, Plymate SR 1998 Overexpression of an inhibitory insulin-like growth factor binding protein (IGFBP), IGFBP-4, delays onset of prostate tumor formation. Endocrinology 139:3456–3464

Devi GR, Sprenger CC, Plymate SR, Rosenfeld RG 2002 Insulin-like growth factor binding protein-3 induces early apoptosis in malignant prostate cancer cells and inhibits tumor formation *in vivo*. Prostate 51:141–152

Fanayan S, Firth SM, Baxter RC 2002 Signaling through the Smad pathway by insulin-like growth factor-binding protein-3 in breast cancer cells. Relationship to transforming growth factor-beta 1 signaling. J Biol Chem 277:7255–7261

Firth SM, Baxter RC 2002 Cellular actions of the insulin-like growth factor binding proteins. Endocr Rev 23:824–854

Gill ZP, Perks CM, Newcomb PV, Holly JM 1997 Insulin-like growth factor-binding protein (IGFBP-3) predisposes breast cancer cells to programmed cell death in a non-IGF-dependent manner. J Biol Chem 272:25602–25607

Giovannucci E, Pollak MN, Platz EA et al 2000 A prospective study of plasma insulin-like growth factor-1 and binding protein-3 and risk of colorectal neoplasia in women. Cancer Epidemiol Biomarkers Prev 9:345–349

Gucev ZS, Oh Y, Kelley KM, Rosenfeld RG 1996 Insulin-like growth factor binding protein 3 mediates retinoic acid- and transforming growth factor beta2-induced growth inhibition in human breast cancer cells. Cancer Res 56:1545–1550

Hankinson SE, Willett WC, Colditz GA et al 1998 Circulating concentrations of insulin-like growth factor-I and risk of breast cancer. Lancet 351:1393–1396

Helle SI, Geisler S, Aas T et al 2001 Plasma insulin-like growth factor binding protein-3 proteolysis is increased in primary breast cancer. Br J Cancer 85:74–77

Hong J, Zhang G, Dong F, Rechler MM 2002 Insulin-like growth factor (IGF)-binding protein-3 mutants that do not bind IGF-I or IGF-II stimulate apoptosis in human prostate cancer cells. J Biol Chem 277:10489–10497

Huynh H, Yang X, Pollak M 1996 Estradiol and antiestrogens regulate a growth inhibitory insulin-like growth factor binding protein 3 autocrine loop in human breast cancer cells. J Biol Chem 271:1016–1021

Hwa V, Oh Y, Rosenfeld RG 1999 The insulin-like growth factor-binding protein (IGFBP) superfamily. Endocr Rev 20:761–787

Jones JI, Clemmons DR 1995 Insulin-like growth factors and their binding proteins: biological actions. Endocr Rev 16:3–34

Kaaks R, Toniolo P, Akhmedkhanov A et al 2000 Serum C-peptide, insulin-like growth factor (IGF)-I, IGF-binding proteins, and colorectal cancer risk in women. J Natl Cancer Inst 92:1592–1600

Kalus W, Zweckstetter M, Renner C et al 1998 Structure of the IGF-binding domain of the insulin-like growth factor-binding protein-5 (IGFBP-5): implications for IGF and IGF-I receptor interactions. EMBO J 17:6558–6572

Kelley KM, Oh Y, Gargosky SE et al 1996 Insulin-like growth factor-binding proteins (IGFBPs) and their regulatory dynamics. Int J Biochem Cell Biol 28:619–637

Khandwala HM, McCutcheon IE, Flyvbjerg A, Friend KE 2000 The effects of insulin-like growth factors on tumorigenesis and neoplastic growth. Endocr Rev 21:215–244

Krajcik RA, Borofsky ND, Massardo S, Orentreich N 2002 Insulin-like growth factor I (IGF-I), IGF-binding proteins, and breast cancer. Cancer Epidemiol Biomarkers Prev 11:1566–1173

Leal SM, Liu Q, Huang SS, Huang JS 1997 The type V transforming growth factor beta receptor is the putative insulin-like growth factor-binding protein 3 receptor. J Biol Chem 272:20572–20576

Lee HY, Chun KH, Liu B et al 2002 Insulin-like growth factor binding protein-3 inhibits the growth of non-small cell lung cancer. Cancer Res 62:3530–3537

Liu B, Lee HY, Weinzimer SA et al 2000 Direct functional interactions between insulin-like growth factor-binding protein-3 and retinoid X receptor-alpha regulate transcriptional signaling and apoptosis. J Biol Chem 275:33607–33613

Longobardi L, Torello M, Buckway C et al 2003 A novel insulin-like growth factor (IGF)-independent role for IGF binding protein-3 in mesenchymal chondroprogenitor cell apoptosis. Endocrinology 144:1695–1702

London SJ, Yuan JM, Travlos GS et al 2002 Insulin-like growth factor I, IGF-binding protein 3, and lung cancer risk in a prospective study of men in China. J Natl Cancer Inst 94:749–754

Lopez-Bermejo A, Buckway CK, Devi GR et al 2000 Characterization of insulin-like growth factor-binding protein-related proteins (IGFBP-rPs) 1, 2, and 3 in human prostate epithelial cells: potential roles for IGFBP-rP1 and 2 in senescence of the prostatic epithelium. Endocrinology 141:4072–4080

Lukanova A, Toniolo P, Akhmedkhanov et al 2001 A prospective study of insulin-like growth factor-I, IGF-binding proteins-1, -2 and -3 and lung cancer risk in women. Int J Cancer 92:888–892

Ma J, Pollak MN, Giovannucci E et al 1999 Prospective study of colorectal cancer risk in men and plasma levels of insulin-like growth factor (IGF)-I and IGF-binding protein-3. J Natl Cancer Inst 91:620–625

Maile LA, Holly JM 1999 Insulin-like growth factor binding protein (IGFBP) proteolysis: occurrence, identification, role and regulation. Growth Horm IGF Res 9:85–95

Mohan S, Baylink DJ 2002 IGF-binding proteins are multifunctional and act via IGF-dependent and -independent mechanisms. J Endocrinol 175:19–31

Muller HL, Oh Y, Gargosky SE et al 1994 Insulin-like growth factor binding protein-3 concentrations and insulin-like growth factor binding protein-3 protease activity in sera of patients with malignant solid tumors or leukemia. Pediatr Res 35:720–724

Oh Y, Muller HL, Pham H, Lamson G, Rosenfeld RG 1992 Non-receptor mediated, post-transcriptional regulation of insulin-like growth factor binding protein (IGFBP)-3 in Hs578T human breast cancer cells. Endocrinology 131:3123–3125

Oh Y, Muller HL, Lamson G, Rosenfeld RG 1993a Insulin-like growth factor (IGF)-independent action of IGF-binding protein-3 in Hs578T human breast cancer cells. Cell surface binding and growth inhibition. J Biol Chem 268:14964–14971

Oh Y, Muller HL, Pham H, Rosenfeld RG 1993b Demonstration of receptors for insulin-like growth factor binding protein-3 on Hs578T human breast cancer cells. J Biol Chem 268:26045–26048

Oh Y, Muller HL, Ng L, Rosenfeld RG 1995 Transforming growth factor-beta-induced cell growth inhibition in human breast cancer cells is mediated through insulin-like growth factor-binding protein-3 action. J Biol Chem 270:13589–13592

Palmqvist R, Hallmans G, Rinaldi S et al 2002 Plasma insulin-like growth factor 1, insulin-like growth factor binding protein 3, and risk of colorectal cancer: a prospective study in northern Sweden. Gut 50:642–646

Perks CM, McCaig C, Holly JM 2000 Differential insulin-like growth factor (IGF)-independent interactions of IGF binding protein-3 and IGF binding protein-5 on apoptosis in human breast cancer cells. Involvement of the mitochondria. J Cell Biochem 80:248–258

Probst-Hensch NM, Yuan JM, Stanczyk SZ, Gao YT, Ross RK, Yu MC 2001 IGF-1, IGF-2 and IGFBP-3 in prediagnostic serum: association with colorectal cancer in a cohort of Chinese men in Shanghai. Br J Cancer 85:1695–1699

Radulescu RT 1994 Nuclear localization signal in insulin-like growth factor-binding protein type 3. Trends Biochem Sci 19:278

Rajah R, Valentinis B, Cohen P 1997 Insulin-like growth factor (IGF)-binding protein-3 induces apoptosis and mediates the effects of transforming growth factor-beta1 on programmed cell death through a p53- and IGF-independent mechanism. J Biol Chem 272:12181–12188

Ricort JM, Binoux M 2002 Insulin-like growth factor-binding protein-3 activates a phosphotyrosine phosphatase. Effects on the insulin-like growth factor signaling pathway. J Biol Chem 277:19448–19454

Ricort JM, Lombet A, Lassarre C, Binoux M 2002 Insulin-like growth factor binding protein-3 increases intracellular calcium concentrations in MCF-7 breast carcinoma cells. FEBS Lett 527:293–297

Scharf JG, Dombrowski F, Ramadori G 2001 The IGF axis and hepatocarcinogenesis. Mol Pathol 54:138–144

Seurin D, Lassarre C, Bienvenu G, Babajko S 2002 Insulin-like growth factor binding protein-6 inhibits neuroblastoma cell proliferation and tumour development. Eur J Cancer 38:2058–2065

Spagnoli A, Hwa V, Horton WA et al 2001 Antiproliferative effects of insulin-like growth factor-binding protein-3 in mesenchymal chondrogenic cell line RCJ3.1C5.18. Relationship to differentiation stage. J Biol Chem 276:5533–5540

Spitz MR, Barnett MJ, Goodman GE, Thornquist MD, Wu X, Pollak M 2002 Serum insulin-like growth factor (IGF) and IGF-binding protein levels and risk of lung cancer: a case-control study nested in the beta-Carotene and Retinol Efficacy Trial Cohort. Cancer Epidemiol Biomarkers Prev 11:1413–1418

Twigg SM, Baxter RC 1998 Insulin-like growth factor (IGF)-binding protein 5 forms an alternative ternary complex with IGFs and the acid-labile subunit. J Biol Chem 273:6074–6079

Weinzimer SA, Gibson TB, Collett-Solberg PF et al 2001 Transferrin is an insulin-like growth factor-binding protein-3 binding protein. J Clin Endocrinol Metab 86:1806–1813

Woodson K, Tangrea JA, Pollak M et al 2003 Serum insulin-like growth factor I: tumor marker or etiologic factor? A prospective study of prostate cancer among Finnish men. Cancer Res 63:3991–3994

Yamanaka Y, Wilson EM, Rosenfeld RG, Oh Y 1997 Inhibition of insulin receptor activation by insulin-like growth factor binding proteins. J Biol Chem 272:30729–30734

Yamanaka Y, Fowlkes JL, Wilson EM, Rosenfeld RG, Oh Y 1999 Characterization of insulin-like growth factor binding protein-3 (IGFBP- 3) binding to human breast cancer cells: kinetics of IGFBP-3 binding and identification of receptor binding domain on the IGFBP-3 molecule. Endocrinology 140:1319–1328

Yu H, Rohan T 2000 Role of the insulin-like growth factor family in cancer development and progression. J Natl Cancer Inst 92:1472–1489

Zeslawski W, Beisel HG, Kamionka M et al 2001 The interaction of insulin-like growth factor-I with the N-terminal domain of IGFBP-5. EMBO J 20:3638–3844

Zhou R, Diehl D, Hoeflich A, Lahm H, Wolf E 2003 IGF-binding protein-4: biochemical characteristics and functional consequences. J Endocrinol 178:177–193
Zumkeller W, Westphal M 2001 The IGF/IGFBP system in CNS malignancy. Mol Pathol 54:227–229

DISCUSSION

LeRoith: You mentioned that some of your patients didn't do too well. I know you meant animals, but there was a confusion. In humans when you give IGF-1 it suppresses GH and IGFBP-3. In all of our animal experiments, every time we have given IGF-1, we have enhanced IGFBP-3 levels because of its post-translational effect. There is no mRNA or gene expression effect in the animals of GH; it is mostly a post-translational effect. Therefore, I would predict that in those animal studies that IGFBP-3 may actually go up and not be suppressed. It will be interesting to see what happens.

Rosenfeld: That is a fair point.

LeRoith: The second issue is that one should not forget that in acromegalics, the IGF-1 and IGFBP-3 levels are both increased. Total IGF-1 goes up, so they are moving up into your quadrant. While it is controversial, there are a number of groups who believe that in acromegalics, the incidence of colonic adenomas (and perhaps even carcinomas) are increased despite the increased IGF-1 and IGFBP-3. Not everyone agrees, but everyone does agree that these patients should be followed with colonoscopy. That means that even those who are not sure are being careful. I am in the school that says that recent data suggest there is an increased incidence of carcinoma or progression from adenoma to carcinoma. This is in a group that has high IGFBP-3/IGF-1. I don't know that we can conclude today that having high IGFBP-3/IGF-1 is protective. It may be that IGFBP-3/IGF-1 complex is actually important for delivering IGF-1 and having some action on an unprotected or susceptible tissue such as the colon.

Rosenfeld: I don't disagree with your points. With respect to the acromegaly issue, if there is an increase in cancer (and this is debated) it seems to be restricted to colonic. This has not been seen for prostate or mammary cancer, for example. Second, while it is correct that the IGFBP-3 levels are increased, their IGF-1 levels are disproportionately increased above IGFBP-3. Third, these are patients who may have a genetic predisposition to cancer to begin with, because they have already developed tumours that have given them acromegaly. They may be a high risk group. I did not by any means want the data I showed you to suggest that the door is closed on this question. I think it needs considerable ongoing investigation.

LeRoith: As Jeff Holly would say, everyone has cancer. Therefore when we think about high GH levels—whether we are giving it or it is because of acromegaly — since everyone has an underlying cancer at some stage we should be careful.

Holly: Ron Rosenfeld said that perhaps IGF-1 is not oncogenic, in that it doesn't accelerate or promote existing tumours. In the human clinical scenario that is the question and that is the problem. When you get into the elderly population, everyone has cancer. The trick is to outlive your cancer. If you accelerate the rate of growth of the tumour without extending your lifespan, the tumour is going to overtake you.

Kaaks: The epidemiological data are not as unequivocal as they may seem. In some epidemiological studies IGFBP-3 was moderately and inversely related with cancer risk, such that when you statistically adjust for the IGFBP-3 level and look at the IGF-1–cancer association, the latter becomes stronger. IGFBP-3 then acts statistically as a negative confounder. Almost all of these studies were done with an ELISA from Diagnostic Systems Laboratories (DSL, Texas). There are, however, a number of other studies where high levels of IGFBP-3 were associated with increased risk of cancer. Virtually all of these studies were done with assays purchased from another company or in-house methods. This discrepancy has led to discussions as to what these assays really measure. It is possible that they are both right but that they don't reflect exactly the same IGFBP-3 varieties. One speculation exists that total IGFBP-3 levels may be higher in terms of overall synthesis or overall amount of IGFBP-3 circulating intact or in fragments, but that it is the intact form which is lower.

Holly: Following Michael Pollak's pioneering work there is now a huge amount of epidemiology. The data for IGF-1 risk association are incredibly robust. Regarding the data for IGFBP-3, if there is nothing in it you would expect maybe a few positives and a few negatives, and for most of the data to aggregate around the null. But this has not happened. There have been a few positives and a few negatives and very few nulls. There is something in this: IGFBP-3 is part of the equation, but we can't be sure whether it is protective or not.

Pollak: These are impressive and expensive experiments designed to be definitive in terms of the safety profile. An effort was seriously made to look at the long term, which is to be applauded. In a sense, though, formally scientifically speaking it is the wrong experiment. You would have to give these animals some other oncological insult and then compare your groups. This is asking the question is IGF-1 carcinogenic? The concern is not from the underlying epidemiology that IGF-1 is a carcinogen; the concern is that it is a progression factor.

Rosenfeld: There are two different questions here, both of which are legitimate and relevant. The question you are asking as an oncologist is different from the question an endocrinologist would be asking. As an oncologist you may say there is a risk in giving oestrogen to a 20 year old hypogonadal woman. As an endocrinologist I might say there is a risk, but there is a rationale for replacing the hormone in that person. As endocrinologists we are asking whether we should consider treating otherwise healthy people with GH or IGF-1. Are we putting them at increased risk of developing cancer or progressing cancer? These kinds of studies are the appropriate kinds of studies. You take 900 rats and you treat them: you don't increase their cancer risk. The truly relevant question from my perspective as an endocrinologist coming out of this meeting isn't going to be whether if you have some predisposed cancer risk IGF-1 is going to be a problem, it is can we begin treating patients with IGF-1?

Pollak: This is why the interdisciplinary interaction here is so important. The notion that the endocrinological replacement therapy is being given to a normal adult who has cancer is the message that we are giving. There is evidence from autopsy series and the recent prostate cancer prevention trial that when healthy men with no clinical symptoms are biopsied, they frequently had cancers. Part of the complexity of looking at the risk–benefit equation is that the very subjects who are 'healthy' and are candidates for hormone replacement therapies of various kinds often have subclinical cancers. The precedent from oestrogen-replacement therapy is telling. There is a risk–benefit equation: women on this therapy get fewer hip fractures but they get more breast cancers.

Lønning: Returning to the issue of binding proteins, a key question is whether binding proteins in general are enhancers of delivery, or prevent delivery of a factor. This is an old discussion: we had it with steroids 30 years ago when Pentii Siterii first proposed that sex hormone binding globulin (SHBG) enhanced oestrogen delivery to the tissue. When we plough through the evidence, it is very difficult to sort out the biochemical effects of binding proteins *invivo* with respect to clinical outcome. I only know one example where we can clearly state that there is no doubt that the binding protein inhibits the action of the ligand. That is, if you look into pregnancy and thyroxine-binding globulin. If thyroxine-binding globulin was an enhancer of delivery of thyroxine, every pregnant woman should suffer from thyrotoxicosis.

LeRoith: I think you are right. Ron brought that up when he said that in many cases IGFBP is often inhibitory, but there are very good examples of where it is also stimulatory. The work of Rob Baxter and myself in MCF-7 cells and in mammary glands of transgenic mice shows that IGFBP-3 enhances the growth. We are not sure whether it is independent, but it may be IGF-dependent. My point is, it could be cell tissue-type specific.

Lønning: I am not denying that. I am taking the perspective of the clinician. If we look at the patients and the clinics, we have only seen one example.

LeRoith: The three of us are in agreement that it is not clear which tissues would respond to which binding proteins and in what manner. In your defence, I want to remind you of the first experiment I showed in my presentation, where we implanted caecum tumours and gave rhIGF-1 and showed growth with high dose but not with lower doses. Ross Clark gave us the rhIGF-1 to do this experiment.

Clark: My interpretation of these data is a little different. I think what these data point towards is the 'bad guy' hormone. Derek LeRoith talked about acromegalics having increased cancer risk. The rat study with IGF-1 is relatively inconclusive. If you had done that same study with GH in rodents, you would probably have got a change of phenotype in mammary tumours, increased number of mammary tumours, and we don't know what else. When we measure IGF in the blood of humans, we have to think about the major factor influencing IGF levels. It is clearly GH. Is this a time to go back and look at the IGF data, and ask whether GH is the bad guy there? This is what the IGF study indicates to me. I am not saying this is what it is, but it makes you think: what are we measuring when we are measuring IGF levels? We are actually getting the integrated exposure to GH.

Laron: I am very happy that now there is agreement that continuous IGF-1 treatment increases BP-3 levels. It doesn't increase much, but it does increase.

LeRoith: In animals.

Laron: No, we found it in our patients (Kanety et al 1997).

Rosenfeld: You are absolutely wrong there!

LeRoith: Just to put this point in perspective, many of us agree that in rodents, IGF-1 increases IGFBP-3. In humans there is a debate about this.

Laron: I have a question and a comment. The rat model is indeed the best model to check the effects of high doses of IGF-1, but in humans we know that with relatively low doses we get hypoglycaemia. When we give it continuously to children and take care of the hypoglycaemia by feeding correctly, we see increased lymphatic tissue. In the cartilage there are changes, such as widening of the nose. These are not seen in the mice. We also know they are less sensitive to IGF-1. The doses used in order to obtain hypoglycaemia are so much higher in the mouse or rat than in human. This reservation should be kept in mind. We know, for instance, than in human, GH has caused deaths when it has been used to treat Prader–Willi syndrome patients, most probably by the increase in lymphatic tissue causing sleep apnoea worse than in patients who have simple obesity. These results observed in rodents are important but should not be translated directly into humans. My question is that you didn't mention IGFBPs: do you have any data on them?

Rosenfeld: IGFBP-1 is a more acutely regulated binding protein than the others. It is affected by insulin, nutrition and IGF-1 administration. I don't have any data of my own on IGFBP-1 and cancer.

Ohlsson: I am struck by the correlation between local *IGF2* expression, organomegaly and increased risk of cancer in Beckwith–Wiedemann syndrome patients. This suggests that IGF-1 administered to the mice or rats could actually have two effects. One is to promote growth of target cells, but it could also involve the immune system. As we know, one of the most decisive events in human cancer is when the immune system is unable to deal with the development of tumours. Has anyone looked at the effects of IGF-1 on the immune system? The point that I am making is that high IGF-1 or IGF-2 expression must be local to have a detrimental effect.

Clark: I published a review in *Endocrine Reviews* some years ago on the human data that IGF-1 can affect lymphoid growth (Clark 1997). It can increase the total bulk of lymphocytes without actually changing the subtypes. It expands the immune system. The logic in that review was that as your bones grow, the amount of bone marrow has to grow with it. As portions of the body increase in size during growth, the immune system has to increase in size. There is a good logic that as part of GH/IGFs overall control of body growth you also control the dimensions and size of the immune system without actually changing the number of cells. We also tested IGF-1 in AIDS patients. They have no immune system and so they are incredibly susceptible to tumour growth. We treated 300–400 AIDS patients and I can recall that there was no dramatic oncological effect. Part of the effect of IGF-1 in rats could be that you are increasing immune surveillance, because the immune system is undoubtedly affected by IGF-1.

LeRoith: We did a study on primates and showed that there was no immune suppression. If anything there was a slight increase in surveillance and immune competence. I don't think it is a loss of the immune system. If anything it is a gain.

Yee: I have a technical question. In terms of rat strains, they differ widely in their susceptibility to mammary carcinogenesis. Which rat did you use?

Clark: It was the traditional animal used in carcinogenicity studies, the Sprague–Dawley strain of rat, where about 60% of the female animals have mammary tumours in their lifetime.

Yee: Sprague–Dawley rats are susceptible to pregnancy promoting a greater incidence of breast cancer.

Clark: These were virgin animals treated at 40 days. They were single housed.

Yee: It would be interesting to see what happens with pregnant animals.

Clark: The large carcinogenicity study was done for regulatory and safety reasons as well as for scientific reasons to really discover what would happen with life-time exposure to IGF-1.

References

Clark R 1997 The somatogenic hormones and insulin-like growth factor-1: stimulators of lymphopoiesis and immune function. Endocr Rev 18:157–179

Kanety H, Silbergeld A, Klinger B, Karasik A, Baxter RC, Laron Z 1997 Long-term effects of insulin-like growth factor (IGF)-I on serum IGF-I, IGF-binding protein-3 and acid labile subunit in Laron syndrome patients with normal growth hormone binding protein. Eur J Endocrinol 137:626–630

The IGF receptor as anticancer treatment target

Valentine M. Macaulay

Cancer Research UK Laboratories, Weatherall Institute of Molecular Medicine, Oxford OX3 9DS, UK

Abstract. The type 1 insulin-like growth factor receptor (IGF-1R) is overexpressed by many tumours and mediates proliferation, motility and apoptosis protection. Tumour growth and metastasis can be blocked by agents that inhibit IGF-1R expression or function, suggesting the IGF-1R as a promising treatment target. We showed that antisense-IGF-1R expression in melanoma cells leads to enhanced radiosensitivity and impaired activation of ATM, required for DNA double-strand break repair. Antisense and dominant negative strategies also enhance tumour cell chemosensitivity, and remarkably, immune protection can be induced by tumour cells killed *in vivo* by IGF-1R-antisense. However, antisense agents cause only modest *IGF1R* down-regulation, and can affect the insulin receptor. Specificity is an important issue for development of both kinase inhibitors and molecular reagents. Using an array-based screen to identify accessible regions of *IGF1R* mRNA, we designed small interfering RNAs (siRNAs) that induce potent *IGF1R* gene silencing without affecting the insulin receptor. These siRNAs block IGF signalling, enhance radio- and chemosensitivity, and show genuine therapeutic potential. The clinical efficacy of IGF-1R targeting will be determined by key factors including the role of the receptor in established tumours, the potency of inhibition achieved *in vivo*, and the extent to which other signalling pathways compensate for IGF-1R loss.

2004 Biology of IGF-1: its interaction with insulin in health and malignant states. Wiley, Chichester (Novartis Foundation Symposium 262) p 235–246

The type 1 insulin-like growth factor receptor (IGF-1R) is frequently upregulated in tumours, and mediates many aspects of the malignant phenotype including proliferation, transformation and apoptosis protection (Baserga 1995, Bohula et al 2003a). These properties make the IGF-1R an attractive anticancer treatment target. This review will outline the rationale for IGF targeting, the strategies available to achieve this, and considerations for clinical testing.

Rationale for targeting the IGF-1R

Two factors underpin the concept of the IGF-1R as anticancer treatment target, relating to the function of the IGF-1R and its pattern of expression. The IGF-1R is expressed on the surface of most normal cells, but it is frequently overexpressed by tumours, including melanoma and cancers of the colon, pancreas, and, as we have shown, prostate (Hellawell et al 2002, Bohula et al 2003a). IGF-1R overexpression transforms NIH-3T3 fibroblasts, and IGF-1R$^{-/-}$ fibroblasts are refractory to transformation by most oncogenes (Baserga 1995). IGFs promote proliferation via the MAP kinase pathway, but can use this same pathway to induce differentiation, perhaps in cells where Shc signalling predominates over IRS1 (Reiss et al 2000). The IGF axis protects from apoptosis induced by a variety of agents including cytotoxic drugs (Bohula et al 2003a). Apoptosis protection occurs principally via IGF-induced activation of PI3K and Akt, and also of MAP kinase and 14-3-3-mediated mitochondrial translocation of Raf-1 (Peruzzi et al 1999). IGFs also influence tumour cell motility and cell–cell adhesion, and are required for hypoxia signalling (Playford et al 2000, Bohula et al 2003a).

The concept of IGF-1R targeting as therapy has been challenged by study of the transgenic adenocarcinoma of mouse prostate (TRAMP) model, in which IGF-1R levels are dramatically down-regulated during progression to metastatic disease (Kaplan et al 1999). It has been suggested that this might be necessary protection against Shc-mediated terminal differentiation in cells that have lost IRS1 expression. IRS1 loss could favour metastatic cell detachment, via impairment of E-cadherin function; in this setting PI3K activation is maintained by loss of function mutation in PTEN (Baserga 1995, McMenamin et al 1999, Reiss et al 2000). However, in our clinical study of paired biopsies of primary prostate cancer and bone metastases, few cases showed this pattern of IGF-1R down-regulation and loss of IRS1 and PTEN. In most cases, IGF-1R and IRS1 expression persisted in the metastases at levels comparable to those detected in the primary. This suggests that IGF-1R down-regulation is not a prerequisite for metastasis (Hellawell et al 2002). Indeed in many studies, IGF-1R activation or overexpression appear to enhance the propensity for invasion and metastasis (Brodt et al 2001, Lopez & Hanahan 2002, Bohula et al 2003a).

IGF-1R inhibitors

IGF signalling can be inhibited by agents designed to block either the expression or function of the IGF-1R.

Inhibitors of IGF-1R function

Small molecule kinase inhibitors

Chemical inhibitors have many advantages as drugs: they can be designed for solubility and stability, and they can often be administered orally with high bioavailability (Drevs et al 2003). Specificity is a major design hurdle for development of IGF-1R inhibitors, given the high degree of homology with the insulin receptor. Recent structural studies reveal regions of divergence within the IGF-1R and insulin receptor kinase domains, suggesting that it may be possible to design specific IGF-1R inhibitors (De Meyts & Whittaker 2002, Garcia-Echeverria et al 2003).

Blocking antibodies

Monoclonal antibodies to the IGF-1R have been shown to inhibit the growth of a range of tumours *in vivo*. Efficacy can be limited by poor penetrance and anti-mouse immune responses, although these problems may be avoided by use of single chain and/or humanized antibodies (Ludwig et al 2003).

Dominant negative proteins

IGF-1R dominant negatives have been constructed as proteins truncated within the β subunit, capable of forming inactive heterodimers of mutant and wild-type receptors unable to transduce downstream signals. Soluble IGF-1R dominant negatives lack the transmembrane region, and compete with wild-type receptors for ligand binding. This strategy has been shown to suppress IGF-1R function, resulting in inhibition of growth and tumorigenicity (reviewed in Bohula et al 2003a).

Inhibitors of IGF-1R expression

Because of difficulties in designing specific small molecule IGF-1R kinase inhibitors we, and others, have used molecular approaches to block IGF-1R expression. Antisense is the best characterized of these, but this is now being superseded by the recent demonstration that profound gene silencing can be induced in mammalian cells by small interfering RNAs (siRNAs; Elbashir et al 2001).

Antisense

Antisense agents are designed to base-pair with target mRNA, causing sequence-specific inhibition of protein synthesis. This can occur via direct obstruction of translation by antisense RNA, or through mRNA digestion by RNAse H, which is activated by the formation of duplexes between mRNA and antisense oligonucleotides (ASOs; Crooke 1999). However many ASOs are ineffective, because intramolecular mRNA folding renders all but 5–10% of most transcripts inaccessible to ASO binding (Stein 2001). Antisense agents are usually designed to target the translation start site, where the transcript generally lacks extensive secondary structure to facilitate translation initiation (Kozak 1991). ASOs have well-recognized sequence-related and -unrelated effects including protein binding, and they may induce down-regulation of proteins in addition to the intended target, because only 4–6 bases of homology are required to induce RNase H activity (Macaulay 1996, Stein 2001).

There are many reports detailing antisense-mediated down-regulation of the IGF-1R in tumour cell lines using AS RNA or ASOs designed to target the IGF-1R translational start site (Resnicoff et al 1994a,b, Bohula et al 2003a). In a wide range of tumour types, antisense-mediated IGF-1R down-regulation effectively blocks survival *in vitro* and tumorigenicity *in vivo*, and can also inhibit metastasis and enhance chemosensitivity (Bohula et al 2003a, Hellawell et al 2003).

Following the demonstration that IGF-1R overexpression is associated with clinical radioresistance in breast cancer (Turner et al 1997), we used antisense-IGF-1R to explore the role of the IGF axis in the DNA damage response. Murine melanoma cells stably expressing antisense-IGF-1R transcripts show increased sensitivity to γ irradiation compared with sense-transfected controls (Macaulay et al 2001). Furthermore, antisense-IGF-1R transfectants display radioresistant DNA synthesis and attenuated post-irradiation p53 response. These features are reminiscent of cells bearing mutation in *ATM* (*A*taxia-*T*elangiectasia *M*utated), which has a key role in the initiation of cell cycle checkpoints and DNA repair pathways after DNA damage (Shiloh 2001). We found that antisense-IGF-1R transfectants show reduced levels of Atm protein, and impaired activation of the Atm kinase after irradiation (Macaulay et al 2001). These findings suggest that the IGF system plays a key role in the cellular response to DNA damage, and also suggest a specific mechanism for antisense-IGF-1R-induced chemosensitization, in addition to the simple removal of apoptosis protection.

Perhaps the most remarkable effect of IGF-1R-antisense has been the demonstration that tumour cells killed *in vivo* following IGF-1R down-regulation can induce a systemic immune response capable of protecting from tumour cell rechallenge (Resnicoff et al 1994b). This approach has been shown to be effective clinically in a pilot study of patients with end-stage malignant astrocytoma (Andrews et al 2001). The use of *ex vivo* transfection avoided the need for systemic administration of IGF-1R ASOs, and there was no apparent normal tissue toxicity. This study provides strong support for further development of IGF-1R targeting as treatment for patients with established tumours.

RNA interference

RNA interference has recently emerged as a potent means of blocking gene expression. In *Caenorhabditis elegans* and *Drosophila melanogaster*, profound gene silencing can be induced by double-stranded RNA (dsRNA), which is cleaved into short duplexes that are incorporated into a nuclease complex that destroys homologous mRNA. However in differentiated mammalian cells, introduction of long dsRNA (>50 bp) activates the interferon response, resulting in generalized suppression of protein synthesis (Hammond et al 2001). Elbashir et al (2001) demonstrated that specific gene silencing can be induced in mammalian cells by short duplexes of 21–23 bp (small interfering RNAs, siRNAs) including 19 bp of homology and 2–3 nt 3′ overhangs. The gene silencing effect appears to be more robust and less variable than that induced by antisense (Elbashir et al 2001). However, only about 50% of siRNAs are effective, and the determinants of activity are unclear.

We previously used ASOs targeting the IGF-1R translation start site, but have been unable to suppress IGF-1R levels to below ~30% of levels in cultures treated with control (scrambled sequence) oligonucleotides (Hellawell et al 2003). Furthermore, phosphorothioate IGF-1R ASOs have significant non-specific toxicity in survival assays (Hellawell et al 2003), and cause modest but detectable suppression of insulin receptor expression (Bohula et al 2003b). We wished to identify alternative sites for molecular targeting, and noted that the complex secondary structure of long mRNAs is difficult to model accurately (Sohail et al 1999). Therefore we conducted an empirical screen, utilizing scanning oligonucleotide arrays to identify regions within *IGF1R* mRNA that are accessible to bind ASOs. We also hybridized the arrays to insulin receptor mRNA, so that we could identify and avoid IGF-1R ASOs that might influence insulin receptor expression. Next we synthesized ASOs and siRNAs homologous to accessible or inaccessible regions of *IGF1R* mRNA, as defined by the array screen, and tested effects on IGF-1R expression in a range of human and murine tumour cells. The results clearly indicated that secondary structure in the *IGF1R* transcript has a major effect on the efficacy, not only of ASOs, but also of siRNAs that mediate *IGF1R* gene silencing (Bohula et al 2003b).

Using siRNAs homologous to accessible regions of *IGF1R* mRNA, we have been able to show that *IGF1R* gene silencing inhibits survival and enhances radio- and chemosensitivity in human and murine tumour cells (Bohula et al 2003b and M. Rochester, V. Macaulay, unpublished work). Unlike single-stranded RNA, which is highly unstable in serum, chemically synthesized siRNAs appear to have stability comparable to that of phosphorothioate DNA (E. Bohula, V. Macaulay, unpublished). This is attributable to the fact that siRNAs are double-stranded and often incorporate DNA, typically deoxythymidine, in the 3′ overhang of each strand (Elbashir et al 2001). Encouragingly, chemically synthesized and plasmid-based siRNAs are now being used *in vivo* (Filleur et al 2003). It seems clear that RNA interference is not only a powerful research tool for studying gene function, but also shows genuine therapeutic potential.

Other molecular approaches

Ribozymes are catalytic RNA molecules that cleave RNA substrates. IGF-1R ribozymes have been shown to reduce retinal neovascularization in a murine model of oxygen-induced retinopathy (Shaw et al 2003). Oligonucleotides have also been designed to block *IGF1R* gene transcription, by induction of triplex formation in the IGF-1R promoter (Rininsland et al 1997). However the triplex approach is limited to purine-rich targets, and the interaction is weak at physiological pH and temperature (Macaulay 1996).

Potential problems of IGF-1R targeting

Normal tissue toxicity

The IGF-1R is virtually ubiquitous, and is clearly important for early development (Baserga 1995), but its role in the adult is less clear. It is possible that IGF-1R inhibitors could cause toxicity to rapidly proliferating tissues, such as the bone marrow and epithelial lining of the gastrointestinal tract. IGFs play an important role in neuronal survival (Garcia-Segura et al 2000), and any impairment of neurological function would be a major problem for this approach. A measure of selectivity may be provided by the fact that normal tissue growth is anchorage-dependent, a mode of growth that is influenced only to a minor extent by IGFs. In contrast neoplastic growth is anchorage-independent, a parameter that is influenced to a much greater extent by the IGF-1R (Baserga 1995). Normal tissue toxicity could be ameliorated by the use of tissue-specific promoters (Erickson 1999), to direct expression of molecular agents to a specific population of cells, or by the approach of Andrews et al (2001) using *ex vivo* transfection of IGF-1R antisense.

Toxicity may also arise from agents that cross-react with the insulin receptor, blocking its expression or function. This is likely to be a significant consideration for small molecule IGF-1R kinase inhibitors, given the similarity between the IGF-1R and insulin receptor kinase domains (De Meyts & Whittaker 2002).

Magnitude of clinical activity

Efficacy is the key factor that will determine whether this approach will be successful in the clinic. At present it is not clear whether the IGF axis is essential for the maintenance of the metastatic phenotype *in vivo*, nor to what extent another growth factor pathway could compensate for loss of IGF signalling. Therapeutic effects are likely to be attenuated in tumour cells expressing the insulin receptor-A splice variant, which generates a mitogenic response to IGF-2 (Frasca et al 1999), and in cells with mutations in signalling intermediates such as PTEN (McMenamin et al 1999). However even here there may be potential therapeutic benefit, given that the IGF-1R can influence survival and metastasis via multiple pathways (Peruzzi et al 1999, Brodt et al 2001).

Preclinical studies suggest that IGF-1R targeting may be effective in a range of tumour types (Bohula et al 2003a, Ludwig et al 2003). Clinical activity may be more limited, for example to tumours with high IGF-1R overexpression. In the first instance it would be reasonable to assess IGF-1R targeting in a wide spectrum of tumours. It will be important to measure IGF-1R levels and activity to allow correlation with clinical response and, hopefully, identification of tumour types/subgroups where this approach is effective.

Conclusion

The next few years will see the introduction of IGF-1R targeting into the clinic. As with all new therapies, the extent of its success will depend upon the balance between antitumour activity and toxicity. The key issues that will determine clinical utility include the potency of IGF-1R inhibition *in vivo*, and the extent to which tumours are able to compensate for loss of IGF signalling.

Acknowledgements

I am grateful to Cancer Research UK for support, and to Payam Mohaghegh for comments on the manuscript.

References

Andrews DW, Resnicoff M, Flanders AE et al 2001 Results of a pilot study involving the use of an antisense oligodeoxynucleotide directed against the insulin-like growth factor type I receptor in malignant astrocytomas. J Clin Oncol 19:2189–2200

Baserga R 1995 The insulin-like growth factor I receptor: a key to tumor growth? Cancer Res 55:249–252

Bohula EA, Playford MP, Macaulay V 2003a Targeting the type 1 insulin-like growth factor receptor as anticancer treatment. Anticancer Drugs 14:669–682

Bohula EA, Salisbury AJ, Sohail M et al 2003b The efficacy of small interfering RNAs targeted to the type 1 IGF receptor is influenced by secondary structure in the IGF1R transcript. J Biol Chem 278:15991–15997

Brodt P, Fallavollita L, Khatib AM, Samani AA, Zhang D 2001 Cooperative regulation of the invasive and metastatic phenotypes by different domains of the type I insulin-like growth factor receptor beta subunit. J Biol Chem 276:33608–33615

Crooke ST 1999 Molecular mechanisms of action of antisense drugs. Biochim Biophys Acta 1489:31–44

De Meyts P, Whittaker J 2002 Structural biology of insulin and IGF1 receptors: implications for drug design. Nat Rev Drug Discov 1:769–783

Drevs J, Medinger M, Schmidt-Gersbach C, Weber R, Unger C 2003 Receptor tyrosine kinases: the main targets for new anticancer therapy. Curr Drug Targets 4:113–121

Elbashir SM, Harborth J, Lendeckel W, Yalcin A, Weber K, Tuschl T 2001 Duplexes of 21-nucleotide RNAs mediate RNA interference in cultured mammalian cells. Nature 411: 494–498

Erickson RP 1999 Antisense transgenics in animals. Methods 18:304–310

Filleur S, Courtin A, Ait-Si-Ali S et al 2003 SiRNA-mediated inhibition of vascular endothelial growth factor severely limits tumor resistance to antiangiogenic thrombospondin-1 and slows tumor vascularization and growth. Cancer Res 63:3919–3922

Frasca F, Pandini G, Scalia P et al 1999 Insulin receptor isoform A, a newly recognized, high-affinity insulin-like growth factor II receptor in fetal and cancer cells. Mol Cell Biol 19: 3278–3288

Garcia-Echeverria C, Brueggen J, Caparo H-G et al 2003 Characterization of potent and selective kinase inhibitors of IGF-IR. Proc Am Assoc Cancer Res 44:1008

Garcia-Segura LM, Cardona-Gomez GP, Chowen JA, Azcoitia I 2000 Insulin-like growth factor-I receptors and estrogen receptors interact in the promotion of neuronal survival and neuroprotection. J Neurocytol 29:425–437

Hammond SM, Caudy AA, Hannon GJ 2001 Post-transcriptional gene silencing by double-stranded RNA. Nat Rev Genet 2:110–119

Hellawell GO, Turner GD, Davies DR, Poulsom R, Brewster SF, Macaulay VM 2002 Expression of the type 1 insulin-like growth factor receptor is up-regulated in primary prostate cancer and commonly persists in metastatic disease. Cancer Res 62: 2942–2950

Hellawell GO, Ferguson DJ, Brewster SF, Macaulay VM 2003 Chemosensitization of human prostate cancer using antisense agents targeting the type 1 insulin-like growth factor receptor. BJU Int 91:271–277

Kaplan P J, Mohan S, Cohen P, Foster BA, Greenberg NM 1999 The insulin-like growth factor axis and prostate cancer: lessons from the transgenic adenocarcinoma of mouse prostate (TRAMP) model. Cancer Res 59:2203–2209

Kozak M 1991 Structural features in eukaryotic mRNAs that modulate the initiation of translation. J Biol Chem 266:19867–19870

Lopez T, Hanahan D 2002 Elevated levels of IGF-1 receptor convey invasive and metastatic capability in a mouse model of pancreatic islet tumorigenesis. Cancer Cell 1:339–353

Ludwig DL, Burtrum D, Lu D et al 2003 A fully human monoclonal antibody to the human IGF-1 receptor that blocks ligand-dependent signaling and inhibits growth of multiple human tumors in nude mice. Proc Amer Assoc Cancer Res 44:761

Macaulay V 1996 Oligonucleotide therapies. In: Yarnold JR, Stratton MR, McMillan TJ (eds) Molecular biology for oncologists. 2nd edn, Chapman and Hall, London, p 275–292

Macaulay V M, Salisbury AJ, Bohula EA, Playford MP, Smorodinsky NI, Shiloh Y 2001 Downregulation of the type 1 insulin-like growth factor receptor in mouse melanoma cells is associated with enhanced radiosensitivity and impaired activation of Atm kinase. Oncogene 20:4029–4040

McMenamin ME, Soung P, Perera S, Kaplan I, Loda M, Sellers WR 1999 Loss of PTEN expression in paraffin-embedded primary prostate cancer correlates with high Gleason score and advanced stage. Cancer Res 59:4291–4296

Peruzzi F, Prisco M, Dews M et al 1999 Multiple signaling pathways of the insulin-like growth factor 1 receptor in protection from apoptosis. Mol Cell Biol 19:7203–7215

Playford MP, Bicknell D, Bodmer WF, Macaulay VM 2000 Insulin-like growth factor 1 regulates the location, stability, and transcriptional activity of beta-catenin. Proc Natl Acad Sci USA 97:12103–12108

Reiss K, Wang JY, Romano G et al 2000 IGF-I receptor signaling in a prostatic cancer cell line with a PTEN mutation. Oncogene 19: 2687–2694

Resnicoff M, Coppola D, Sell C, Rubin R, Ferrone S, Baserga R 1994a Growth inhibition of human melanoma cells in nude mice by antisense strategies to the type 1 insulin-like growth factor receptor. Cancer Res 54:4848–4850

Resnicoff M, Sell C, Rubini M et al 1994b Rat glioblastoma cells expressing an antisense RNA to the insulin-like growth factor-1 (IGF-1) receptor are nontumorigenic and induce regression of wild-type tumors. Cancer Res 54: 2218–2222

Rininsland F, Johnson TR, Chernicky CL, Schulze E, Burfeind P, Ilan J 1997 Suppression of insulin-like growth factor type I receptor by a triple-helix strategy inhibits IGF-I transcription and tumorigenic potential of rat C6 glioblastoma cells. Proc Natl Acad Sci USA 94:5854–5859

Shaw LC, Afzal A, Lewin AS, Timmers AM, Spoerri PE, Grant MB 2003 Decreased expression of the insulin-like growth factor 1 receptor by ribozyme cleavage. Invest Ophthalmol Vis Sci 44:4105–113

Shiloh Y 2001 ATM and ATR: networking cellular responses to DNA damage. Curr Opin Genet Dev 11: 71–77

Sohail M, Akhtar S, Southern EM 1999 The folding of large RNAs studied by hybridization to arrays of complementary oligonucleotides. RNA 5:646–655

Stein CA 2001 The experimental use of antisense oligonucleotides: a guide for the perplexed. J Clin Invest 108:641–644

Turner BC, Haffty BG, Narayanan L et al 1997 Insulin-like growth factor-I receptor overexpression mediates cellular radioresistance and local breast cancer recurrence after lumpectomy and radiation. Cancer Res 57:3079–3083

DISCUSSION

Carbone: You have to be a little careful about concluding that IGF-1R blockade sensitizes only to DNA-damaging agents. Your data are very likely to be model dependent. Prostate cancer cells may not have an apoptotic response to 5-fluorouracil (5-FU). In our model system receptor blockade dramatically sensitizes to 5-FU in gastrointenstinal tumours. Different tumours respond to different therapeutics in different ways, and I think that it is likely that it would be pro-apoptotic for other chemotherapies in the setting of a tumour that responds.

Macaulay: I saw your results with 5-FU. Taking your *in vitro* result, if you plot it as a percentage of the untreated, do you see relative enhancement of survival? Sure, you can increase the effect with 5-FU, but as a percentage of the untreated there may not necessarily be any chemosensitization.

Carbone: It depends on how you measure efficacy. Efficacy is increased, but we didn't do the careful dose ranging study in the animals that you showed in your system.

Macaulay: It would be great if one could use this approach to chemosensitize to a wider range of agents.

Roberts: I think the fact that you got the R4 to work well was probably good luck. You were doing the array scan with an *in vitro* synthesized fragment of the *IGF1R* mRNA. We don't know what conformation it assumes *in vivo*. Predicting on the basis of that is very difficult. It is almost as easy to make things and see which ones work.

Macaulay: We did use a fragment of the mRNA. There is quite a lot of evidence that mRNAs fold as they are transcribed, they don't come out like a stick. There is experimental evidence that the folding of the 5′ fragment is virtually identical, whether you have the full length or just one or two kilobases of sequence. However if you remove more than about 200 nucleotides from the 5′ end, then you do get a significant change in secondary structure. We incorporated the 5′ end so we were confident that the conformation of that transcript was comparable to the full-length mRNA. This conclusion was supported by the fact that we got such a good correlation between the intensity of hybridization of the array-selected oligos to *IGF1R* mRNA, and the effect in cells. This was despite the fact that array was obviously very unphysiological: the mRNAs were tethered at their 3′ ends, and the hybridizations were performed in 1 M salt. But even so, there was an excellent correlation.

Roberts: The second point is that there have been recent disturbing reports of off-target regulation by siRNAs (Jackson et al 2003). It has been found that an siRNA with a single base mismatch will bind a 3′ UTR very effectively, preventing translation (Saxena et al 2003). Any single siRNA can potentially target any gene that can match with a single mismatch with a 3′UTR. In the future reviewers are going to require that any effect be seen with two completely different siRNAs. A further correlate of this is that the commercial efforts to get people to buy a mixture of four siRNAs to guarantee targeting of one gene also ensures that there will be a lot of off-target regulation. The therapeutic use of siRNAs is going to be a problem because any specific sequence you pick will have quite a number of potentially unrelated target genes.

Macaulay: I accept that. We also have found that a single base mismatch does not abolish activity of siRNA. Other people have reported that it does, and have suggested that this could be used to target mutant oncogenes (Borkhardt 2002). In terms of crude survival, the results I presented earlier indicate that our control duplexes do not detectably affect genes that influence survival. We are now probing some antibody arrays to assess which other proteins are down-regulated by *IGF1R* siRNAs. So far we haven't seen significant effects on protein levels above and beyond what we'd expect from the downstream effects of IGF receptor knock-down.

LeRoith: Charles Roberts made the good point that your work as proof of principle is wonderful, but for the rest of us to find the right siRNA it may be best for us to just do the quick and dirty trawl to find one or two that work.

Macaulay: I agree—no one else is going to use our array strategy. It was simply that we had the tools to measure secondary structure in the *IGF1R* transcript. We didn't know what was affecting siRNA efficacy, and this was a way to address it.

LeRoith: I'd like to comment on your ATM story. We have recently been studying checkpoint molecules in MCF7 cells. We have found that IGF-1 specifically up-regulates the expression of p53. We haven't looked at ATM, but perhaps we should. In our case, when we stimulate with IGF-1 we see increased p53. In your case, when you inhibit the receptor function you lose apoptosis. This could be one occasion where you and I agree on the same result!

Macaulay: You have also shown effects of IGF-1 on p21, which is an inevitable downstream consequence of that.

LeRoith: We have shown that IGF can up-regulate p21, which is fairly unusual because p21 is thought to be an inhibitor of cell cycle progression. But there have been other reports that support p21 being an enhancer of cell cycle, not an inhibitor. It could be cell type specific.

Macaulay: Also, if you want to invoke a checkpoint, which is in the end going to be protective, it is an advantage to up-regulate the inhibitor.

LeRoith: We think it is an enhancer because when we did antisense to p21 we blocked our chief effect. We think it is acting in a way that is different from what is described generally as being an inhibitor. The same goes with the story of the motility. We did this in MCF-7 cells; you used different cells. When we inhibit the IGF receptor we get more motility. Eva Surmacz (2000) showed that when she did the opposite, enhancing the IGF-1 receptor in the same cell line, motility was inhibited. Again, it may be cell type specific.

Lønning: When p21 binds to cyclin D the current concept is that it stabilizes the complex, while it inhibits cyclin E. One of the theories about why p16 knockout is dangerous is that this stabilizes p21 in the cyclin D complex, leaving the cyclin E alone. If you are looking at p21, you need to also assess p27 and p16, and you need to look at cyclin D and cyclin E status. With the PTEN mutation status, are you sure that these mutations knock out PTEN function?

Macaulay: DU145 cells contain one wild-type *PTEN* allele and a second variant allele, and produce functional PTEN protein. PC3 cells have a homozygous *PTEN* gene deletion, and LNCaP have a deletion of one *PTEN* allele and mutation of the other, so neither PC3 nor LNCaP cells express detectable PTEN protein (McMenamin et al 1999, Davies et al 1999). As a consequence, Akt phosphorylation is deregulated.

LeRoith: We have re-expressed PTEN in PC3 cells. It had an effect downstream, but it also interfered with IGF-1R expression. This may be another mechanism whereby it can interfere with the downstream signalling. We think that gene expression was at the translational level.

Yee: When you did the chemotherapy and radiation survival curves, did you do that with and without IGF-1? That is, when you show that you down-regulate IGF-1R, is that only in cells exposed to IGF-1?

Macaulay: These experiments are all done in serum.

Yee: The reason I am asking is that we have talked a little about how IGF-2 has effects on the insulin receptor. Your model system will allow you to address this.

Tyrosine kinase inhibitor, even in our hands, down-regulates the insulin receptor, as do almost all of the antibodies directed against the IGF-1R. If you do these experiments in defined media with and without both IGF-1 and IGF-2, this may help decide whether IGF-1R by itself is the only target.

Macaulay: We could try this, but colony assays take at least a week. Will MDA-MB-231 grow for that long in serum-free medium?

Yee: The 231s will grow serum free in a colony assay.

References

Borkhardt A 2002 Blocking oncogenes in malignant cells by RNA interference — new hope for a highly specific cancer treatment? Cancer Cell 2:167–168

Davies MA, Koul D, Dhesi H et al 1999 Regulation of Akt/PKB activity, cellular growth, and apoptosis in prostate carcinoma cells by MMAC/PTEN. Cancer Res 59:2551–2556

Jackson AL, Bartz SR, Schelter J et al 2003 Expression profiling reveals off-target gene regulation by RNAi. Nat Biotechnol 21:635–637

McMenamin ME, Soung P, Perera S, Kaplan I, Loda M, Sellers WR 1999 Loss of PTEN expression in paraffin-embedded primary prostate cancer correlates with high Gleason score and advanced stage. Cancer Res 59:4291–4296

Saxena S, Jonsson ZO, Dutta A 2003 Small RNAs with imperfect match to endogenous mRNA repress translation. Implications for off-target activity of small inhibitory RNA in mammalian cells. J Biol Chem 278:44312–44319

Surmacz E 2002 Function of the IGF-I receptor in breast cancer. J Mammary Gland Biol Neoplasia 5:95–105

Nutrition, insulin, IGF-1 metabolism and cancer risk: a summary of epidemiological evidence

Rudolf Kaaks

International Agency for Research on Cancer, Lyon, France

Abstract. A Western lifestyle — characterized by low physical activity, and high dietary intake, animal protein, saturated fats and rapidly digestible carbohydrates — is associated with increased risks of many cancers. It has been postulated that, at least in part, these increases may be mediated by alterations in the metabolism of insulin and insulin-like growth factors (IGFs), related to nutritional lifestyle. Insulin regulates energy metabolism and increases the bio-activity of IGF-1 by enhancing its synthesis and by decreasing several of its binding proteins (IGFBP-1 and 2). Insulin and IGF-1 both stimulate anabolic processes as a function of available energy and elementary substrates (e.g. amino acids). The anabolic signals by insulin or IGF-1 can promote tumour development by inhibiting apoptosis, and by stimulating cell proliferation. Epidemiological evidence is accumulating and suggests that the risk of cancers of the colon, pancreas, endometrium, breast and prostate are related to circulating levels of insulin, IGF-1, or both. Nutritional energy balance, macronutrient composition of the diet and physical activity levels appear to be major determinants of IGF-1 bioactivity.

2004 Biology of IGF-1: its interaction with insulin in health and malignant states. Wiley, Chichester (Novartis Foundation Symposium 262) p 247–264

In industrially developed parts of the world, notably Western Europe, North America or Australia, age-standardized incidence rates of cancers of the colorectum, pancreas, breast, endometrium and prostate are up to 10-fold higher than in rural regions of Africa or South East Asia (Cancer Incidence in Five Continents 2002). Increases in the incidence rates of these cancers in migrants moving from low-risk to high-risk areas, and the strong increases in the incidence rates in western countries during the course of the 20th century, indicate that the risks of these cancers depend largely on environmental (i.e. non-genetic) risk factors, including lifestyle.

In particular, nutritional lifestyle factors — such as a Western diet rich in total and saturated fats, rapidly digestible carbohydrates and animal protein — have been implicated in the aetiology of each of these various forms of cancer. Excess body weight (adiposity), reflecting an excessive energy intake relative to total energy expenditure, is associated with an increased risk of cancers of the colon, endometrium, pancreas, breast (among postmenopausal women), kidney (renal cell carcinoma) and several other tumours (IARC Prevention Handbooks 2002). By contrast, physical activity has been clearly established to be protective against cancers of the breast and colon, and possibly endometrium and other organs. Animal experiments have shown a strongly protective effect of chronic energy restriction against tumour development (Weindruch 1992, Kritchevsky 1999).

Although physiological mechanisms relating excess weight, lack of physical activity or diet to cancer have not been entirely elucidated, evidence is increasing that, at least in part, this relationship is due to alterations in endogenous hormone metabolism. Initially, sex steroids (androgens, oestrogens, progesterones) were a particular focus as factors potentially playing a role in carcinogenesis through their regulatory effects on cellular differentiation, mitosis and apoptosis (Henderson et al 1982, Dickson & Stancel 2000, Key & Pike 1988). Besides the sex steroids, there has recently also been increasing interest in the possible roles of insulin, insulin-like growth factor 1 (IGF-1) and IGF-binding proteins, as factors that may favour tumour development.

Insulin and IGF-1 both have mitogenic and anti-apoptotic effects in normal and neoplastic cells of various tissue origins (Khandwala et al 2000, Werner & LeRoith 1996), influence cellular (de-)differentiation, and have been documented to favour neoplastic transformation (Benito et al 1996, Khandwala et al 2000, Stewart & Rotwein 1996, Werner & LeRoith 1996). *In vitro* studies have clearly established that both insulin and IGF-1 act as growth factors, enhancing cell proliferation and inhibiting apoptosis (Khandwala et al 2000, Lawlor & Alessi 2001, Ish-Shalom et al 1997, LeRoith 2000). Experiments with insulin-deficient (diabetic) animals have shown *in vivo* that insulin promotes tumour growth and development in xenograft models and in chemical models of carcinogenesis (Shafie & Grantham 1981, Shafie & Hilf 1981, Heuson & Legros 1970, 1972, Cocca et al 1998, 2003). Likewise, animal experiments have also shown reduced tumour growth after inactivation of the IGF-1 receptor, or after manipulations to reduce circulating or tissue IGF-1 levels (Khandwala et al 2000, LeRoith & Roberts 2003). Finally, endogenous levels of insulin and IGF-1 depend on nutritional factors such as energy balance, and amounts and types of proteins, carbohydrates and fats in the diet (see discussion below). Taken together, these various observations indicate that dysregulations in the metabolism of insulin or IGF-1 might form a metabolic link between a Western lifestyle and high incidence rates of various forms of cancer that are frequent in industrially developed societies.

Obesity, physical inactivity and insulin resistance

Excess weight and lack of physical activity both generally cause a diminished sensitivity of tissues (especially skeletal muscle, liver and adipose tissue) to the physiological actions of insulin. To compensate for such insulin resistance, and to maintain blood glucose levels within acceptable limits, plasma insulin levels are increased in fasting as well as non-fasting states. Thus, body mass index (BMI) generally shows a direct linear relationship with insulin levels. In addition, insulin-resistant subjects tend to have increased glucose concentrations, both in the fasting state and after the consumption of a given amount of carbohydrate, and often also have increased fasting and non-fasting levels of triglycerides and very-low density lipoproteins (VLDLs), and low levels of high-density lipoprotein (HDL) cholesterol. This constellation of metabolic characteristics is often referred to as the 'insulin resistance syndrome', or 'metabolic syndrome' (Reaven 1988, Grundy et al 2004).

Nutritionally-induced insulin resistance can be seen as a metabolic adaptation to increase hepatic and muscular uptake and oxidation of fatty acids, which needs to be compensated for by a reduced capacity of these tissues to absorb, store and metabolize glucose (Kraegen et al 2001, Randle 1998, DeFronzo 1988). The cellular and molecular mechanisms leading to insulin resistance include reductions in cellular insulin receptor levels and reduced responsiveness of some intracellular transduction pathways mediating the effects of insulin binding to its receptor. Especially increased intra-abdominal body fat stores (Abate 1996), from which free fatty acids are easily mobilized and regularly released into the circulation, are a strong determinant of insulin resistance. In addition to free fatty acids, all adipose tissue compartments release a number of endocrine signalling factors, such as tumour necrosis factor (TNF)α, adiponectin, leptin and resistin, which all also have some role in the regulation of insulin sensitivity in liver, skeletal muscle and other tissues (Hotamisligil 2000, Steppan & Lazar 2002, Trayhurn & Beattie 2001, Kahn & Flier 2000).

Physical activity generally improves insulin sensitivity (Grimm 1999, Henriksen 2002). One mechanism through which this may occur is the limitation of weight gain or reduction of excess weight. However, physical activity also improves insulin sensitivity through mechanisms that are independent of body weight, as evidenced by the fact that, in previously sedentary subjects, physical activity generally improves insulin sensitivity and decreases plasma insulin levels within a few days. Mechanisms that may mediate such effects include reductions of intramuscular triglyceride stores (Pan et al 1997), increased muscular phosphatidylinositol-3 kinase activity (Houmard et al 1999), and an increased capacity of skeletal muscle to metabolize or store glucose (Goodyear & Kahn 1998, Hargreaves et al 1998, Perseghin et al 1996).

Besides a degree of adiposity and physical activity levels, diet can also have an influence on insulin sensitivity. In particular, the types and amounts of fats and carbohydrates are important. Thus saturated fats have been shown to reduce insulin sensitivity, whereas sensitivity can be improved by *n*-3 polyunsaturated fatty acids (Storlien et al 2001).

Chronic hyperinsulinaemia and cancer risk

Epidemiological associations of colon cancer risk with documented nutritional determinants of insulin resistance and postprandial hyperinsulinaemia — excess weight, physical inactivity, a diet rich in saturated fats and rapidly digestible carbohydrates, and poor in *n*-3 fatty acids — have led to the hypothesis that chronically elevated insulin levels might be a causal factor in the aetiology of colon cancer (McKeown-Eyssen 1994, Giovannucci 1995). Similar hypotheses have been formulated for cancers of the breast (Kaaks 1996, Stoll 1999), pancreas (Weiderpass et al 1998) and endometrium (Kaaks et al 2002a).

Risks of cancers of the colon (Giovannucci 1995, McKeown-Eyssen 1994, Hu et al 1999), endometrium (Kaaks et al 2002a), pancreas (Weiderpass et al 1998, Everhart & Wright 1995) and kidney (Coughlin et al 1997, Lindblad et al 1999, Wideroff et al 1997) are increased in subjects with type II diabetics, a metabolic disorder that is associated with prolonged periods of severe insulin resistance and hyperinsulinaemia both before and after its onset.

In addition to studies relating cancer risk to the previous diagnoses of type II diabetes, prospective cohort studies have also directly shown increased risks of several cancer types with prediagnostic levels of insulin, or associated markers. A prospective study in New York showed an approximate fourfold increase in colon cancer risk among women who were in the top quartile, compared to the bottom quartile, of C-peptide (a marker for pancreatic insulin secretion) (Kaaks et al 2000a). This finding was recently replicated in another US cohort (Ma et al 2004), and confirmed findings by of a previous cohort study in which colorectal cancer risk was related to fasting glucose, or insulin measured two hours after absorption of a standard oral dose of glucose (Schoen et al 1999).

For endometrial cancer, one case–control study (Troisi et al 1997) and one prospective study combining data and blood samples from three different cohorts in New York, Umeå (Northern Sweden) and Milan also showed a direct relationship between cancer risk and prediagnostic C-peptide levels, and an inverse relationship of cancer risk and blood levels of insulin-like growth factor binding proteins (IGFBPs) 1 and 2 (Lukanova et al 2004). The tumour-enhancing effects of insulin might be either directly mediated by insulin receptors in the (pre)neoplastic target cells, or might be due to related changes in endogenous hormone metabolism, such as an increase in IGF-1 bioactivity or alterations in sex steroid synthesis and bioavailability. In particular, elevated insulin can enhance ovarian, and possibly also adrenal, androgen synthesis, and in some premenopausal women, who probably also have some specific genetic susceptibility, can cause the development of polycystic ovary syndrome (PCOS). PCOS is characterized by ovarian hyperandrogenism, chronic anovulation, and progesterone deficiency (Ehrmann et al 1995, Dunaif 1997), and is a relatively frequent syndrome, with an estimated prevalence of around 4–6% of premenopausal women. Substantial evidence indicates that among premenopausal women progesterone deficiency is a key risk factor for endometrial cancer (Kaaks et al 2002a).

With regard to breast cancer, several case–control studies (Bruning et al 1992, Del Giudice et al 1998, Hirose et al 2003) but not all (Schairer et al 2004), showed an increase in risk among both pre- and postmenopausal women with elevated blood insulin concentrations, but these findings were not confirmed by several prospective studies, (Kaaks et al 2002b, Keinan-Boker et al 2003, Muti et al 2002, Toniolo et al 2000), even though a majority of studies do clearly show a moderate, direct relationship of BMI with postmenopausal breast cancer risk. No consistent relationship has been found between type II diabetes and breast cancer risk (Kaaks 1996). Finally, there is no clear relationship of *prostate* cancer risk with excess weight or pre-existing type II diabetes (Kaaks et al 2000b), and one prospective cohort study showed no clear relationship of prostate cancer with plasma levels of (fasting) insulin, IGFBP-1 and IGFBP-2 (Stattin et al 2000).

Energy balance and the IGF-1 system

IGF-1 and at least six different IGF-binding proteins are synthesized in most, perhaps all, major tissue types. Most (>80%) IGF-1 and IGFBPs in the circulation, however, are synthesized in the liver. The biological activity of IGF-1 depends on the binding of IGF-1 from endocrine, paracrine and autocrine sources, with cellular receptors. IGF-1 bioactivity is strongly modulated by IGFBPs, which control the size of the circulating and tissue IGF-1 pools, regulate the efflux of IGF-1 from the circulation towards target tissues, and within tissues regulate binding of IGF-1 to its tissue receptors (Jones & Clemmons 1995, Wetterau et al 1999).

In liver, and many other tissues, the principal stimulus for the synthesis of IGF-1 is provided by growth hormone (GH), although IGF-1 synthesis can be modulated by many other physiological factors (Le Roith et al 2001). In some tissues, the principal stimulus is not GH; for example, in endometrium the synthesis of IGF-1 appears to be mostly under the control of oestrogens (Murphy & Ghahary 1990, Rutanen 1998). In addition to GH, insulin appears to be central to the regulation of IGF-1 bioactivity as a function of energy from diet or body fat stores (Thissen et al 1994, Straus 1994). Insulin enhances GH-stimulated

IGF-1 synthesis by increasing GH receptor (GHR) levels in the liver (Tollet et al 1990, Baumann & Mercado 1993), and possibly also in other tissues, and by enhancing cellular protein synthesis in general (Thissen et al 1994, Straus 1994, Proud 2004). Besides these permissive effects of insulin on the GH-stimulated synthesis of IGF-1, insulin augments IGF-1 bioactivity by inhibiting the production of IGFBP-1 and IGFBP-2 in the liver and in other tissues (Suikkari et al 1988, Boni-Schnetzler et al 1990).

During prolonged fasting, as well as in insulin-dependent diabetes mellitus (IDDM), low endogenous production (and hence hepatic concentrations) of insulin causes resistance to the GH stimulation of IGF-1 synthesis because of reductions in GH receptor levels (Baxter et al 1981, Baumann & Mercado 1993, Mercado & Baumann 1995), and thus decreases in plasma IGF-1 levels (Clemmons & Underwood 1991, Thissen et al 1994, Straus 1994, Dunger & Cheetham 1996). In compensation for GH-resistance, pituitary secretion and circulating levels of GH rise (Clemmons & Underwood 1991, Thissen et al 1994, Straus 1994, Dunger & Cheetham 1996). Hypo-insulinaemic states are also associated with increases in levels of IGFBP-1 and IGFBP-2 (Counts et al 1992, Bereket et al 1995, Dunger & Cheetham 1996, Argente et al 1997, Bereket et al 1999). Low IGF-1 levels, but elevated levels of IGFBP-1 and IGFBP-2, result in reduced plasma concentrations of free IGF-1, a small fraction of IGF-1 that is not bound to any IGFBP, and that may be indicative of the bioavailability of circulating IGF-1 to target tissues.

In chronically hyperinsulinaemic states, such as obesity, but also (type II) non-insulin-dependent diabetes mellitus (NIDDM), inverse effects are observed, compared to the hypoinsulinaemic state, but with one major exception. GH receptor levels are generally increased, and levels of GH reduced (Cordido et al 1991, Prelevic et al 1992, Frystyk et al 1995, Veldhuis et al 1995, Bernardi et al 1998). Furthermore, chronic hyperinsulinaemia leads to reductions in IGFBP-1 and IGFBP-2 (Clemmons & Underwood 1991, Thissen et al 1994, Frystyk et al 1995, Argente et al 1997, Nam et al 1997, Nyomba et al 1997), and therefore increases in free IGF-1 (Frystyk et al 1995, Nam et al 1997, Nyomba et al 1997). Compared to normal-weight and non-diabetic subjects, however, the plasma total IGF-1 levels of obese and hyperinsulinaemic subjects either remain stable (Cordido et al 1991, Frystyk et al 1995, Nam et al 1997) or are actually decreased, just as in insulin-deficient states (Copeland et al 1990, Marin et al 1993, Veldhuis et al 1995).

Reduced levels of circulating IGF-1 in both undernourished and obese states, compared to normal-weight subjects, suggests a non-linear relationship of IGF-1 with adiposity. Several recent cross-sectional studies indeed confirmed this, showing increasing IGF-1 levels with increasing BMI, with the maximum concentrations at a BMI of about 25–26 kg/m^2, and decreasing levels of IGF-1 when BMI rises further (Lukanova et al 2002, Allen et al 2003, Lukanova et al 2004, Holmes et al 2002).

Experimental studies have clearly demonstrated a strong dependence of circulating IGF-1 levels on dietary intakes and body reserves of energy providing nutrients, and intakes of protein, particularly of animal sources (Clemmons & Underwood 1991, Thissen et al 1994, Noguchi 2000). Several recent cross-sectional studies showed a direct relationship of circulating IGF-1 with dietary intake levels of animal protein (Allen et al 2002, Allen et al 2003, Giovannucci et al 2003), dairy products (Giovannucci et al 2003, Ma et al 2004), calcium, and other nutrients (Estivariz & Ziegler 1997, Straus 1994, Thissen et al 1994) .

The effects of physical activity on IGF-1 levels is unclear. In several studies, a short bout of exercise, at least in adults, caused an acute transient increase in IGF-1 and a dramatic increase in IGFBP1, and in some, but not all studies prolonged physical training was also found to increase total circulating IGF-1 levels (Elias et al 2000, Bermon et al 1999). Prolonged exercise that results in a strongly negative energy balance for a number of days, such as marathon running, may decrease IGF-1 levels for at least a number of days afterwards (Koistinen et al 1996).

IGF-1, IGFBP-3 and cancer risk

A substantial number of studies have recently addressed the question as to whether circulating levels of IGF-1 and its major plasma binding protein, IGFBP-3, were associated with the risk of developing cancer.

Several case–control studies (Bohlke et al 1998, Bruning et al 1995, Li et al 2001, Peyrat et al 1993) and prospective cohort studies (Hankinson et al 1998, Toniolo et al 2000, Muti et al 2002) showed an increased risk among women with elevated plasma or serum IGF-1, and especially for breast cancers diagnosed at a young, premenopausal age. However this finding was not confirmed in a third prospective study, combining two cohorts in Northern and Southern Sweden (Kaaks et al 2002b) and in three other case–control studies (Del Giudice et al 1998, Ng et al 1998, Petridou et al 2000). In several studies, the association with IGF-1 was stronger after adjustment for levels of IGFBP-3 (Hankinson et al 1998), or when IGF-1 levels were expressed as molar ratios to IGFBP-3 (Bruning et al 1995). The latter suggested that risk may be related more strongly to increased bioavailability or bioactivity of IGF-1, due to comparatively low IGFBP-3 levels, or might also point to a direct protective effect of IGFBP-3 through its proper cellular binding sites.

For *colorectal* cancer, studies have also indicated an increased risk. Patients with acromegaly — a pathology due to GH excess and associated with elevated IGF-1 levels — have an increased risk of developing colonic polyps and colon cancer (Cats et al 1996, Colao et al 1997). Furthermore, several prospective cohort studies (Kaaks et al 2000a, Giovannucci et al 2000, Ma et al 1999, Probst-Hensch et al 2001, Palmqvist et al 2002) showed increases in risk either of colon cancer, or of colon and rectal cancers combined, among men and women who have elevated blood concentrations of IGF-1. In only one of these studies (Palmqvist et al 2002) was the association with absolute circulating levels of IGF-1 statistically significant, but for colon cancer only. In two of the five prospective studies (Giovannucci et al 2000, Ma et al 1999), the association of colon cancer risk with IGF-1 became much stronger, and statistically significant, only after adjustment for IGFBP-3. A similar effect of IGFBP-3 adjustment was seen in studies on other cancer types conducted by the same (Harvard) group (Chan et al 1998, Hankinson et al 1998). In all of these studies, IGFBP-3 had been measured by an ELISA, from Diagnostic Systems Laboratories (DSL; Webster, Texas). In all other studies, IGFBP-3 had been measured by various other assays, and elevated IGFBP-3 was systematically found to be associated with an increased risk of colon cancer.

With regard to *prostate* cancer, case–control (Mantzoros et al 1997, Wolk et al 1998) and prospective cohort (Chan et al 1998, Harman et al 2000, Stattin et al 2000) studies have shown an increase in prostate cancer risk in men with comparatively elevated absolute levels of IGF-1 (Harman et al 2000, Mantzoros et al 1997, Wolk et al 1998), or with elevated levels of IGF-1, either as absolute concentrations or relative to levels of IGFBP-3 (Chan et al 1998). There is some evidence that this relationship may be stronger for tumours that are more advanced or aggressive, at the time of diagnosis (Chan et al 2002, Stattin et al 2004).

Taken together, it appears that elevated plasma IGF-1, as absolute concentrations or relative to levels of IGFBP-3, may be a risk factor for a number of different tumours that are frequent in Western societies. It is possible that the elevated IGF-1 levels in men or women who subsequently develop cancer is due to increased pituitary GH secretion, and further studies are needed to address that question.

Conclusions

In many developing countries with low incidence rates of cancers of the breast, colon, prostate, and ovary, the average BMI is (or used to be) below 22 kg/m^2 for the vast majority of the population, whereas in industrially developed societies the median BMI may lie around 25 kg/m^2 or above (IARC Prevention Handbooks, 2002). Furthermore, low-risk countries have generally much lower intakes of animal protein.

As summarized in this chapter, increasing BMI is associated with increasing fasting and non-fasting insulin levels. In addition, up to a level of about 25–26 kg/m^2, BMI also appears to be directly related with blood concentrations of IGF-1. Elevated insulin levels clearly appear to be a risk factor for cancer of the colon and endometrium, and possibly of other organs (e.g., pancreas, renal cell tumours), whereas elevated IGF-1 is associated with increased risks of cancers of the colorectum, prostate and most likely breast (especially premenopausal women).

Taken together, these data suggest that differences in circulating insulin IGF-1 levels may at least partially explain the large differences in cancer risk observed between economically developed and less developed parts of the world.

References

Abate N 1996 Insulin resistance and obesity. The role of fat distribution pattern. Diabetes Care 19:292–294

Allen N, Appleby P, Davey G, Kaaks R, Rinald S, Key TJ 2002 The associations of diet with serum insulin-like growth factor I and its main binding proteins in 292 women meat-eaters, vegetarians, and vegans. Cancer Epidemiol Biomarkers Prev 11:1441–1448

Allen N, Appleby P, Kaaks R et al 2003 Lifestyle determinants of serum insulin-like growth-factor-I (IGF-I), C-peptide and hormone binding protein levels in British women. Cancer Causes Control 14:65–74

Argente J, Caballo N, Barrios V et al 1997 Multiple endocrine abnormalities of the growth hormone and insulin-like growth factor axis in patients with anorexia nervosa: effect of short- and long-term weight recuperation. J Endocrinol Metab 82:2084–2092

Baumann G, Mercado M 1993 Growth hormone-binding proteins in plasma. Nutrition 9: 546–553

Baxter R, Bryson J, Turtle J 1981 The effect of fasting on liver receptors for prolactin and growth hormone. Metabolism 30:1086–1090

Benito M, Valverde A, Lorenzo M 1996 IGF-I: a mitogen also involved in differentiation processes in mammalian cells. Int J Biochem Cell Biol 28:499–510

Bereket A, Lang C, Wilson T 1999 Alterations in the growth hormone-insulin-like growth factor axis in insulin dependent diabetes mellitus. Horm Metab Res 31:172–181

Bereket A, Lang C, Blethen S et al 1995 Effect of insulin on the insulin-like growth factor system in children with new-onset insulin-dependent diabetes mellitus. J Clin Endocrinol Metab 80:1312–1317

Bermon S, Ferrari P, Bernard P, Altare S, Dolisi C 1999 Responses of total and free insulin-like growth factor-I and insulin-like growth factor binding protein-3 after resistance exercise and training in elderly subjects. Acta Physiol Scand 165:51–56

Bernardi F, Petraglia F, Seppala M et al 1998 Somatotropic axis and body weight in pre-menopausal and post-menopausal women: evidence for a neuroendocrine derangement, in absence of changes of insulin-like growth factor binding protein concentrations. Hum Reprod 13:279–284

Bohlke K, Cramer D, Trichopoulos D, Mantzoros C 1998 Insulin-like growth factor-I in relation to premenopausal ductal carcinoma *in situ* of the breast. Epidemiology 9:570–573

Boni-Schnetzler M, Schmid C, Mary J et al 1990 Insulin regulates the expression of the insulin-like growth factor binding protein 2 mRNA in rat hepatocytes. Mol Endocrinol 4:1320–1326

Bruning P, Bonfrer J, van Noord P et al 1992 Insulin resistance and breast-cancer risk. Int J Cancer 52:511–516

Bruning P, Van Doorn J, Bonfrer J et al 1995 Insulin-like growth-factor-binding protein 3 is decreased in early-stage operable pre-menopausal breast cancer. Int J Cancer 62:266–270

Cancer incidence in five continents 2002 In: Cancer incidence in five continents. IARC Sci Publ, p 1–781

Cats A, Dullaart R, Kleibeuker J et al 1996 Increased epithelial cell proliferation in the colon of patients with acromegaly. Cancer Res 56:523–526

Chan J, Stampfer M, Ma J et al 2002 Insulin-like growth factor-I (IGF-I) and IGF binding protein-3 as predictors of advanced-stage prostate cancer. J Natl Cancer Inst 94:1099–1106

Chan J, Stampfer M, Giovannucci E et al 1998 Plasma insulin-like growth factor-I and prostate cancer risk: a prospective study. Science 279:563–566

Clemmons D, Underwood L 1991 Nutritional regulation of IGF-I and IGF binding proteins. Annu Rev Nutr 11:393–412

Cocca C, Gutierrez A, Nunez M et al 2003 Suppression of mammary gland tumorigenesis in diabetic rats. Cancer Detect Prev 27:37–46

Cocca C, Martin G, Rivera E et al 1998 An experimental model of diabetes and cancer in rats. Eur J Cancer 34:889–894

Colao A, Balzano A, Ferone D et al 1997 Increased prevalence of colonic polyps and altered lymphocyte subset pattern in the colonic lamina propria in acromegaly. Clin Endocrinol (Oxf) 47:23–28

Copeland K, Colletti R, Devlin J, McAuliffe T 1990 The relationship between insulin-like growth factor-I, adiposity, and aging. Metabolism 39:584–587

Cordido F, Casanueva F, Vidal J, Dieguez C 1991 Study of insulin-like growth factor I in human obesity. Horm Res 36:187–191

Coughlin S, Neaton J, Randall B, Sengupta A 1997 Predictors of mortality from kidney cancer in 332,547 men screened for the Multiple Risk Factor Intervention Trial. Cancer 79:2171–2177

Counts D, Gwirtsman H, Carlsson L, Lesem M, Cutler G J 1992 The effect of anorexia nervosa and refeeding on growth hormone-binding protein, the insulin-like growth factors (IGFs), and the IGF-binding proteins. J Clin Endocrinol Metab 75:762–767

DeFronzo R 1988 Lilly lecture 1987. The triumvirate: beta-cell, muscle, liver. A collusion responsible for NIDDM. Diabetes 37:667–687

Del Giudice M, Fantus I, Ezzat S et al 1998 Insulin and related factors in premenopausal breast cancer risk. Breast Cancer Res Treat 47:111–120

Dickson R, Stancel G 2000 Estrogen receptor-mediated processes in normal and cancer cells. J Natl Cancer Inst Monogr (27):135–145

Dunaif A 1997 Insulin resistance and the polycystic ovary syndrome: mechanism and implications for pathogenesis. Endocr Rev 18:774–800

Dunger D, Cheetham T 1996 Growth hormone insulin-like growth factor I axis in insulin-dependent diabetes mellitus. Horm Res 46:2–6

Ehrmann D, Barnes R, Rosenfield R 1995 Polycystic ovary syndrome as a form of functional ovarian hyperandrogenism due to dysregulation of androgen secretion. Endocr Rev 16:322–353

Elias A, Pandian M, Wang L et al 2000 Leptin and IGF-I levels in unconditioned male volunteers after short-term exercise. Psychoneuroendocrinology 25:453–461

Estivariz C, Ziegler T 1997 Nutrition and the insulin-like growth factor system. Endocrine 7: 65–71

Everhart J, Wright D 1995 Diabetes mellitus as a risk factor for pancreatic cancer. A meta-analysis. J Am Med Assoc 273:1605–1609

Frystyk J, Vestbo E, Skjaerbaek C, Mogensen C, Orskov H 1995 Free insulin-like growth factors in human obesity. Metabolism 44(suppl 10):37–44

Giovannucci E 1995 Insulin and colon cancer. Cancer Causes Control 6:164–179

Giovannucci E, Pollak M, Liu Y et al 2003 Nutritional predictors of insulin-like growth factor I and their relationships to cancer in men. Cancer Epidemiol Biomarkers Prev 12:84–89

Giovannucci E, Pollak M, Platz E et al 2000 A prospective study of plasma insulin-like growth factor-1 and binding protein-3 and risk of colorectal neoplasia in women. Cancer Epidemiol Biomarkers Prev 9:345–349

Goodyear L, Kahn B 1998 Exercise, glucose transport, and insulin sensitivity. Annu Rev Med 49:235–261

Grimm J 1999 Interaction of physical activity and diet: implications for insulin-glucose dynamics. Public Health Nutr 2:363–368

Grundy S, Brewer HJ, JI C et al 2004 Definition of metabolic syndrome: Report of the National Heart, Lung, and Blood Institute/American Heart Association conference on scientific issues related to definition. Circulation 109:433–438

Hankinson S, Willett W, Colditz G et al 1998 Circulating concentrations of insulin-like growth factor-I and risk of breast cancer. Lancet 351:1393–1396

Hargreaves M, McKenna M, Jenkins D et al 1998 Muscle metabolites and performance during high-intensity, intermittent exercise. J Appl Physiol 84:1687–1691

Harman S, Metter E, Blackman M et al 2000 Serum levels of insulin-like growth factor I (IGF-I), IGF-II, IGF-binding protein-3, and prostate-specific antigen as predictors of clinical prostate cancer. J Clin Endocrinol Metab 85:4258–4265

Henderson B, Ross R, Pike M, Casagrande J 1982 Endogenous hormones as a major factor in human cancer. Cancer Res 42:3232–3239

Henriksen E 2002 Effects of acute exercise and exercise training on insulin resistance. J Appl Physiol 93:788–796

Heuson J, Legros N 1970 Effect of insulin and of alloxan diabetes on growth of the rat mammary carcinoma in vivo. Eur J Cancer 6:349–351

Heuson J, Legros N 1972 Influence of insulin deprivation on growth of the 7,12-dimethylbenz(a)anthracene-induced mammary carcinoma in rats subjected to alloxan diabetes and food restriction. Cancer Res 32:226–232

Hirose K, Toyama T, Iwata H et al 2003 Insulin, insulin-like growth factor-I and breast cancer risk in Japanese women. Asian Pac J Cancer Prev 4:239–246

Holmes M, Pollak M, Hankinson S 2002 Lifestyle correlates of plasma insulin-like growth factor I and insulin-like growth factor binding protein 3 concentrations. Lifestyle correlates of plasma insulin-like growth factor I and insulin-like growth factor binding protein 3 concentrations 11:862–867

Hotamisligil G 2000 Molecular mechanisms of insulin resistance and the role of the adipocyte. Int J Obes Relat Metab Disord 24(suppl 4):S23–S27

Houmard J, Shaw C, Hickey M, Tanner C 1999 Effect of short-term exercise training on insulin-stimulated PI 3-kinase activity in human skeletal muscle. Am J Physiol 277:E1055–1060

Hu FB, Manson JE, Liu S et al 1999 Prospective study of adult onset diabetes mellitus (type 2) and risk of colorectal cancer in women. J Natl Cancer Inst 81:542–547

Ish-Shalom D, Christoffersen C, Vorwerk P et al 1997 Mitogenic properties of insulin and insulin analogues mediated by the insulin receptor. Diabetologia 40(suppl 2): S25–S31

IARC Handbooks of Cancer Prevention. Vol 6: Weight control and physical activity. IARC press, France

Jones J, Clemmons D 1995 Insulin-like growth factors and their binding proteins: biological actions. Endocr Rev 16:3–34

Kaaks R 1996 Nutrition, hormones, and breast cancer: is insulin the missing link? Cancer Causes Control 7:605–625

Kaaks R, Toniolo P, Akhmedkhanov A et al 2000a Serum C-peptide, insulin-like growth factor (IGF)-I, IGF-binding proteins, and colorectal cancer risk in women. J Natl Cancer Inst 92:1592–1600

Kaaks R, Lukanova A, Sommersberg B 2000b Plasma androgens, IGF-1, body size, and prostate cancer risk: a synthetic review. Prostate Cancer Prostatic Dis 3:157–172

Kaaks R, Lukanova A, Kurzer M 2002a Obesity, endogenous hormones, and endometrial cancer risk: a synthetic review. Cancer Epidemiol Biomarkers Prev 11:1531–1543

Kaaks R, Lundin E, Rinaldi S et al 2002b Prospective study of IGF-I, IGF-binding proteins, and breast cancer risk, in northern and southern Sweden. Cancer Causes Control 13:307–316

Kahn B, Flier J 2000 Obesity and insulin resistance. J Clin Invest 106:473–481

Keinan-Boker L, Bueno De Mesquita H, Kaaks R et al 2003 Circulating levels of insulin-like growth factor I, its binding proteins -1,-2, -3, C-peptide and risk of postmenopausal breast cancer. Int J Cancer 106:90–95

Key T, Pike M 1988 The dose-effect relationship between 'unopposed' oestrogens and endometrial mitotic rate: its central role in explaining and predicting endometrial cancer risk. Br J Cancer 57:205–212

Khandwala H, McCutcheon I, Flyvbjerg A, Friend K 2000 The effects of insulin-like growth factors on tumorigenesis and neoplastic growth. Endocr Rev 21:215–244

Koistinen H, Koistinen R, Selenius L, Ylikorkala Q, Seppala M 1996 Effect of marathon run on serum IGF-I and IGF-binding protein 1 and 3 levels. J Appl Physiol 80:760–764

Kraegen E, Cooney G, Ye J, Thompson A 2001 Triglycerides, fatty acids and insulin resistance — hyperinsulinemia. Exp Clin Endocrinol Diabetes 109:S516–S526

Kritchevsky D 1999 Caloric restriction and experimental carcinogenesis. Toxicol Sci 52(suppl 2):13–16

Lawlor M, Alessi D 2001 PKB/Akt: a key mediator of cell proliferation, survival and insulin responses? J Cell Sci 114:2903–2910

Le Roith D, Bondy C, Yakar S, Liu J, Butler A 2001 The somatomedin hypothesis: 2001. Endocr Rev 22:53–74

LeRoith D 2000 Insulin-like growth factor I receptor signaling — overlapping or redundant pathways? Endocrinology 141:1287–1288

LeRoith D, Roberts CJ 2003 The insulin-like growth factor system and cancer. Cancer Lett 195:127–137

Li B, Khosravi M, Berkel H et al 2001 Free insulin-like growth factor-I and breast cancer risk. Int J Cancer 91:736–739

Lindblad P, Chow W, Chan J et al 1999 The role of diabetes mellitus in the aetiology of renal cell cancer. Diabetologia 42:107–112

Lukanova A, Soderberg S, Stattin P et al 2002 Nonlinear relationship of insulin-like growth factor (IGF)-I and IGF-I/IGF-binding protein-3 ratio with indices of adiposity and plasma insulin concentrations (Sweden). Cancer Causes Control 13:509–516

Lukanova A, Zeleniuch-Jacquotte A, Lundin E et al 2004 Prediagnostic levels of C-peptide, IGF-I, IGFBP -1, -2 and -3 and risk of endometrial cancer. Int J Cancer 108:262–268

Ma J, Pollak M, Giovannucci E et al 1999 Prospective study of colorectal cancer risk in men and plasma levels of insulin-like growth factor (IGF)-I and IGF-binding protein-3. J Natl Cancer Inst 91:620–625

Ma J, Giovannucci E, Pollak M et al 2004 A prospective study of plasma C-peptide and colorectal cancer risk in men. J Natl Cancer Inst 96:546–553

Mantzoros C, Tzonou A, Signorello L et al 1997 Insulin-like growth factor 1 in relation to prostate cancer and benign prostatic hyperplasia. Br J Cancer 76:1115–1118

Marin P, Kvist H, Lindstedt G, Sjostrom L, Bjorntorp P 1993 Low concentrations of insulin-like growth factor-I in abdominal obesity. Int J Obes Relat Metab Disord 17:83–89

McKeown-Eyssen G 1994 Epidemiology of colorectal cancer revisited: are serum triglycerides and/or plasma glucose associated with risk? Cancer Epidemiol Biomarkers Prev 3:687–695

Mercado M, Baumann G 1995 Characteristics of the somatotropic axis in insulin dependent diabetes mellitus. Arch Med Res 26:101–109

Murphy L, Ghahary A 1990 Uterine insulin-like growth factor-1: regulation of expression and its role in estrogen-induced uterine proliferation. Endocr Rev 11:443–453

Muti P, Quattrin T, Grant B et al 2002 Fasting glucose is a risk factor for breast cancer: a prospective study. Cancer Epidemiol Biomarkers Prev 11:1361–1368

Nam S, Lee E, Kim K et al 1997 Effect of obesity on total and free insulin-like growth factor (IGF)-1, and their relationship to IGF-binding protein (BP)-1, IGFBP-2, IGFBP-3, insulin, and growth hormone. Int J Obes Relat Metab Disord 21:355–359

Ng E, Ji C, Tan P et al 1998 Altered serum levels of insulin-like growth-factor binding proteins in breast cancer patients. Ann Surg Oncol 5:194–201

Noguchi T 2000 Protein nutrition and insulin-like growth factor system. Br J Nutr 84(suppl 2):S241–S244

Nyomba B, Berard L, Murphy L 1997 Free insulin-like growth factor I (IGF-I) in healthy subjects: relationship with IGF-binding proteins and insulin sensitivity. J Clin Endocrinol Metab 82:2177–2181

Palmqvist R, Hallmans G, Rinaldi S et al 2002 Plasma insulin-like growth factor 1, insulin-like growth factor binding protein 3, and risk of colorectal cancer: a prospective study in northern Sweden. Gut 50:642–646

Pan D, Lillioja S, Kriketos A et al 1997 Skeletal muscle triglyceride levels are inversely related to insulin action. Diabetes 46:983–988

Perseghin G, Price T, Petersen K et al 1996 Increased glucose transport-phosphorylation and muscle glycogen synthesis after exercise training in insulin-resistant subjects. N Engl J Med 335:1357–1362

Petridou E, Papadiamantis Y, Markopoulos C et al 2000 Leptin and insulin growth factor I in relation to breast cancer (Greece). Cancer Causes Control 11:383–388

Peyrat J, Bonneterre J, Hecquet B et al 1993 Plasma insulin-like growth factor-1 (IGF-1) concentrations in human breast cancer. Eur J Cancer 29A:492–497

Prelevic G, Wurzburger M, Balint-Peric L, Ginsburg J 1992 Twenty-four-hour serum growth hormone, insulin, C-peptide and blood glucose profiles and serum insulin-like growth factor-I concentrations in women with polycystic ovaries. Horm Res 37:125–131

Probst-Hensch N, Yuan J, Stanczyk F et al 2001 IGF-1, IGF-2 and IGFBP-3 in prediagnostic serum: association with colorectal cancer in a cohort of Chinese men in Shanghai. Br J Cancer 85:1695–1699

Proud C 2004 mTOR-mediated regulation of translation factors by amino acids. Biochem Biophys Res Commun 313:429–436

Randle P 1998 Regulatory interactions between lipids and carbohydrates: the glucose fatty acid cycle after 35 years. Diabetes Metab Rev 14:263–283

Reaven G 1988 Banting Lecture 1988. Role of insulin resistance in human disease. Nutrition 13:65–66

Rutanen E 1998 Insulin-like growth factors in endometrial function. Gynecol Endocrinol 12:399–406

Schairer C, Hill D, Sturgeon S et al 2004 Serum concentrations of IGF-I, IGFBP-3 and c-peptide and risk of hyperplasia and cancer of the breast in postmenopausal women. Int J Cancer 108:773–779

Schoen R, Tangen C, Kuller L et al 1999 Increased blood glucose and insulin, body size, and incident colorectal cancer. J Natl Cancer Inst 91:1147–1154

Shafie S, Grantham F 1981 Role of hormones in the growth and regression of human breast cancer cells (MCF-7) transplanted into athymic nude mice. J Natl Cancer Inst Monogr 67:51–56

Shafie S, Hilf R 1981 Insulin receptor levels and magnitude of insulin-induced responses in 7,12-dimethylbenz(a)anthracene-induced mammary tumors in rats. Cancer Res 41:826–829

Stattin P, Bylund A, Rinaldi S et al 2000 Plasma insulin-like growth factor-I, insulin-like growth factor-binding proteins, and prostate cancer risk: a prospective study. J Natl Cancer Inst 92:1910–1917

Stattin P, Rinaldi S, Biessy C, Hallmans G, Kaaks R 2004 High levels of circulating insulin-like growth factor-I increase prostate cancer risk. A prospective study. J Clin Oncol, in press

Steppan C, Lazar M 2002 Resistin and obesity-associated insulin resistance. Trends Endocrinol Metab 13:18–23
Stewart C, Rotwein P 1996 Growth, differentiation, and survival: multiple physiological functions for insulin-like growth factors. Physiol Rev 76:1005–1026
Stoll B 1999 Western nutrition and the insulin resistance syndrome: a link to breast cancer. Eur J Clin Nutr 53:83–87
Storlien L, Tapsell L, Fraser A et al 2001 Insulin resistance. Influence of diet and physical activity. World Rev Nutr Diet 90:26–43
Straus D 1994 Nutritional regulation of hormones and growth factors that control mammalian growth. FASEB J 8:6–12
Suikkari A, Koivisto V, Rutanen E et al 1988 Insulin regulates the serum levels of low molecular weight insulin-like growth factor-binding protein. J Clin Endocrinol Metab 66:266–272
Thissen J, Ketelslegers J, Underwood L 1994 Nutritional regulation of the insulin-like growth factors. Endocr Rev 15:80–101
Tollet P, Enberg B, Mode A 1990 Growth hormone (GH) regulation of cytochrome P-450IIC12, insulin-like growth factor-I (IGF-I), and GH receptor messenger RNA expression in primary rat hepatocytes: a hormonal interplay with insulin, IGF-I, and thyroid hormone. Mol Endocrinol 4:1934–1942
Toniolo P, Bruning P, Akhmedkhanov A et al 2000 Serum insulin-like growth factor-I and breast cancer. Int J Cancer 88:828–832
Trayhurn P, Beattie J 2001 Physiological role of adipose tissue: white adipose tissue as an endocrine and secretory organ. Proc Nutr Soc 60:329–339
Troisi R, Potischman N, Hoover R, Siiteri P, Brinton L 1997 Insulin and endometrial cancer. Am J Epidemiol 146:476–482
Veldhuis J, Liem A, South S et al 1995 Differential impact of age, sex steroid hormones, and obesity on basal versus pulsatile growth hormone secretion in men as assessed in an ultrasensitive chemiluminescence assay. J Clin Endocrinol Metab 80:3209–3222
Weiderpass E, Partanen T, Kaaks R et al 1998 Occurrence, trends and environment etiology of pancreatic cancer. Scand J Work Environ Health 24:165–174
Werner H, LeRoith D 1996 The role of the insulin-like growth factor system in human cancer. Adv Cancer Res 68:183–223
Wetterau L, Moore M, Lee K, Shim M, Cohen P 1999 Novel aspects of the insulin-like growth factor binding proteins. Mol Genet Metab 68:161–181
Wideroff L, Gridley G, Mellemkjaer L et al 1997 Cancer incidence in a population-based cohort of patients hospitalized with diabetes mellitus in Denmark. J Natl Cancer Inst 89:1360–1365
Wolk A, Mantzoros C, Andersson S et al 1998 Insulin-like growth factor 1 and prostate cancer risk: a population-based, case–control study. J Natl Cancer Inst 90:911–915

DISCUSSION

Lønning: You said that you had used the C peptide because you used non-fasting blood samples. At the same time you recorded IGFBP-1. IGFBP-1 is clearly influenced by diet, and whether you are taking fasting or non-fasting samples. Could you comment on this?

Kaaks: Immediately after a meal, insulin goes up and there is an acute decrease in IGFBP-1. However, in the fasting state there are also very clear cross-sectional negative correlations between the blood levels of insulin and IGFBP-1. In that particular study that you refer to there were strong correlations between BMI and C peptide in the order of 0.50. There was also a fairly strong inverse correlation between BMI and IGFBP-1. I suspect that not all of these women were fasting, but a large proportion of them may have been very close to fasting. We also had some data on time since last food consumption confirming this. But it was not a formal requirement in this study to be fasting.

Lønning: My second comment concerns sex hormone binding globulin (SHBG). It is correct that you need to assess SHBG when you study total oestrogen levels. But I am doubtful of the concept that any influence on SHBG would influence sex hormone disposition. If you increase SHBG you increase the bound fraction. But if you assume that the delivery from the protein remains unchanged, and that the free fraction available for metabolism and biological function on the target is the same unbound hormones, you would just increase the total amount and not influence the free fraction, so you should not influence the amount available to the tissue. This has been a long debate in steroid metabolism. If you change SHBG you just change the nominal parameter and it will not influence biology.

Kaaks: This is a complex debate. I know there are these two opposing opinions, but I don't know who is right. With regard to breast cancer, I would probably agree with the view that circulating levels of total or bioavailable oestrogens may not be the key determinant of tissue levels. There is a very high amount of oestrogen synthesis in the adipose tissue of the breast. In endometrial cancer, I am less certain. Endometrial tissue is more sensitive to an oestrogenic stimulus, and may respond more directly than breast tissue to variations in circulating levels.

Laron: It does not mean that if a certain hormone is high or low that there is a causal effect with whatever one tests. IGF-1 is more stable during the day. Insulin changes a great deal according to exercise and nutrition. The same may be true of secondary influences by insulin. The differences you showed were often quite minimal: do they have any real value? Also there was a lot of variance from day to day in these patients.

Kaaks: If there was a large day-to-day variation in insulin levels, this would translate into a random error in the exposure measurements that we have, as compared to the long term average which should really matter with respect to chronic disease development. In this case, one would expect a weakening of the association observed with risk. In this case, the associations we find are underestimates of the true degree of association.

Laron: Or the opposite.

Kaaks: No. There is no bias in these studies. The cases and control subjects come from the same cohort. All their blood was given years before the tumour developed. The controls were randomly chosen in a representative way from those who didn't develop cancer. There is no reason why random errors in exposure should have led to higher levels in the cases than the controls, or the other way round. If anything, it would dilute the relationship.

Laron: Has anyone followed ballet dancers, athletes and other people who watch their diet and weight very carefully? Do they have less or more cancer?

Kaaks: They have less breast cancer. I am not sure how strong the evidence is, but women who are physically very active young in life have a reduced breast cancer risk.

Laron: What happens in male athletes?

Pollak: I don't think this has been studied in great detail. It is very hard to quantitate exercise among the normal distribution of exercise, and then severely fit athletes are relatively rare. I have a question. We had an unpublished result from a study looking at IGF-1 as a risk factor for colon cancer. In colon cancer, high BMI is itself a risk factor. When we excluded the fatter people from the analysis for this reason, it strengthened the relationship. In other words, the obese people had an IGF-1-independent elevated risk. When you leave these out the IGF-1 seems to be a stronger risk factor. Have you had the opportunity to check this kind of thing in any of your studies?

Kaaks: No, but it would fit the non-linear relationship that we were looking at. The obese subjects might have a higher risk because of higher insulin levels, but they would have lower IGF-1 levels than the rest of the population. You would get some negative confounding from this, and by leaving out the obese group we might get a stronger relationship.

Pollak: Perhaps in obese people it is more insulin or insulin-related binding protein alterations that are important, and the IGF-1 as a single factor is more important for the thin people who have a lower baseline risk. One of the reasons we didn't publish that is because it is a trend but it doesn't achieve statistical significance, because our group is small enough that when we remove obese people we are left with a rather small group.

Holly: Following on from that we should always remember what we understand about the physiology of the system. Certainly, there is measurement noise, and as Rudolf correctly says, that should attenuate any association. We have been talking about the assay problems. We know that this is a factor in our studies and the associations we see are probably stronger in reality than what we are measuring, because of this noise. When we measure a concentration of IGF-1 we are measuring a circulating store. Within that there is a huge complexity in terms of the bioavailability and the different binding proteins and so on. Derek LeRoith's liver-specific knockout shows that you can have big changes in concentration without any effect in terms of the bioassay of somatic growth. Our data with bioassays show that huge variations in IGFBP-1 give acute changes in activity without any changes in total IGF concentration. The result is that what we are measuring has assay noise, but it is also a very crude measure of what is a potentially incredibly complex system. If we knew how to measure the relevant component the disease association could be far stronger than what we are actually seeing.

Kaaks: And for obesity measured by BMI this is an important comment. It is a very imperfect measure of body fat. The correlation of BMI with body fat mass measurements based on underwater weighing are only in the order of 0.6 or 0.7. This implies a huge amount of attenuation of that relationship as well. The classification of BMI up to 25 being normal weight and 25–30 being overweight is very crude. If I calculate for myself what weight gain I would need to reach a BMI of 25, it would be 14 kg more than I currently weigh. Metabolically speaking I am convinced that I would be obese if I put this weight on. For other people who are more muscular this would not be the case.

Laron: What do we know about follow-up of girls who had precocious puberty? Do they have more breast and endometrial cancer?

Pollak: For sure. Even before people started measuring any hormones in the classic oncology literature there has always been a fairly strong positive relationship between age of menarche and breast cancer risk. The earlier you begin to menstruate, the higher the lifelong breast cancer risk. The more you menstruate the higher the breast cancer risk.

Holly: Added to that, IGF-1 levels in 60 year olds correlates tightly with peak height velocity. If you develop early you have a higher IGF-1, and you still have a higher IGF-1 concentration 50 years later on.

Lønning: Early menarche correlates with breast cancer risk, but the increase is moderate. If you look at early compared with late menarche, there's a 2:1 difference in risk. If you have early menarche, you are also likely to have a later menopause. So is it the early menarche and late menopause that is the risk factor, or is this reflecting a genetic trend for higher oestrogen levels? We don't know.

Laron: At the beginning Dr Pollak said that it is important to have an early high IGF-1 level, which subsequently influences longevity. Thus there might be a pre-programming of risk for cancer if you have high levels of IGF-1 or oestrogen early on. If this is true, policies for GH treatment especially in short non-GH children may have to be reconsidered.

Pollak: What I find unexpected and interesting is the correlation between early life growth in mice and life expectancy in the mice. Something happens at the end of life that can be predicted by something going on early in life. In this work we are not talking about any particular disease, we are just talking about lifespan. The notion that lifespan is shorter if you mature earlier, independent of any particular disease is quite fascinating. It is shown in lots of mice models, where the early growers have shorter lifespan. This relates to the discussion about evolutionary selection: there would have been strong selection for early growth and fertility. Even if you achieve fertility at the expense of life expectancy, it would still be selected for because there is no reproductive fitness gain in living a long life whereas there is strong selection for fertility early in life. Then the question is, could it be that a particularly robust GH–IGF axis is a really good thing to have to maximize your reproductive potential early in life? Then we have to acknowledge that the same 'fitness' early in life may have a certain liability in the circumstances of Western society where we have long lives. People talk about the rate of living hypothesis where people run out of cell divisions. One of the recent papers in *Nature* showing the partial deletion of the IGF-1 receptor being associated with the extension of lifespan is giving the message in the same direction (Holzenberger et al 2003). I think this represents an interesting coming together of experimental and population data.

Laron: If I remember correctly, there were data on dietary fibre from a doctor on the British railway in India. He showed that the incidence of colon cancer was reduced with a certain fibre intake. Is this anything to do with your theory, Rudolf Kaaks?

Kaaks: The fibre hypothesis is an old one that dates back 30 or 40 years. Denis Burkett was one of the most important proponents of it. It focuses on the idea that a diet insufficient in plant wall material, which increases faecal bulk, would lead to enhanced colon cancer risk. People don't agree how fibre should be defined in chemical terms. People have thought of fibre as bulking agents or metabolic fuel for the colonic flora which would dilute carcinogen concentrations or have effects on transport. But there is another concept which is more interesting: the fibre in a fibre-rich diet represents a marker for food rich in plant material with intact cell structures. It is perhaps the accessibility of carbohydrates to digestion enzymes and the glycaemic responses after consumption that are very important. One may wonder whether fibre itself would be a protective agent if it is added to a diet rich in highly refined carbohydrates as an additive. It might be inversely associated with this risk because it is a correlate of a diet rich in whole plant food materials such as whole grain foods. This links up with the insulin hypothesis.

Jenkins: I thought some of the fibre story had been recently debunked. You mentioned the bile acid story. Isn't that an important aspect of this, with the anaerobic conversion to the toxic bile acids? If one extrapolates in the acromegalic story with the increased risk of colorectal cancer, which we know is partially related to IGF-1, we also suspect this is due to differences in bile acids. Acromegalics have increased amounts of the toxic deoxycholic acid in the right side of the bowel. *In vitro*, this bile acid is apoptotic and IGF-1 counteracts these apoptotic effects. It is possible that there is a dual effect of IGF-1 and bile acids acting in opposite directions, which in conjunction with the mitogenic effects of IGF-1, results in a hyperproliferative epithelium and increased chance of survival of DNA damaged cells.

Reference

Holzenberger M, Dupont J, Ducos B et al 2003 IGF-1 receptor regulates lifespan and resistance to oxidative stress in mice. Nature 421:182–187

Final discussion

De Meyts: We have pretty much discussed the insulin-like growth factor 1 receptor (IGF-1R) as a monotherapy. It is clear that it is probably more permissive than oncogenic. There has been no discussion of the possible application of IGF-1 as an adjunct in combined therapies with other agents. Is this something we should discuss?

Macaulay: I think that is a good point. If we block the IGF receptor by whatever strategy, it is highly likely that some other growth factor pathway will attempt to compensate. Perhaps we could look at the effects of blocking the IGF receptor on epidermal growth factor (EGF) receptor activity, for example? Perhaps in defined tumour types we should block multiple receptors, for example the EGF receptor, HER2 and the IGF receptor in breast cancer.

Pollak: Coming at this from the opposite direction, we have blocked the HER2/neu receptor and found that you could get resistance to the benefit by accelerating the signal through the IGF receptor. By extension, if you block the IGF receptor it is quite possible that you will get resistance by means of a different receptor substituting it. If that hypothesis, which unfortunately is quite plausible, is true, it is not particularly bad news for targeting the IGF receptor—rather, it is bad news for the entire approach of receptor blockade. It may not be a fatal flaw because it doesn't limit utility. For example, where we have the most experience, with oestrogen receptor blockade or castration for prostate cancer, we have treatments that are useful but imperfect. Perhaps from that experience we might predict that if there is utility to block the IGF-1R, it will be some small or medium step forward rather than a cure for cancer. This is quite plausible.

Lønning: I think we have some important and serious lessons to learn from breast cancer, with respect to combined therapy in general. 40 years ago someone proposed that by giving different types of chemotherapy in concert we should be able to avoid chemoresistance. So, for 40 years we have done this, despite the fact that everyone sees that it doesn't work. It is the emperor's new clothes. The same thing applies to combining endocrine therapy. Combining tamoxifen and an aromatase inhibitor was detrimental compared with aromatase inhibitor alone. We need to show for each therapy whether it works as a monotherapy first, and then we can evaluate the potential combinations *in vivo*. We have to move carefully here.

Holly: Countering that, if you are trying to target homeostatic biological mechanisms, for example by blocking androgens in the prostate or oestrogens in the breast, we are eventually selecting out a resistance. The system is compensating, which is what it is designed to do. If you are blocking EGF or IGF you are turning on homeostatic mechanisms to compensate for this. Rather than viewing it as trying to block that support, the problem with radio or chemotherapy that some cells survive inappropriately, and if you view these mechanisms as the reason why some cells may survive then the problem with radiotherapy and chemotherapy is that they are not too specific in that they have adverse effects in the host as well as the tumour. This is dose limiting, because if you push them too hard then the patient does worse than the disease does. If you sensitize cells to those agents, however, then it might allow more efficient killing by blocking the escape routes for the tumour cells.

Lønning: I take your point well, but there is also a dark heritage there. People have tried in breast cancer in an adjuvant setting to give tamoxifen and chemotherapy in concert. In most centres, patients are given six months of chemotherapy adjuvant before they use tamoxifen. There are some data that giving the two in concert could be detrimental, slowing down the growth rate and desensitizing the cells to chemotherapy. The message is that whatever we are doing we are talking about so much redundancy in the biology and there are so many escape doors for each type of therapy. You have to test it in the *in vivo* situation based on a current hypothesis, but we always need to be very careful and be prepared for the unexpected.

Pollak: That is true. Nothing will substitute for the trials or the experiments. There is a concern that co-treatment with tamoxifen and chemotherapy might be counter-productive, as you say, but in the case of herceptin and chemotherapy herceptin is rarely given alone because it is best used in combination with chemotherapy. Therefore, it is hard to predict the future from the past and nothing will substitute for a careful clinical trial.

Yee: I would argue that as these drugs come forward, it is not going to be in our hands as to how they are developed. The companies will develop them the way they will develop them, with our input at some level. I would argue for those of you who have influence in this area that you should make sure that tissues and biomarkers are collected. The last thing you want to do is to be like Astra-Zeneca who did a huge clinical trial of Iressa (gefitinib) in addition to chemotherapy, with no benefit for the addition of Iressa. It is not clear why this happened. You have to collect the tissues and understand the biomarkers for response. As smart as everyone is, we still don't know exactly what is going to happen if we start giving these drugs to people. We need to have all the bases covered to interpret the trial once it is done.

Jenkins: Carrying on from that point, to make the assumption that all chemoresistance can be explained by just one pathway is also a bit simplistic. Now with microarrays and proteomics we should be able to tease out the precise mechanisms in individual patients who have developed resistance. Once we start getting individual passports for patients then we can use more targeted therapy.

Lønning: I don't agree completely with that. In the microarrays we have done we have tried to look at the predictive value. We find something like 75% correct prediction, as seen by others (Chang et al 2003). What we are focusing on now are the functional pathway characteristics instead. Among clinicians, people are a little too optimistic about the microarrays.

Jenkins: I agree that 60–70% specificity is not very good. But David Carbone is suggesting that he gets 95–98% specificity with his proteomics.

Yee: We need to think about the clinical trials in the way that we set up the experiments. In the lab you would like to know the array pattern before and after exposure to the drug, and in the clinic we never have these data.

Pollak: Whether it is antibodies or kinase inhibitors or whatever strategy for targeting the IGF-1R, we are interested in the results. It would be nice if these trials could be among the best conducted methodologically. Even for people who have no particular interest in the IGF-1R, it would be nice if industry could collect the samples and learn some biology as well as learning a response rate. Traditionally in a phase I/II trial you don't ask anything about 'why?', you just look at whether it works or not. This is not the way to do the trial.

Holly: We should always remember that the companies are working under their own pressures in a very different world. People pushing IGF-1 tyrosine kinase inhibitors are competing for resources in a company with a whole bunch of other people pushing other therapies, and they need to get a quick answer before they can get resources from the company to do the nice science we would like to see.

Werner: We have to be very careful regarding over-simplifications. Although IGF-1 and IGF-2 are important growth factors, there are about 50 or so other growth factors with defined roles in growth processes. In addition, there are complex interactions between IGFs and other growth factors.

Laron: I have been asked to sum up this meeting. I am not sure who has seen the play *Jumpers* by Tom Stoppard. It features a university professor who is in a dilemma as to what is good or bad. The question that came up repeatedly at this meeting is whether IGF and insulin are good or whether they are a risk factor for cancer. At the beginning of the meeting Derek LeRoith posed the question, 'Are there differences between IGF-1 and insulin signalling?' We have agreed that there are major differences. We don't know why certain levels of insulin have a certain effect and IGF-1 another effect. We don't know much about the role of the hybrid receptor. This is a field where the answers remain elusive but the direction of further research has been clarified. The second question was whether IGF-1 and insulin are proven growth factors. It is clear that in genetic IGF-1 deficiency there is a reduction in growth, but not a complete stop of growth. Thus there must be other intrauterine growth factors. The animal models grow less than humans in this situation. This was one of the examples of the differences between the animal models used in the laboratory and the experience in humans. We can't extrapolate everything from animals to humans. One of the other major questions was: is IGF-1 a causative factor for cancer, or an innocent bystander? There is no good evidence that it is causative, but it is also not an innocent bystander. Certain levels of IGF-1 at a specific stage of life may be a risk factor for subsequent development of cancer. There is agreement that most tumorous tissues have an increased number of IGF-1 receptors, although we don't yet know why. In certain cancers elevated levels of IGF-1 have active effects on the cancer process. This explains why anti-IGF-1 or anti-growth hormone (GH) drugs can slow down certain malignancies in humans and experimental animals. So the big question is, if indeed we can influence the secretion of IGF-1 and the binding protein release of IGF-1, will this either prevent the cancer development or influence its progress? The next question is whether hyperinsulinaemia is a risk factor for cancer. At present we can only say that that hyperinsulinaemia and obesity are certainly detrimental to health.

To conclude, we have discussed at this meeting up-to-date knowledge on the possible links between IGF-1, its binding proteins and insulin with malignancies. We have exchanged information, views and beliefs. Even if many questions have not been answered, we now know better what the future steps should be in researching the roles of IGF-1 and insulin in the pathophysiology of the malignant state and whether to use them or their analogues in the treatment of cancer. To end, I wish to thank the organizers, the speakers and all the discussants.

Reference

Chang JC, Wooten EC, Tsimelzon A et al 2003 Gene expression profiling for the prediction of therapeutic response to docetaxel in patients with breast cancer. Lancet 362:362–369

Index of contributors

Non-participating co-authors are indicated by asterisks. Entries in bold indicate papers; other entries refer to discussion contributions.

P

R

S

T

W

Y

Z

Subject index

Page numbers in *italic* indicate tables.

D

E

F

G

H

J

K

L

V

W